Essentials of Nuclear Medicine Physics, Instrumentation, and Radiation Biology

Dedication

In memory of my parents, Rhoda and Edward Powsner, for all of their love, support, and guidance throughout the years.

R.A.P.

To the memory of my father, Ivan George Palmer, who would have said, "Well, what's all this then?"

M.R.P.

Essentials of Nuclear Medicine Physics, Instrumentation, and Radiation Biology

FOURTH EDITION

Rachel A. Powsner, MD

Clinical Professor of Radiology
Boston University School of Medicine
Director, Division of Nuclear Medicine
Department of Radiology
Boston Veterans Administration Healthcare System
Boston, MA, USA

Matthew R. Palmer, PhD

Director of Medical Imaging Physics
Department of Radiology
Beth Israel Deaconess Medical Center
Assistant Professor of Radiology
Harvard Medical School
Boston, MA, USA

Edward R. Powsner, MD*

Former Chief, Nuclear Medicine Service Veterans Administration Hospital
Allen Park, MI, USA
Former Professor and Associate Chairman
Department of Pathology
Michigan State University
East Lansing, MI, USA
Deceased

WILEY Blackwell

Registered Office(s)
John Wiley & Sons, Inc., 111 River Street, Hoboken, NJ 07030, USA
John Wiley & Sons Ltd, The Atrium, Southern Gate, Chichester, West Sussex, PO19 8SQ, UK

Editorial Office
9600 Garsington Road, Oxford, OX4 2DQ, UK

For details of our global editorial offices, customer services, and more information about Wiley products visit us at www.wiley.com.

Wiley also publishes its books in a variety of electronic formats and by print-on-demand. Some content that appears in standard print versions of this book may not be available in other formats.

Library of Congress Cataloging-in-Publication Data

Names: Powsner, Rachel A. author. | Palmer, Matthew R., 1958- author. |
   Powsner, Edward R., 1926- author.
Title: Essentials of nuclear medicine physics, instrumentation, and
   radiation biology / Rachel A. Powsner, Matthew R. Palmer, Edward R. Powsner.
Other titles: Essentials of nuclear medicine physics
Description: Fourth edition. | Hoboken, NJ : Wiley-Blackwell, 2022. |
   Preceded by: Essentials of nuclear medicine physics and instrumentation
   / Rachel A. Powsner, Matthew R. Palmer, Edward R. Powsner. Third
   edition. Chichester, West Sussex, UK : Wiley-Blackwell, 2013. | Includes
   bibliographical references and index.
Identifiers: LCCN 2021032438 (print) | LCCN 2021032439 (ebook) | ISBN 9781119620990 (paperback)
   | ISBN 9781119621003 (adobe pdf) | ISBN 9781119621010 (epub)
Subjects: MESH: Nuclear Medicine | Nuclear Medicine–instrumentation |
   Nuclear Physics | Radiation, Ionizing | Radiation Effects | Radioactive
   Hazard Release–prevention & control
Classification: LCC R896.7 (print) | LCC R896.7 (ebook) | NLM WN 440 |
   DDC 616.07/575–dc23
LC record available at https://lccn.loc.gov/2021032438
LC ebook record available at https://lccn.loc.gov/2021032439

Cover Design: Wiley
Cover Image: © Courtesy of Rachel A. Powsner

Set in 9/12pt PhotinaMTStd by Straive, Pondicherry, India

Contents

Preface

After many years of postgraduate training, many physicians have forgotten some (or most) of their undergraduate and high school physics and may find submersion into nuclear physics somewhat daunting. This book begins with a very basic introduction to nuclear physics and the interactions of radiation and matter. It then proceeds with a discussion of the methods for production of nuclides and the instrumentation used for dose measurement, surveying radioactivity, and imaging. The imaging section has been expanded to cover MRI and PET-MRI in addition to SPECT, PET, and PET-CT. The final chapters of the book focus on radiation biology, radiation safety, radiopharmaceutical therapy, and radiation accidents.

Numerous illustrations are included. They are highly schematic and are designed to illustrate concepts rather than represent scale models of their subjects. This text is intended for radiology residents, cardiology fellows, nuclear medicine residents and fellows, nuclear medicine technology students, and others interested in an introduction to concepts in nuclear medicine physics and instrumentation.

Rachel A. Powsner
Matthew R. Palmer

Acknowledgments

The authors would like to thank the following experts for their help with this edition: Larry Panych, PhD for his in-depth critique and suggestions for the MRI chapter, Annick Van Den Abbeele, MD, FACR, and Kun Huang, MD, for their review and corrections of the chapters on radiopharmaceutical therapy and radiation biology, respectively, and Chad Smith, PhD for his review of radiation safety and dosimetry. We are grateful for the assistance of Arda Konik, PhD for his guidance on interpretation of GE PET QC images as well as Mr. Brandon Clifton and Jeanette Y. Kleier, RT (R)(N), CNMT for help with understanding Philips PET and SPECT QC images and Stephen Baker for his aid with Siemens PET QC images. In addition, Mr. Mitchell Kruzel from Nuclear Fields provided helpful information on current utility of collimator designs.

Since this edition is built upon information included in prior editions, the authors would like to thank the following individuals for their help on the third edition: Anupma Jati, MD for critiquing the CT dosimetry section of the text, Gary Murphy, RT, for help with CT QC questions and Kandace Craft, RTN and Chris Lindsey, FSE for information about PET-CT. P. Satish Nair, PhD generously made comments on the dosimetry chapter. David Drum, MD answered numerous questions about radiation safety and dosimetry. J. Anthony Parker, MD was helpful on the topic of cancer induction from low-dose ionizing radiation as well as serving as a reference for an assortment of other specific questions.

For the second edition the following individuals were most generous with information: Stephen Moore, PhD on the topic of SPECT processing including iterative reconstruction, Fred Fahey, DSc on PET instrumentation, and Robert Zimmerman, MSEE on gamma camera quality control and the physics of crystal scintillators. In addition, Dr. Frank Masse generously reviewed the material on radiation accidents and Mark Walsh, CHP critiqued the radiation safety text.

We would also like to thank the following individuals for their help in reviewing portions of the first edition during its preparation: David Rockwell, MD, Maura Dineen-Burton, CNMT, Dipa Patel, MD, Alfonse Taghian, MD, Hernan Jara, PhD, Susan Gussenhoven, PhD, John Shaw, MS, Michael Squillante, PhD, Kevin Buckley, CHP, Jayne Caruso, Victor Lee, MD, Toby Wroblicka, MD, Dan Winder, MD, Dennis Atkinson, MD, and Inna Gazit, MD. Thanks to Peter Shomphe, ARRT, CNMT, Bob Dann, PhD, and Laura Partriquin, MD for wading through the manuscript in its entirety. We greatly appreciate the patience shown at that time by Robert Zimmerman, MSEE, Kevin Buckley, CHP, John Widman, PhD, CHP, Peter Waer, PhD, Stephen Moore, PhD, Bill Worstell, PhD, and Hernan Jara, PhD while answering our numerous questions. Thanks to Delia Edwards, Milda Pitter, and Paul Guidone, MD for taking time to pose as models. The authors would also like to thank Rhoda M. Powsner, MD for her assistance in reviewing sections of the text and for proofreading the review questions.

CHAPTER 1

Basic Nuclear Medicine Physics

Properties and structure of matter

Matter has several fundamental properties. For our purposes the most important are mass and charge (electric). We recognize mass by the force gravity exerts on a material object (commonly referred to as its weight) and by the object's inertia, which is the "resistance" we encounter when we attempt to change the position or motion of a material object.

Similarly, we can, at least at times, recognize charge by the direct effect it can have on us, or that we can observe it to have on inanimate objects. For example, we may feel the presence of a strongly charged object when it causes our hair to move or even to stand on end. More often than not, however, we are insensitive to charge. But whether grossly detectable or not, its effects must be considered here because of the role charge plays in the structure of matter.

Charge is generally thought to have been recognized first by the ancient Greeks. They noticed that some kinds of matter, an amber rod for example, can be given an electric charge by rubbing it with a piece of cloth. Their experiments convinced them that there are two kinds of charge: opposite charges, which attract each other, and like charges, which repel. One kind of charge came to be called positive, the other negative. We now know that the negative charge is associated with electrons. The rubbing transferred some of the electrons from the atoms of the matter in the rod to the cloth. In a similar fashion, electrons can be transferred from a cat's fur to a hand. After petting, the cat will have a net positive charge and the person a net negative charge

(Figure 1.1). With these basic properties in mind, we can look at matter in more detail.

Matter is composed of molecules. In any chemically pure material, the molecules are the smallest units that retain the characteristics of the material itself. For example, if a block of salt were to be broken into successively smaller pieces, the smallest fragment with the properties of salt would be a single salt molecule (Figure 1.2). With further fragmentation, the molecule would no longer be salt. Molecules, in turn, are composed of atoms. Most molecules consist of more than one kind of atom—salt, for example, is made up of atoms of chlorine and atoms of sodium. The atoms themselves are composed of smaller particles, the subatomic particles, which are discussed later.

The molecule is held together by the chemical bonds among its atoms. These bonds are formed by the force of electrical attraction between oppositely charged parts of the molecule. This force is often referred to as the Coulomb force after Charles A. de Coulomb, the physicist who characterized it. This is the force involved in chemical reactions such as the combining of hydrogen and oxygen to form water. The electrons of the atom are held by the electrical force between them and the positive nucleus. The nucleus of the atom is held together by another type of force—nuclear force—which is involved in the release of atomic energy. Nuclear forces are magnitudes greater than electrical forces.

Elements

There are more than 100 species of atoms. These species are referred to as **elements**. Most of the

Essentials of Nuclear Medicine Physics, Instrumentation, and Radiation Biology, Fourth Edition.
Rachel A. Powsner, Matthew R. Palmer, and Edward R. Powsner.
© 2022 John Wiley & Sons Ltd. Published 2022 by John Wiley & Sons Ltd.

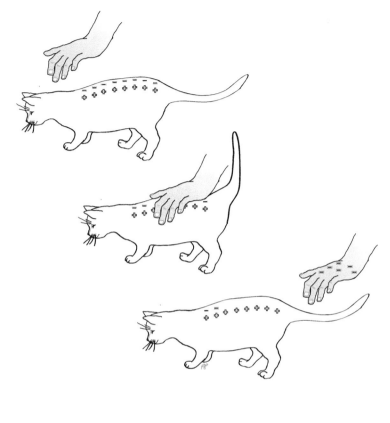

Figure 1.1 Electrostatic charge.

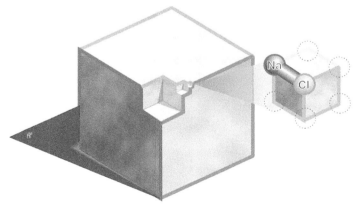

Figure 1.2 The NaCl molecule is the smallest unit of salt that retains the characteristics of salt.

known elements—for example, mercury, helium, gold, hydrogen, and oxygen—occur naturally on earth; others are not usually found in nature but are made by humans—for example, europium and americium. A reasonable explanation for the absence of some elements from nature is that if and when they were formed they proved too unstable to survive in detectable amounts into the present.

All the elements have been assigned symbols or abbreviated chemical names: gold, Au, mercury, Hg; helium, He. Some symbols are obvious abbreviations of the English name; others are

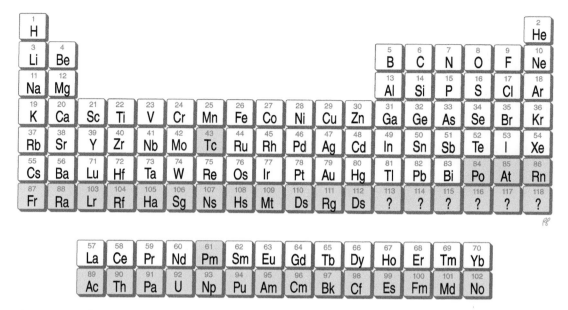

Figure 1.3 Periodic table.

derived from the original Latin name of the element, for example, Au is from aurum, the Latin word for gold.

All of the known elements, both natural and those made by humans, are organized in the **periodic table**. In Figure 1.3, the elements that have a stable state are shown in white boxes; those that occur only in a radioactive form are shown in gray boxes. The number appearing above each element's abbreviation is referred to as the atomic number, which will be discussed later in this chapter.

The elements in the periodic table are arranged in columns (called groups) and rows (called periods). In general, elements within groups demonstrate similar properties. This is because elements in a group often have similar numbers of electrons in their outer shell; outer shell electron configurations are more important in determining how an atom interacts with other elemental atoms. The lanthanides and actinides are special groups of elements, conventionally shown in rows, separated and placed below the table. These two groups have the same number of outer-shell electrons and share many common properties.

Atomic structure

Atoms initially were thought of as no more than small pieces of matter. Our understanding that

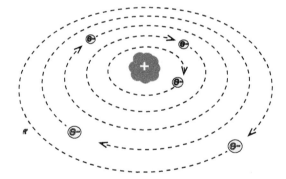

Figure 1.4 Flat atom. The standard two-dimensional drawing of atomic structure.

they have an inner structure has its roots in the observations of earlier physicists that the atoms of which matter is composed contain **electrons** of negative charge. In as much as the atom as a whole is electrically neutral, it seemed obvious that it must also contain something with a positive charge to balance the negative charge of the electrons. Thus, early attempts to picture the atom, modeled on our solar system, showed the negatively charged electrons orbiting a central group of particles, the positively charged **nucleus** (Figure 1.4).

Electrons

In our simple solar-system model of the atom, the electrons are viewed as orbiting the nucleus at high speeds. They have a negative charge and the nucleus has a positive charge. The electrical charges of the atom are "balanced," that is, the total negative charge of the electrons equals the positive charge of the nucleus. As we shall see in a moment, this is simply another way to point out that the number of orbital electrons equals the number of nuclear protons.

Electron shells and binding energy: By adding a third dimension to our model of the atom, we can depict the electron orbits as the surfaces of spheres (called **shells**) to suggest that, unlike the planets orbiting the sun, electrons are not confined to a circular orbit lying in a single plane but may be more widely distributed (Figure 1.5). Although it is convenient for us to talk about distances and diameters of the shells, distance on the atomic scale does not have quite the same meaning it does with everyday objects. The most significant characteristic of a shell is its energy level. The "closer" an electron is to the nucleus, the more tightly it is bound to the nucleus. In saying this, we mean that more work (energy) is required to remove an inner-shell electron than an outer one. The energy that must be put into the atom to separate an electron is called the **electron binding energy**. It is usually expressed in **electron volts (eV)**. The electron binding energy varies from a few thousand electron volts (keV) for inner-shell electrons to just a few eV for the less tightly bound outer-shell electrons.

Electron volt

The electron volt is a special unit defined as the energy required to move one electron against a potential difference of one volt. Conversely it is also the amount of kinetic (motion) energy an electron acquires if it "falls" through a potential difference of one volt. It is a very small unit on the everyday scale, at only 1.6×10^{-19} joules (J), but a very convenient unit on the atomic scale. One joule is the Système International (SI) unit of work or energy. For comparison, 1 J equals 0.24 small calories (as opposed to the kcal used to measure food intake).

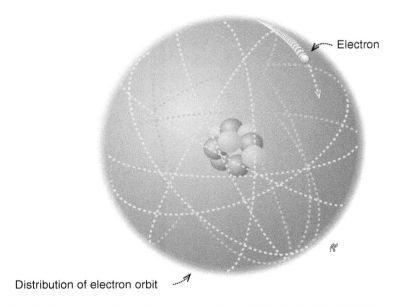

Electron

Distribution of electron orbit

Figure 1.5 An electron shell is a representation of the energy level associated with an atomic electron.

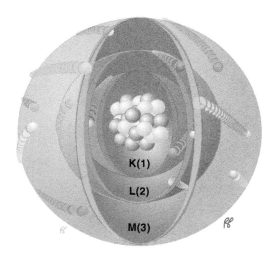

Figure 1.6 K, L, and M electron shells.

Quantum numbers: The atomic electrons in their shells are usually described by their quantum numbers, of which there are four types. The first is the **principal quantum number (*n*)**, which identifies the shell. The first three shells (K, L, and M) are depicted in Figure 1.6. The electron binding energy is greatest for the innermost shell (K) and is progressively less for the outer shells. Larger atoms have more shells.

The second (azimuthal), third (magnetic), and fourth (spin) quantum numbers refer to other physical properties of the electron. Each electron within an atom has a unique combination of the four quantum numbers.

The maximum number of electrons associated with each energy shell is $2n^2$, where n is the shell number. The first shell (the K shell) can contain a maximum of two electrons, the second shell (the L shell) can contain a maximum of eight electrons, the third shell (the M shell) can contain a maximum of 18 electrons, and so on.

Representation of electron distribution: Most of the diagrams (for example Figure 1.6) in this chapter reflect what is referred to as the **Bohr model** of the atom and as such all electrons within each shell are depicted as moving along the surface of a sphere, each shell represented as one such sphere with a distinct radial distance from a centrally located nucleus. The radius of these spheres increases with principal quantum number. This model of the atom

is frequently used for teaching purposes because the radial distance of an electron from the nucleus is used to depict with how tightly bound it is to the atom—the closest electrons being most tightly bound.

A more accurate quantum mechanical description of electron distribution uses a sequence of **orbitals**. Orbitals are mathematical functions that describe the probability of finding an electron in a region of space near the nucleus. For each principal quantum number (each shell) there is a spherical orbital denoted by the principal quantum number followed by the letter "s". This orbital contains two electrons (Figure 1.7a). This is the only orbital for the K shell which contains at maximum two electrons and this orbital is called the **1s orbital.** The neutral atom with a full K shell is the helium atom.

The next shell, the L shell ($n = 2$), also has a spherical orbital, denoted 2s (also depicted as Figure 1.7a) which contains two electrons, as well as three **sub-orbitals**, denoted $2p_x$, $2p_y$, $2p_z$. Each sub-orbital has a shape like a dumb-bell or three-dimensional figure eight (see Figure 1.7b). The three sub-orbitals are oriented along three orthogonal axes as shown in Figure 1.7c. Each sub-orbital is filled by two electrons and the neutral atom with completely filled orbitals for $n = 1$ and $n = 2$ is Neon.

For the higher order orbitals, $n > 2$, the sub-orbitals associated with higher azimuthal quantum number become even more complicated in structure and will not be discussed here.

Quantum numbers

The term **quantum** means, literally, amount. It acquired its special significance in physics when Bohr and others theorized that physical quantities such as energy and light could not have a range of values as on a continuum, but rather could have only discrete, step-like values. The individual steps are so small that their existence escaped the notice of physicists until Bohr postulated them to explain his theory of the atom. We now refer to Bohr's theory as **quantum theory** and the resulting explanations of motion in the atomic scale as **quantum mechanics** to distinguish it from the classical mechanics described by Isaac Newton, which is still needed for everyday engineering.

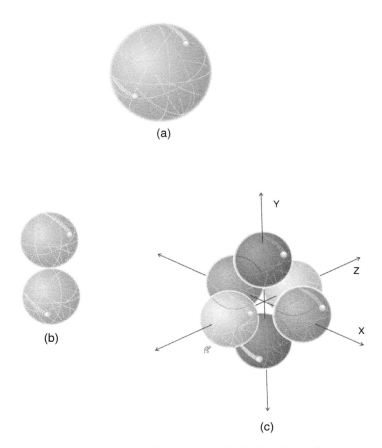

Figure 1.7 Electron orbitals and sub-orbitals. (a) s orbital, (b) p suborbital, (c) p suborbitals, p_x, p_y, p_z.

Stable electron configuration: Just as it takes energy to remove an electron from its atom, it takes energy to move an electron from an inner shell to an outer shell, which can also be thought of as the energy required to pull a negative electron away from the positively charged nucleus. Any vacancy in an inner shell creates an unstable condition often referred to as an **excited state**.

The electrical charges of the atom are balanced, that is, the total negative charge of the electrons equals the total positive charge of the nucleus. This is simply another way of pointing out that the number of orbital electrons equals the number of nuclear protons. Furthermore, the electrons must fill the shells with the highest binding energy first. At least in the elements of low atomic number, electrons within the inner shells have the highest binding energy.

If the arrangement of the electrons in the shells is not in the stable state, they will undergo rearrangement in order to become stable, a process often referred to as **de-excitation**. Because the stable configuration of the shells always has less energy than any unstable configuration, the de-excitation releases energy as X-rays and electrons (this will be discussed in more detail later in this chapter in the section on internal conversion).

Nucleus

Like the atom itself, the atomic nucleus also has an inner structure (Figure 1.8). Experiments showed that the nucleus consists of two types of particles: **protons**, which carry a positive charge, and **neutrons**, which carry no charge. The general term for protons and neutrons is **nucleons**. The nucleons have a much greater mass than electrons. Table 1.1 reviews the properties of the various subatomic particles.

A simple but useful model of the nucleus is a tightly bound cluster of protons and neutrons. Protons naturally repel each other since they are positively charged; however, there is a powerful binding force called the **nuclear force** that holds the nucleons together very tightly (Figure 1.9).

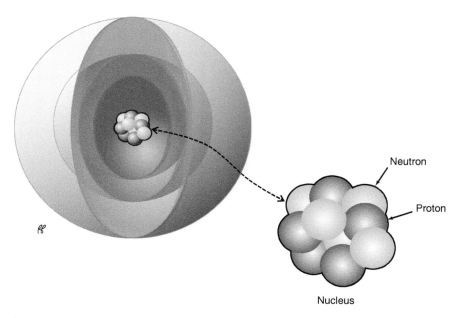

Figure 1.8 The nucleus of an atom is composed of protons and neutrons.

Table 1.1 Properties of the subatomic particles

Name(s)	Symbol	Mass[a]	Charge
Neutron	N	1839	None
Proton	P	1836	Positive (+)
Electron	e⁻	1	Negative (−)
Beta particle (beta minus particle, electron)[b]	B−	1	Negative (−)
Positron (beta plus particle, positive electron)	β+	1	Positive (+)
Gamma ray (photon)	γ	None	None
X-ray	X-ray	None	None
Neutrino	ν	Near zero	None
Antineutrino	$\overline{\nu}$	Near zero	None

[a] Relative to an electron.
[b] There is no physical difference between a beta particle and an electron; the term beta particle is applied to an electron that is emitted from a radioactive nucleus. The symbol β without a minus or plus sign attached always refers to a beta minus particle or electron.

The work (energy) required to overcome the nuclear force, the work to remove a nucleon from the nucleus, is called the **nuclear binding energy**. Typical binding energies are in the range of 2 million

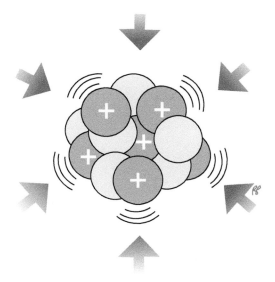

Figure 1.9 Nuclear binding force is strong enough to overcome the electrical repulsion between the positively charged protons.

to 9 million electron volts (MeV) (approximately one thousand to one million times the electron binding force). The magnitude of the binding energy is related to another fact of nature: the measured mass of a nucleus is always less than the mass expected from the sum of the masses of its neutrons and protons. The "missing" mass is called the **mass defect**, the energy equivalent of which is equal to the nuclear binding energy. This inter-changeability of mass and energy was immortalized in Einstein's equation $E = mc^2$.

Isotopes, isotones, and isobars: Each atom of any sample of an element has the same number of protons (the same **Z**: atomic number) in its nucleus. Lead

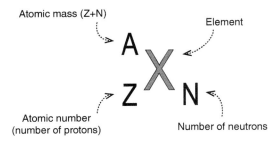

Atomic mass (Z+N)

Element

Atomic number (number of protons)

Number of neutrons

Figure 1.10 Standard atomic notation.

found anywhere in the world will always be composed of atoms with 82 protons. The same does not apply, however, to the number of neutrons in the nucleus.

An **isotope** of an element is a particular variation of the nuclear composition of the atoms of that element. The number of protons (**Z**: atomic number) is unchanged, but the number of neutrons (**N**) varies. Since the number of neutrons changes, the total number of neutrons and protons (**A**: the atomic mass) changes. The chemical symbol for each element can be expanded to include these three numbers (Figure 1.10).

Two related entities are **isotones** and **isobars**. Isotones are atoms of different elements that contain identical numbers of neutrons but varying numbers of protons. Isobars are atoms of different elements with identical numbers of nucleons. Examples of these are illustrated in Figure 1.11.

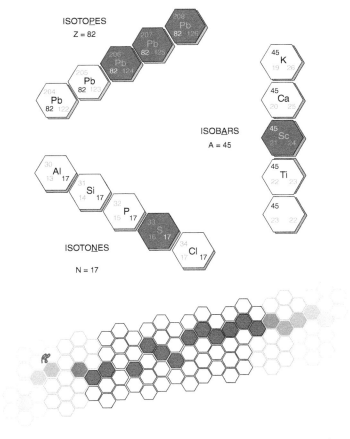

Figure 1.11 Nuclides of the same atomic number but different atomic mass are called isotopes, those of an equal number of neutrons are called isotones, and those of the same atomic mass but different atomic number are called isobars. Stable nuclear configurations are shaded gray, radioactive configurations are white. (Adapted from Brucer, M. Trilinear Chart of the Nuclides, Mallinkrodt Inc, 1979.)

Nuclide is a general term for the composition of a nucleus and includes isotopes, isotones, isobars, and other nuclear configurations.

The stable nucleus: Not all elements have stable isotopes; they do exist for most of the light and midweight elements, those with atomic numbers (number of protons) up to and including bismuth (Z = 83). However, there are no stable isotopes of technetium (Z = 43), promethium (Z = 61), or for all elements with atomic numbers higher than 83. Prominent examples are radium (Z = 88) and uranium (Z = 92), which are found naturally as a mix of isotopic forms that are all radioactive.

For those nuclei with a stable state there is an optimal ratio of neutrons to protons. For the lighter elements this ratio is approximately 1:1; for increasing atomic weights, stability is more likely when the number of neutrons exceeds the number of protons. A plot depicting the number of neutrons as a function of the number of protons is called the **line of stability** (Figure 1.12).

Stability

Strictly speaking, stability is a relative term. We call a nuclide stable when its half-life is so long as to be practically immeasurable—say greater than 100 years. An isotope of potassium, ^{40}K for example, which makes up about 1% of the potassium found in nature is considered stable but actually has a half-life of 10^9 years.

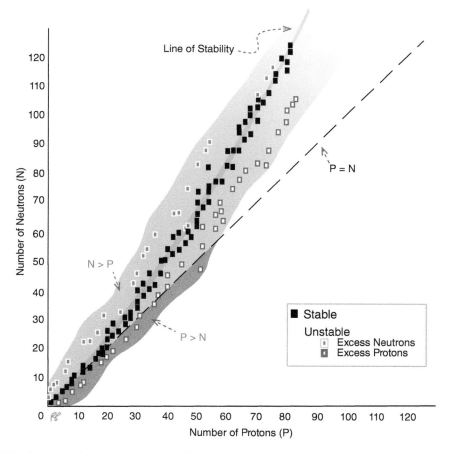

Figure 1.12 Combinations of neutrons and protons that can coexist in a stable nuclear configuration all lie within the gray shaded regions.

Radioactivity

The unstable nucleus and radioactive decay

A nucleus which is not in its stable state will adjust itself until it is more stable either by ejecting portions of its nucleus or by emitting energy in the form of photons (gamma rays). This process is referred to as **radioactive decay**. The type of decay depends on which of the following rules for nuclear stability is violated.

Excessive nuclear mass

Alpha decay: Very large unstable atoms, atoms with high atomic mass, may split into nuclear fragments. The smallest stable nuclear fragment that is emitted is the particle consisting of two neutrons and two protons, equivalent to the nucleus of a helium atom. Because it was one of the first types of radiation discovered, the emission of a helium nucleus is called **alpha radiation**, and the emitted helium nucleus an **alpha particle** (Figure 1.13).

Fission: Under some circumstances, the nucleus of the unstable atom may break into larger fragments, a process usually referred to as **nuclear fission**. During fission two or three neutrons are emitted (Figure 1.14).

Unstable Neutron–Proton Ratio

Too many neutrons—beta decay: Nuclei with excess neutrons can achieve stability by a process that amounts to the conversion of a neutron into a proton and an electron. The proton remains in the nucleus, but the electron is emitted. This is called **beta radiation**, and the electron itself a **beta particle** (Figure 1.15). The process and the emitted electron were given these names to contrast with the alpha particle before the physical nature of either was discovered. The beta particle generated in this decay will become a free electron until it finds a vacancy in an electron shell either in the atom of its origin or in another atom.

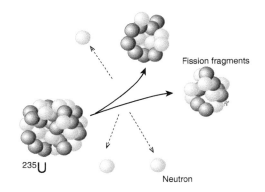

Figure 1.14 Fission of a ^{235}U nucleus.

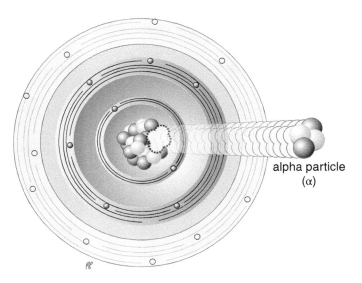

Figure 1.13 Alpha decay.

Antineutrino $\bar{\nu}$

Beta particle (β^-)

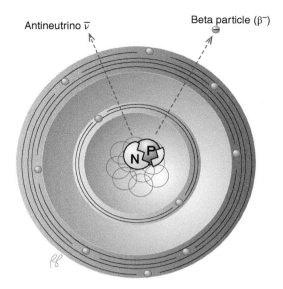

Figure 1.15 $\beta-$ (negatron) decay.

Neutrino ν

Positron (β^+)

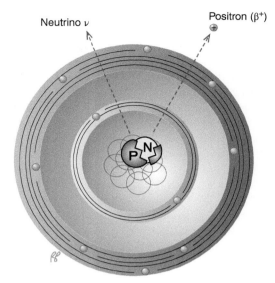

Figure 1.16 $\beta+$ (positron) decay.

Careful study of beta decay suggested to physicists that the conversion of neutron to proton involved more than the emission of a beta particle (electron). Beta emission satisfied the rule for conservation of charge in that the neutral neutron yielded one positive proton and one negative electron; however, it did not appear to satisfy the equally important rule for conservation of energy. Measurements showed that most of the emitted electrons simply did not have all the energy expected. To explain this apparent discrepancy, the emission of a second particle was postulated and that particle was later identified experimentally. Called an **antineutrino** (neutrino for small and neutral), it carries the "missing" energy of the reaction.

Too many protons—positron decay and electron capture: In a manner analogous to that for excess neutrons, an unstable nucleus with too many protons can undergo a decay that has the effect of converting a proton into a neutron. There are two ways this can occur: positron decay and electron capture. In general, these proton rich nuclei decay by a combination of these two processes.

Positron decay: A proton can be converted into a neutron and a **positron**, which is an electron with a positive, instead of negative, charge (Figure 1.16).

The positron is also referred to as a positive beta particle or positive electron or anti-electron. In positron decay, a **neutrino** is also emitted. In many ways, positron decay is the mirror image of beta decay: positive electron instead of negative electron, neutrino instead of antineutrino. Unlike the negative electron, the positron itself survives only briefly. It quickly encounters an electron (electrons are plentiful in matter), and both are **annihilated** (see Chapter 8, Figure 8.1). This is why it is considered an anti-electron. Generally speaking, antiparticles react with the corresponding particle to annihilate both. During the annihilation reaction, the combined mass of the positron and electron is converted into two photons of energy equivalent to the mass destroyed, each with an energy of 511 keV or a total of 1.022 MeV. Following ejection of a positron from a nucleus the atom must also shed an orbital electron to keep the overall charge of the atom neutral. So, in essence, the atom is losing the mass equivalent of two electrons (remember positrons are basically positively charged electrons). Positron emission will only occur when the difference in mass between the parent (original) and daughter atoms is at minimum the mass of two electrons, which, as we will see in Chapter 2, Figure 2.12 is equal to 1.02 MeV of energy.

Energy of beta particles and positrons

Although the total energy emitted from an atom during beta decay or positron emission is constant, the relative distribution of this energy between the beta particle and antineutrino (or positron and neutrino) is variable. For example, the total amount of available energy released during beta decay of a phosphorus-32 atom is 1.7 MeV. This energy can be distributed as 0.5 MeV to the beta particle and 1.2 MeV to the antineutrino, or 1.5 MeV to the beta particle and 0.2 MeV to the antineutrino, or 1.7 MeV to the beta particle and no energy to the antineutrino, and so on. In any group of atoms the likelihood of occurrence of each of such combinations is not equal. It is very uncommon, for example, that all of the energy is carried off by the beta particle. It is much more common for the particle to receive less than half of the total amount of energy emitted. This is illustrated by Figure 1.17, a plot of the number of beta particles emitted at each energy from zero to the maximum energy released in the decay. $E_{\beta max}$ is the maximum possible energy that a beta particles can receive during beta decay of any atom, $\overline{E}_\beta$ is the average energy of all beta particles for decay of a group of such atoms. The average energy is approximately one-third of the maximum energy or

$$\overline{E}_\beta \cong \tfrac{1}{3}E_{\beta max}$$

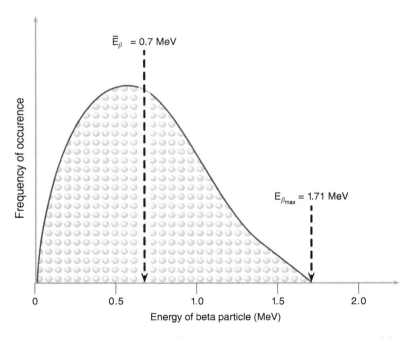

Figure 1.17 Beta emissions (both β⁻ and β⁺) are ejected from the nucleus with energies between 0 and their maximum possible energy ($E_{\beta max}$). The average energy ($\overline{E}_\beta$) is equal to approximately one third of the maximum energy.

Electron capture: Through a process that competes with positron decay, a nucleus can combine with one of its inner orbital electrons to achieve the net effect of converting one of the protons in the nucleus into a neutron (Figure 1.18). An outer-shell electron then fills the vacancy in the inner shell left by the captured electron. The energy lost by the "fall" of the outer-shell electron to the inner shell isemitted as an X-ray.

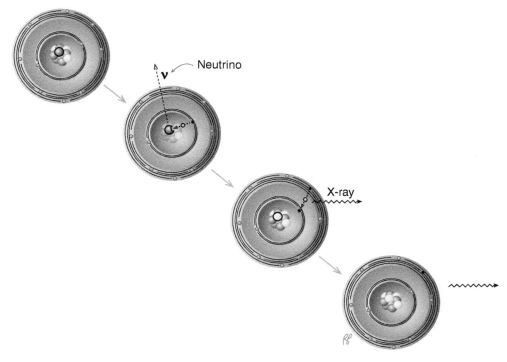

Figure 1.18 Electron capture.

Appropriate numbers of nucleons, but too much energy

Isomeric transition: Following alpha and beta decay and electron capture, the nucleus has a more favorable physical configuration of nucleons but usually contains an excess of energy. The nucleus is said to be in an excited state when the energy of the nucleus is greater than its resting level. This excess energy is shed by **isomeric transition**. This may occur by either or both of two competing reactions: gamma emission or internal conversion. Most isomeric transitions occur as a combination of these two reactions.

Gamma emission: In this process, excess nuclear energy is emitted as a gamma ray (Figure 1.19). The name gamma was given to this radiation, before its physical nature was understood, because it was the third (alpha, beta, gamma) type of radiation discovered. A gamma ray is a photon (energy) emitted by an excited nucleus. Despite its unique name, it cannot be distinguished from photons of the same energy from different sources, for example X-rays.

Internal conversion: The excited nucleus can transfer its excess energy to an orbital electron (generally an inner-shell electron) causing the electron to be ejected from the atom. This can only occur if the excess energy is greater than the binding energy of the electron. This electron is called a **conversion electron**. The resulting inner orbital vacancy is rapidly filled with an outer-shell electron (as the atom assumes a more stable state, inner orbitals are filled before outer orbitals). The energy released as a result of the "fall" of an outer-shell electron to an inner shell is emitted as an X-ray (Figure 1.20a) or as a free electron, an **Auger electron** (Figure 1.20b). The emitted X-ray is called a **characteristic X-ray** because its energy always equals the difference in binding energies between the electron shells.

Decay notation

Decay from an unstable parent nuclide to a more stable daughter nuclide can occur in a series of steps, with the production of particles and photons characteristic of each step. A standard notation is used to describe these steps (Figure 1.21). The uppermost level of the schematic is the state with

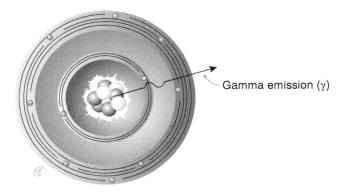

Figure 1.19 Isomeric transition. Excess nuclear energy is carried off as a gamma ray.

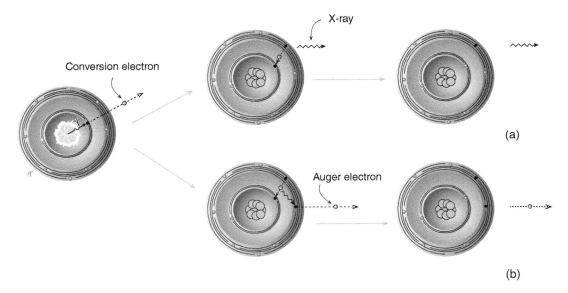

Figure 1.20 Internal conversion. As an alternative to gamma emission, it can lead to emission of either an X-ray (a) or an Auger electron (b).

the greatest energy. As the nuclide decays by losing energy and/or particles, lower horizontal levels represent states of relatively lower energy. Directional arrows from one level to the next indicate the type of decay. By convention, an oblique line angled downward and to the left indicates electron capture; downward and to the right, beta emission; and a vertical arrow, an isomeric transition. The dogleg is used for positron emission. A dogleg with a "Z" denotes alpha decay. Notice that a pathway ending to the left, as in electron capture or positron emission, corresponds to a decrease in atomic number. On the other hand, a line ending to the right, as in

beta emission, corresponds to an increase in atomic number.

Figure 1.22 depicts specific decay schemes for ^{99m}Tc, ^{111}In, ^{131}I, and ^{226}Ra (this is not the isotope used for treatment in nuclear medicine, ^{223}Ra, which will be discussed in detail in Chapter 18). The "m" in ^{99m}Tc stands for **metastable**, which refers to an excited nucleus with an appreciable lifetime ($>10^{-12}$ seconds) prior to undergoing isomeric transition.

Half-life

It is not possible to predict when an individual nuclide atom will decay, just as in preparing

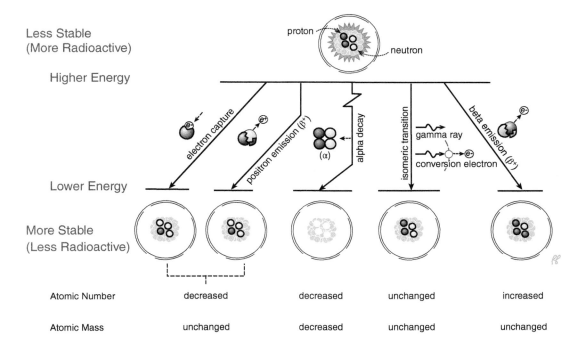

Less Stable
(More Radioactive)

Higher Energy

proton

neutron

electron capture

positron emission (β⁺)

alpha decay
(α)

isomeric transition

gamma ray

conversion electron

beta emission (β⁺)

Lower Energy

More Stable
(Less Radioactive)

Atomic Number	decreased	decreased	unchanged	increased
Atomic Mass	unchanged	decreased	unchanged	unchanged

Figure 1.21 Decay schematics.

popcorn one cannot determine when any particular kernel of corn will open. However, the average behavior of a large number of the popcorn kernels is predictable. From experience with microwave popcorn, one knows that half of the kernels will pop within 2 minutes and most of the bag will be done in 4 minutes. In a like manner, the average behavior of a radioactive sample containing billions of atoms is predictable. The time it takes for half of these atoms to decay is called (appropriately enough) the **half-life**, or in scientific notation $T_{1/2}$ pronounced "T one-half"). It is not surprising that the time it takes for half of the remaining atoms to decay is also $T_{1/2}$. This process continues until the number of nuclide atoms eventually comes so close to zero that we can consider the process complete. A plot of **A(t)**, the activity remaining, is shown in Figure 1.23.

This curve, and therefore the average behavior of the sample of radioactivity, can be described by the **decay equation:**

$$A(t) = A(0)e^{-0.693t/T_{1/2}}$$

where **A(0)** is the initial number of radioactive atoms.

A commonly used alternative form of the decay equation employs the **decay constant** (λ), which is approximately 0.693 divided by the half-life ($T_{1/2}$):

$$\lambda = 0.693/T_{1/2}$$

The decay equation can be rewritten as

$$A(t) = A(0)e^{-\lambda t}$$

The amount of activity of any radionuclide may be expressed as the number of decays per unit time. Common units for measuring radioactivity are the **curie** (after Marie Curie) or the SI unit, the **becquerel** (after another nuclear pioneer, Henri Becquerel). One becquerel is defined as one radioactive decay per second. Nuclear medicine doses are generally a million times greater and are more easily expressed in megabecquerels (MBq). One curie (Ci) is defined as 3.7×10^{10} decays per second (this was picked because it is approximately equal to the radioactivity emitted by 1 g of radium in equilibrium with its daughter nuclides). A partial list of conversion values is provided in Table 1.2.

A related term that is frequently confused with decay is the **count**, which refers to the registration of a single decay by a detector such as a Geiger counter.

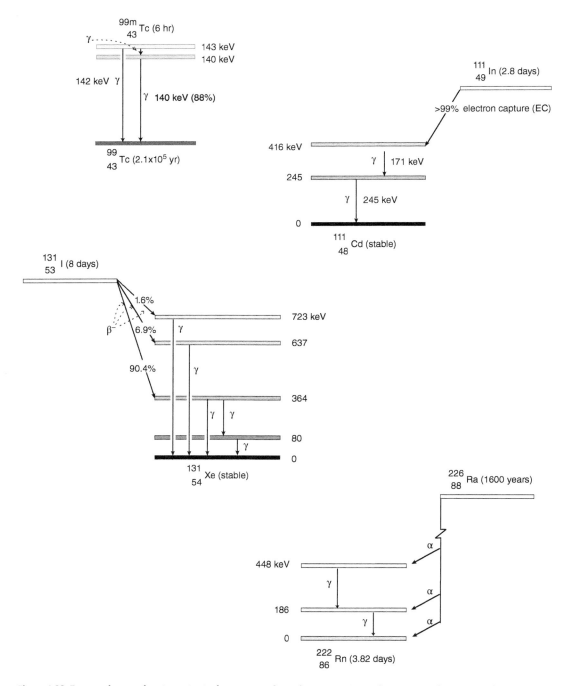

Figure 1.22 Decay schemes showing principal transitions for technetium-99m, indium-111, iodine-131 and radium-226. Energy levels are rounded to three significant figures.

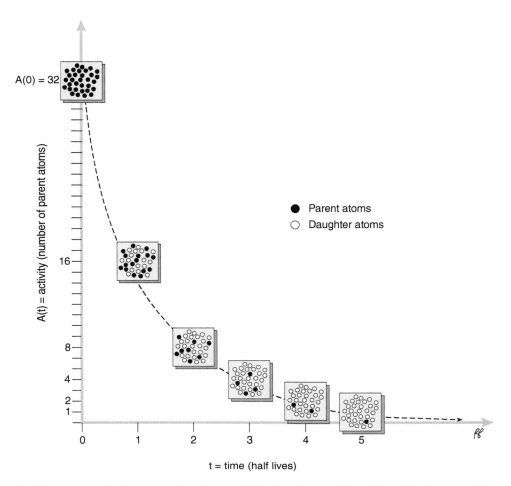

Figure 1.23 Decay curve. Note the progressive replacement of radioactive atoms (parent) by relatively more stable atoms (daughter) as shown schematically in each box.

Table 1.2 Conversion values for units of radioactivity

One curie (Ci) =		*1×10^3 mCi*	*1×10^6 μCi*	*37×10^9 Bq*	*37×10^3 MBq*
One millicurie (mCi) =	1×10^{-3} Ci		1×10^3 μCi	37×10^6 Bq	37 MBq
One microcurie (μCi) =	1×10^{-6} Ci	1×10^{-3} mCi		37×10^3 Bq	37×10^{-3} MBq
One bequerel (Bq)* =	27×10^{-12} Ci	27×10^{-9} mCi	27×10^{-6} μCi		1×10^{-6} MBq
One megabequerel (MBq) =	27×10^{-6} Ci	27×10^{-3} mCi	27 μCi	1×10^6 Bq	

* One bequerel = 1 decay per second.

Most of the detectors used in nuclear medicine detect only a fraction of the decays, principally because the radiation from many of the decays is directed away from the detector. Count rate refers to the number of decays actually counted in a given time, usually counts per minute. All things being equal, the count rate will be proportional to the decay rate, and it is a commonly used, if inexact, measure of radioactivity.

Questions

1. The chemical interactions between various elements are mainly determined by:
   (a) The number of protons.
   (b) The number of neutrons.
   (c) The number of electrons in the outermost shell.
   (d) The number of protons minus the number of electrons.

2. For each of the five terms below, choose the best definition:
   (1) Isobars.
   (2) Isoclines.
   (3) Isomers.
   (4) Isotones.
   (5) Isotopes.
      (a) Atoms of the same element (equal Z) with different numbers of neutrons (N).
      (b) Atoms of the same element (equal Z) with different numbers of protons.
      (c) Atoms of different elements (different Z) with equal numbers of neutrons (N).
      (d) Atoms of different elements with equal atomic mass (A).

3. Which of the following statements are correct?
   (a) There is a stable isotope of technetium.
   (b) Atoms with atomic numbers (Z) > 83 are inherently unstable.
   (c) For lighter elements nuclear stability is achieved with equal numbers of protons and neutrons; for heavier elements the number of neutrons exceeds the number of protons.

4. For internal conversion to occur, the excess energy of the excited nucleus must equal or exceed:
   (a) 511 keV.
   (b) 1.022 MeV.
   (c) The internal conversion coefficient.
   (d) The average energy of the Auger electrons.
   (e) The binding energy of the emitted electron.

5. For an atom undergoing beta decay, the average energy of the emitted beta particles is approximately:
   (a) 511 keV.
   (b) 0.551 times the loss of atomic mass.
   (c) One half of the total energy released for the individual event.

   (d) One third of the maximum energy of the emitted beta particles.
   (e) Equal to the average energy of the accompanying antineutrinos.

6. You receive a dose of ^{99m}Tc measuring 370 MBq from the radiopharmacy at 10 am. Your patient does not arrive in the department until 2 pm. How much activity, in mCi, remains? (The $T_{1/2}$ of ^{99m}Tc is 6 hours. The constant e = 2.718).

7. Rank the following binding energies from greatest to least:
   (1) Electron binding energy for outer shell electrons.
   (2) Nuclear binding energy.
   (3) Electron binding energy for inner shell electrons.

8. True or false: The term metastable refers to an intermediate state of nuclear decay lasting longer than 10^{-12} seconds prior to undergoing isomeric transition.

9. Which of the following is true regarding beta decay of a specific radioisotope:
   (1) The energy of the emitted beta particle is always the same.
   (2) The energy of the emitted antineutrino is always the same.
   (3) The summed energy of the emitted beta particle and antineutrino is always the same.

10. Which unit of measurement for radioactivity is defined as one radioactive decay per second?
    (1) Bequerel.
    (2) Millicurie.
    (3) Megabequerel.

11. 10 mCi equals how many MBq?
    (1) 2.7 MBq.
    (2) 37 MBq.
    (3) 270 MBq.
    (4) 370 MBq.

12. Lighter nuclides (Z < 83) with an excess of neutrons tend to decay by:
    (1) Gamma emission.
    (2) Beta minus decay.
    (3) Isomeric transition.
    (4) Positron emission.
    (5) Alpha emission.

13. Which of the following statements are true?
    (1) An alpha particle is the same thing as a helium nucleus.
    (2) Neutrinos have the same charge as an electron.
    (3) X-rays always have lower energies than gamma rays.
    (4) The terms "activity" and "count rate" are the same—they express a measurement of photons per second.

14. When orbital electrons move from an outer shell to an inner-shell, which of the following is **not** true
    (a) Characteristic X-rays can be emitted.
    (b) Auger electrons can be emitted.
    (c) The atom becomes more stable.
    (d) A mixture of gamma rays and internal conversion electrons can be emitted.

Answers

1. (c)
2. (1) d. (2) None of the above; usually used as a geological term. (3) None of the above; in nuclear medicine it refers to an element whose nucleus is in an unstable (excited) state. (4) (c). (5) (a).
3. (b) and (c) are true. (a) is false; technetium does not have a stable form; ^{99}Tc has a $T_{1/2}$ of 2.1×10^5 year.
4. (e).
5. (d).
6. 6.3 mCi.
7. Nuclear binding energy, electron binding energy for inner shell electrons, electron binding energy for outer shell electrons.
8. True.
9. (3).
10. Bequerel.
11. 370 MBq.
12. (2) Beta minus decay.
13. (1) only.
14. (d).

CHAPTER 2

Interaction of Radiation with Matter

When radiation strikes matter, both the nature of the radiation and the composition of the matter affect what happens. The process begins with the transfer of radiation energy to the atoms and molecules, heating the matter or even modifying its structure.

If all the energy of a bombarding particle or photon is transferred, the radiation will appear to have been stopped within the irradiated matter. Conversely, if the energy is not completely deposited in the matter, the remaining energy will emerge as though the matter were transparent or at least translucent. This said, we will now introduce some of the physical phenomena involved as radiation interacts with matter, and in particular we shall consider, separately at first, the interactions in matter of both photons (gamma rays and X-rays) and charged particles (alpha and beta particles).

Interaction of photons with matter

As they pass through matter, photons interact with atoms. The type of interaction is a function of the energy of the photons and the atomic number (Z) of elements composing the matter.

Types of photon interactions in matter

In the practice of nuclear medicine, where gamma rays with energies between 50 keV and 550 keV are used, **Compton scattering** is the dominant type of interaction in materials with lower atomic numbers, such as human tissue (Z = 7.5). The **photoelectric effect** is the dominant type of interaction in materials with higher atomic numbers, such as lead (Z = 82). A third type of interaction of photons with

matter, **pair production**, only occurs with very high photon energies (greater than 1020 keV) and is therefore not important in clinical nuclear medicine. Figure 2.1 depicts the predominant type of interaction for various combinations of incident photons and absorber atomic numbers.

Compton scattering

In Compton scattering the incident photon transfers part of its energy to an outer shell or (essentially) "free" electron, ejecting it from the atom. Upon ejection this electron is called the **Compton electron**. The photon, which has lost energy in the interaction, is scattered (Figure 2.2) at an angle that depends on the amount of energy transferred from the photon to the electron. The scattering angle can range from nearly 0° to 180°. Figure 2.3 illustrates scattering angles of 135° and 45°.

Photoelectric effect

An incident photon may also transfer its energy to an orbital (generally inner-shell) electron. This process is called the **photoelectric effect** and the ejected electron is called a **photoelectron** (Figure 2.4). This electron leaves the atom with an energy equal to the energy of the incident gamma ray diminished by the binding energy of the electron. An outer-shell electron then fills the inner-shell vacancy and the excess energy is emitted as an X-ray.

$$E_{photoelectron} = E_{photon} - E_{binding}$$

Table 2.1 lists the predominant photon interactions in some common materials.

Essentials of Nuclear Medicine Physics, Instrumentation, and Radiation Biology, Fourth Edition.
Rachel A. Powsner, Matthew R. Palmer, and Edward R. Powsner.
© 2022 John Wiley & Sons Ltd. Published 2022 by John Wiley & Sons Ltd.

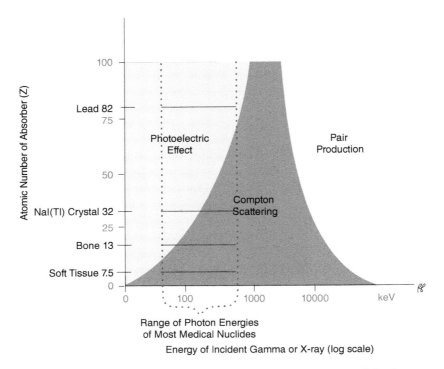

Figure 2.1 Predominant type of interaction for various combinations of incident photons and absorber atomic numbers.

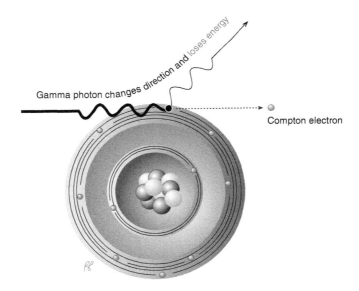

Figure 2.2 Compton scattering.

Attenuation of photons in matter

As the result of the interactions between photons and matter, the **intensity** of the **beam** (stream of photons), that is, the number of photons remaining in the beam, decreases as the beam passes through matter (Figure 2.5). This loss of photons is called **attenuation**; the matter through which the beam passes is referred to as the **attenuator**. Specifically, attenuation is the ratio of intensity at the point the beam exits the attenuator, I_{out}, to the intensity it had where it entered, I_{in}. Attenuation is an exponential function of the thickness, x, of the attenuator in centimeters. That the function is exponential can be understood to mean that if half of the beam is lost in traversing the first centimeter of material, half of the remainder will be lost traversing the next centimeter, and so on. This resembles the exponential manner in which radioactivity decays with time. Expressed symbolically,

$$I_{out}/I_{in} = e^{-\mu x}$$

where μ, the **linear attenuation coefficient** is a property of the attenuator. When, as is usually the case, thickness is given in centimeters, the linear attenuation coefficient is expressed as "per centimeter" or "cm^{-1}". As might be expected, the linear attenuation coefficient is greater for dense tissue

such as bone than for soft tissue such as fat. In general, the linear attenuation coefficient depends on both the energy of the photons and on the average atomic number (Z) and thickness of the attenuator. The lower the energy of the photons or the greater the average atomic number or thickness of the attenuator, the greater the attenuation (Figure 2.6).

A separate term, the **mass attenuation coefficient** (μ/ρ), is the linear attenuation coefficient divided by the density of the attenuator. When the density of a material is given in grams/cm^3 the units of the mass attenuation coefficient are cm^2/gram.

Absorption of radiation describes another aspect of the process of attenuation. Attenuation describes the weakening of the beam as it passes through matter. Absorption describes the transfer of energy from the beam to the matter.

Half-value and tenth-value layers

A material's effectiveness as a photon attenuator is described by the attenuation coefficient. An alternative descriptor, one that is the more easily visualized,

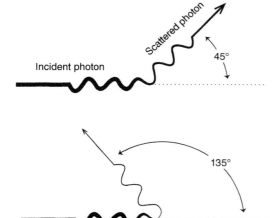

Figure 2.3 Angle of photon scattering.

Table 2.1 Predominant photon interactions in common materials at diagnostic energies

Material	Atomic number (Z)	Density (gm/cm³)	Predominant interaction
H$_2$O	7.4	1.0	Compton scatter
Soft tissue	7.5	1.0	Compton scatter
Glass (silicon)	14	2.6	Compton scatter
O$_2$ (gas)	16	0.0014	Compton scatter
NaI (crystal)	32	3.7	Photoelectric effect
Lead	82	11.4	Photoelectric effect
Leaded glass	14, 82	4.8–6.2	Photoelectric effect

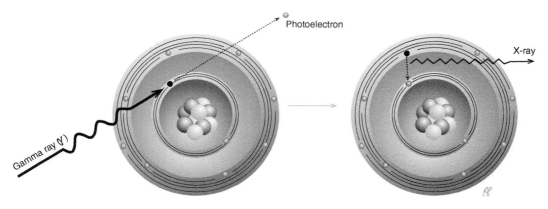

Figure 2.4 Photoelectric effect.

is the "half-value layer" (**HVL**) which is simply the thickness of a slab of the attenuator that will remove exactly one half of the radiation of a beam. A second slab of the same thickness will remove half of the remainder (see comment below regarding monoenergetic beams), leaving one quarter of the original beam, and so forth. For a gamma photon of 100 keV, the HVL in soft tissue is about 4 cm [1].

For any attenuator the HVL can be determined experimentally using a photon source and a suitable detector. For calculations involving attenuation of high-intensity radiation beams, an entirely similar concept, the tenth-value layer

(**TVL**), is useful. The TVL is the thickness of the attenuator that will transmit only one tenth of the photons in the beam. For a monoenergetic beam (containing photons of identical energies) directed at a material, two such thicknesses will transmit only one hundredth of the beam. If, however, the beam contains photons of different energies this rule is not applicable (see text box on beam hardening).

Table 2.2 lists half and tenth value layer of lead for photons emitted by some common medical radionuclides.

For a monoenergetic beam of photons, the linear attenuation coefficient, μ, is related to the HVL as follows:

$$\mu = 0.693 / \mathrm{HVL}$$

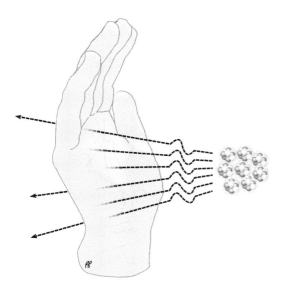

Figure 2.5 Attenuation.

Beam hardening

When a beam contains photons of different energies such as an X-ray beam, it is termed **polychromatic.** As a polychromatic beam penetrates a material, lower energy photons are extinguished or scattered preferentially over higher energy photons and the result is that, while the overall intensity is diminished, the average energy of the transmitted fraction of the beam is increased. This phenomenon is known as **beam hardening**. A hardened beam is more penetrating and so a second HVL or TVL will be slightly thicker than the first.

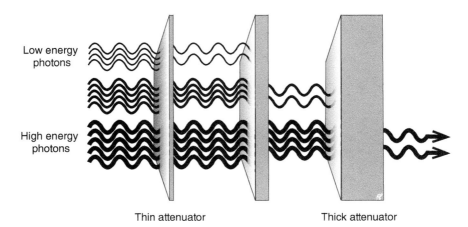

Low energy photons

High energy photons

Thin attenuator   Thick attenuator

Figure 2.6 The amount of attenuation of a photon beam is dependent on the photon energy and the thickness (and/or atomic number) of the attenuator.

Table 2.2 HVL and TVL of lead for photons of common medical nuclides

Nuclide	Gamma energy (keV)	Half-value layer (cm)	Tenth-value layer (cm)
^{99m}Tc	140	0.03	0.09
^{67}Ga	93, 185, 300, 393	0.07	0.41
^{123}I	159	0.04	0.12
^{131}I	364	0.3	1
^{18}F	511	0.39	1.3
^{111}In	172, 245	0.023	0.2

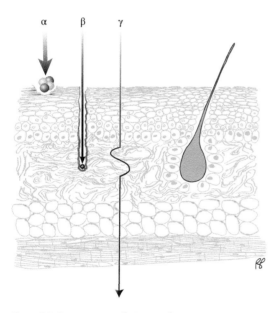

Figure 2.7 Penetrating radiation and nonpenetrating radiation.

The term **penetrating radiation** may be used to describe X-ray and gamma radiation, as they have the potential to penetrate considerable thickness of a material. Although we have just described some of the many ways photons interact with matter, the likelihood of any of these interactions occurring over a short distance is small. An individual photon may travel several centimeters or farther into tissue before it interacts. In contrast, charged particles (alpha, beta) undergo many closely spaced interactions. This sharply limits their penetration (Figure 2.7).

Interaction of charged particles with matter

Because of the strong electrical force between a charged particle and the atoms of an absorber, charged particles can be stopped by matter with relative ease. Compared to photons, they transfer a greater amount of energy in a shorter distance and come to rest more rapidly. For this reason, they are referred to as **nonpenetrating radiation** (see depiction of alpha and beta particles in Figure 2.7). In contrast to a photon of 100 keV which has a HVL of 4 cm in soft tissue, an electron of this energy would penetrate less than 0.00014 cm in soft tissue [1].

Excitation

Charged particles (alphas, betas, and positrons) interact with the electrons surrounding the atom's nucleus by transferring some of their kinetic energy to the electrons. The energy transferred from a low-energy particle is often only sufficient to bump an electron from an inner to an outer shell of the atom. This process is called excitation. Following excitation, the displaced electron promptly returns to the lower-energy shell, releasing its recently acquired energy as an X-ray in a process called de-excitation (Figure 2.8). Because the acquired energy is equal to the difference in binding energies of the electron shells and the binding energies of the electron shells are determined by the atomic structure of the element, the X-ray is referred to as a **characteristic X-ray**.

Ionization

Charged particles of sufficient energy may also transfer enough energy to an electron (generally one in an outer shell) to eject the electron from the atom. This process is called **ionization** (Figure 2.9). This hole in the outer shell is rapidly filled with an unbound electron. If an inner shell electron is ionized (a much less frequent occurrence) an outer shell electron will "drop" into the inner shell hole and a characteristic X-ray will be emitted. Ionization is not limited to the interaction of charged particles and matter, the photoelectric effect and Compton interactions are examples of photon interactions with matter that produce ionization.

Specific ionization

When radiation causes the ejection of an electron from an atom of the absorber, the resulting positively

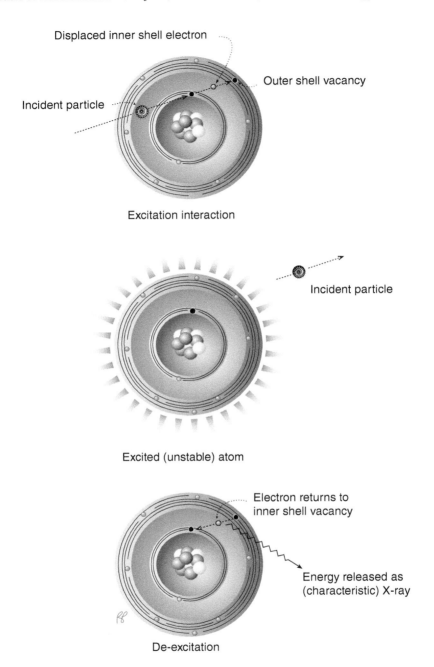

Figure 2.8 Excitation and de-excitation.

charged atom and free negatively charged electron are called an **ion pair** (Figure 2.9). The amount of energy transferred per ion pair created, **W**, is characteristic of the materials in the absorber. For example, approximately 33 eV (range 25 to 40 eV) is transferred to the absorber for each ion pair created in air or water. It is often convenient to refer to the number of ion pairs created per unit distance the radiation travels as its **specific ionization (SI)**.

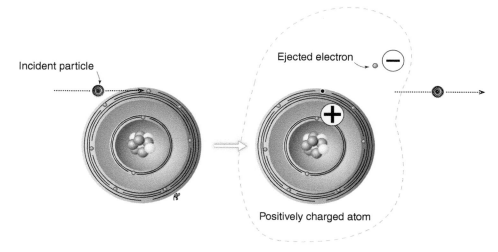

Figure 2.9 Ionization. The ejected electron and the positively charged atom are called an "ion pair" (demarcated by dashed line).

Particles with more charge (alpha particles) have a higher specific ionization than lighter particles (electrons).

Linear energy transfer

Linear energy transfer **(LET)** is the amount of energy transferred in a given distance by a particle moving through an absorber. Linear energy transfer is related to specific ionization:

$$LET = SI \times W$$

Alpha particles are classified as high LET radiation, beta particles and photons as low LET radiation.

Range

Range is the distance radiation travels through the absorber. Particles that are lighter, have less charge (such as beta particles), and/or have greater energy travel farther than particles that are heavier, have a greater charge (such as alpha particles), and/or have less energy (Figure 2.10).

In traversing an absorber, an electron loses energy at each interaction with the atoms of the absorber. The energy loss per interaction is variable. Therefore, the total distance traveled by electrons of the same energy can vary by as much as 3% to 4%. This variation in range is called the **straggling of the ranges**. The heavier alpha particles are not affected to a significant degree and demonstrate very little straggling of range.

Annihilation

This interaction in matter most often involves a positron (positive electron) and an electron (negatron). After a positron has transferred most of its kinetic energy by ionization and excitation, it combines with a free or loosely bound negative electron. Recall that electrons and positrons have equal mass but opposite electric charge. This interaction is explosive, as the combined mass of the two particles is instantly converted to energy in the form of two oppositely directed photons, each of 511 keV. This is referred to as an **annihilation reaction** (Figure 2.11). It is another example of the interchangeability of mass and energy described in Einstein's equation: energy equals mass times the speed of light squared, or $E = mc^2$ (Figure 2.12).

Bremsstrahlung

Small charged particles such as beta particles (electrons and positrons) may be deflected by nuclei as they pass through matter, which may be attributed to the positive charge of the atomic nuclei. As the electron or positron is deflected it also loses speed (decelerates) and this interaction generates X-radiation known as bremsstrahlung (Figure 2.13), which in German means "braking radiation." The energy of the X-ray is equal to the loss of the kinetic

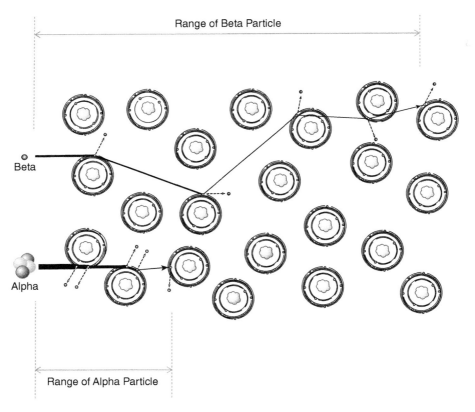

Figure 2.10 Particle range in an absorber.

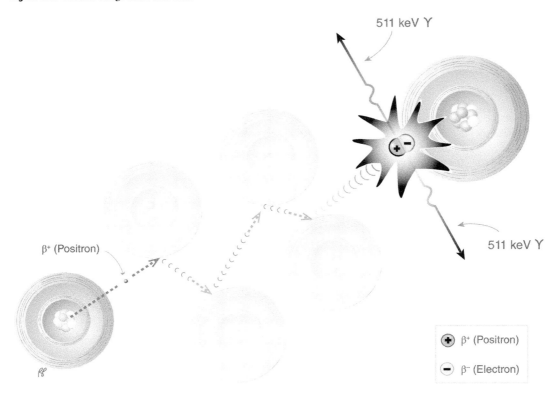

Figure 2.11 Annihilation reaction.

energy of the incident electron or proton as it decelerates (see section on kinetic energy). The greater the speed of the incident particle, the greater the charge of the nucleus, and the closer the incident

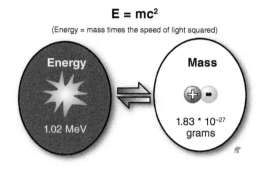

E = mc²

(Energy = mass times the speed of light squared)

Energy

1.02 MeV

Mass

1.83 * 10⁻²⁷ grams

Figure 2.12 Einstein's theory of the equivalence of energy and mass.

particle is to the nucleus the greater the energy of the generated X-ray (Figure 2.14). Since the proximity of the incident particle to the nucleus is random, the X-rays produced by a stream of particles will have a range of energies from near zero up to the kinetic energy of the incident particle (the maximum value is generated when the incident particle is completely stopped by the atomic nucleus). Figure 2.15 illustrates the bremsstrahlung X-ray spectrum for ⁹⁰Yttrium which has a maximum X-ray energy equal to the maximum beta particle energy of 2280 keV.

Reference

1. Shapiro, J. Radiation Protection. A *Guide for Scientists, Regulators, and Physicians*, 4th edn. Cambridge MA: Harvard University Press, 2002, pp. 42 and 53.

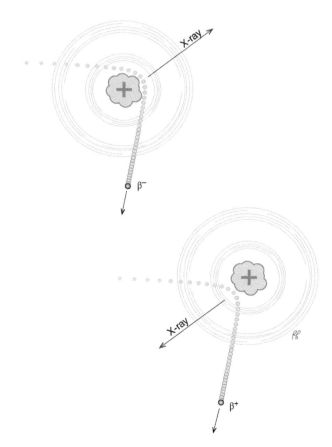

Figure 2.13 Bremsstrahlung. Beta particles (β⁻) and positrons (β⁺) that travel near the nucleus will be attracted or repelled by the positive charge of the nucleus generating X-rays in the process.

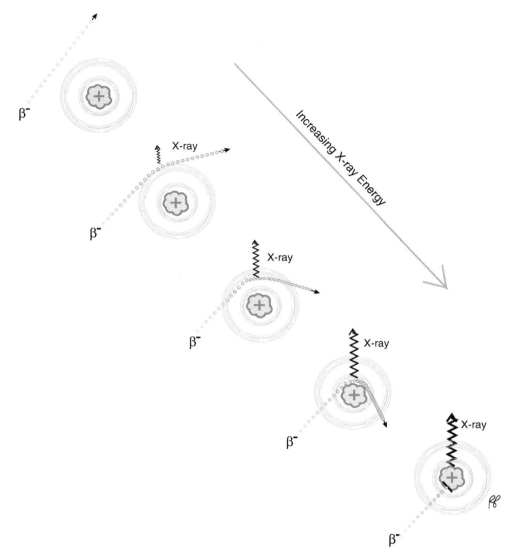

Figure 2.14 Bremsstrahlung X-ray energies increase with increasing proximity of the beta particle to the atomic nucleus (illustrated), greater incident beta particle energy, and greater nucleus charge.

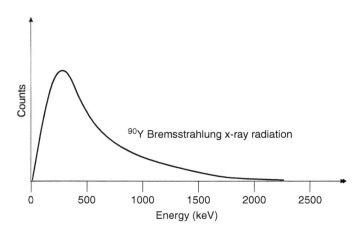

Figure 2.15 Bremsstrahlung X-ray energies vary from near zero to the maximum incident beta particle energy.

Questions

1. Which of the following is true of the interaction of charged particles with matter?
   (a) Alpha particles have a higher LET than beta particles.
   (b) The range of alpha particles is generally greater than beta particles.
   (c) Alpha particles have a higher specific ionization than beta particles.

2. True or false: Bremsstrahlung is X-ray radiation emitted as a moving electron or positron decelerates and changes direction in close proximity to a nucleus.

3. True or false: The photoelectric effect is the dominant type of photon interaction in tissue for radionuclides used in the practice of nuclear medicine.

4. For each of the terms listed here, select the appropriate definition:
   (1) HVL (half value layer).
   (2) TVL (tenth value layer).
   (3) μ (mu) (linear attenuation coefficient).
      (a) Thickness of an attenuator that will reduce the intensity (number of photons) in a monoenergetic beam by 90%.
      (b) Thickness of an attenuator that will reduce the intensity (number of photons) in a monoenergetic beam by 50%.
      (c) 0.693/HVL.

5. Which of the following occur during photon interactions with matter (more than one answer may apply)?
   (a) Excitation.
   (b) Pair production.
   (c) Ionization.
   (d) Compton scattering.
   (e) Bremsstrahlung.
   (f) Photoelectric effect.
   (g) Annihilation reaction.

6. Which of the following occur during charged particle interactions with atoms (more than one answer may apply)?
   (a) Excitation.
   (b) Pair production.
   (c) Ionization.
   (d) Compton scattering.
   (e) Bremsstrahlung.
   (f) Photoelectric effect.
   (g) Annihilation reaction.

7. Which of the following are true about annihilation reaction?
   (a) The conversion of the mass of the positron and electron into energy is an example of the interchangeability of mass and energy as described by Einstein's famous equation $E = mc^2$.
   (b) Two oppositely opposed 450 keV photons are emitted as a result of the annihilation reaction.
   (c) Both (a) and (b).

8. Which of the following are referred to as non-penetrating radiation?
   (a) Positrons.
   (b) Gamma photons.
   (c) X-rays.
   (d) Alpha particles.
   (e) Beta particles.

9. Which term refers to the loss of photons from a beam of radiation as it passes through matter?
   (a) Attenuation.
   (b) Absorption.

10. Which term is used to describe the transfer of energy from radiation to surrounding matter?
    (a) Attenuation.
    (b) Absorption.

11. You shield a sample of ^{99m}Tc using a 1 mm-thick sheet of lead. What fraction of the photons will be transmitted through the lead? The linear attenuation coefficient, μ, of lead for 140 keV photons is 23.1 cm^{-1}.

Answers

1. (a) and (c) are true, (b) is false; alpha particles have a shorter range than beta particles.
2. True.
3. False: Compton scattering is the dominant interaction.
4. (a) 2, (b) 1, (c) 3.
5. (b), (c), (d), (f).

6. (a), (c), (e), (g).
7. (a).
8. (a), (d), (e).
9. (a).
10. (b).
11. 0.1 (transmitted fraction $= I_{out} / I_{in} = e^{-\mu x} = e^{-2.31} = 0.1$).

CHAPTER 3

Formation of Radionuclides

Many radionuclides exist in nature. An example is ^{14}C, which decays slowly with a half-life of 5700 years and is used to date fossils. The nuclides we use in nuclear medicine, however, are not naturally occurring but rather are made either by bombarding stable atoms or by splitting massive atoms. There are three basic types of equipment that are used to make medical nuclides: generators, cyclotrons, and nuclear reactors.

Generators

Generators are units that contain a radioactive **"parent" nuclide** with a relatively long half-life that decays to a short-lived **"daughter" nuclide**. The most commonly used generator is the technetium-99m (^{99m}Tc) generator (Figure 3.1), which consists of a heavily shielded column with molybdenum-99 (^{99}Mo; parent) bound to the alumina of the column. The ^{99m}Tc (daughter) is "milked" (eluted) by drawing sterile saline through the column into the vacuum vial. The parent ^{9}Mo (small gray circles) remains on the column, but the daughter ^{99m}Tc (white circles) is washed away in the saline.

A generator like the one just described is frequently called a **cow**, the elution of the daughter nuclide is referred to as **milking**, and the surrounding lead is called a **pig**, a term used for any crude cast-metal container. Another generator that is used extensively for cardiac imaging is the ^{82}Sr–^{82}Rb generator. Its design and construction is very similar to the ^{99}Mo–^{99m}Tc generator but due to the 75 second half-life of ^{82}Rb, the generator must be located on site—usually right next to the PET scanner where the generator is eluted and the solution is infused into the patient in one automated step.

Table 3.1 describes the features of three common generators.

Activity curves for generators

The formal mathematical description of time-activity behavior for parent and daughter radionuclides is complicated because it involves the competition between the accumulation (caused by decay of the parent) and decay of the daughter. The plot of the curve describing the amount of daughter nuclide in a generator following elution has two segments. The first segment traces the period of rapid accumulation of the daughter nuclide and lasts for approximately four half-lives of the daughter nuclide (which for ^{99m}Tc is approximately 24 hours). The second segment of the curve traces what is called the period of **equilibrium**, during which time the amount of daughter nuclide decreases as the parent nuclide decays.

Medical radionuclide generator systems, for practical reasons, have parent half-lives longer than their daughters—in most cases much longer. We classify generators into two groups: those in which the parent half-life is 10 to 100 times that of the daughter and those in which the parent half-life is more than 100 times that of the daughter. In the first group, the activity of the daughter during equilibrium decreases perceptibly over time (when time is measured in units of daughter half-lives). This is called **transient equilibrium**. On the other hand, the equilibrium segment of the curve for the second group is relatively flat. This is called **secular equilibrium**.

Essentials of Nuclear Medicine Physics, Instrumentation, and Radiation Biology, Fourth Edition.
Rachel A. Powsner, Matthew R. Palmer, and Edward R. Powsner.
© 2022 John Wiley & Sons Ltd. Published 2022 by John Wiley & Sons Ltd.

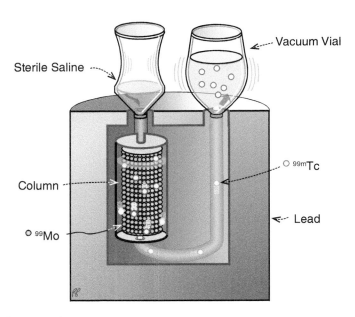

Figure 3.1 ^{99m}Technetium generator.

Table 3.1 Characteristics of three commonly used generators

Generator (Parent–Daughter)	Clinical uses of daughter nuclide	Half-life of parent ($T_{1/2p}$)	Half-life of daughter ($T_{1/2d}$)	$T_{1/2p}/T_{1/2d}$
^{99}Mo–^{99m}Tc (molybdenum-99–technetium-99m)	Used in most radiopharmaceuticals for nuclear studies	66 h	6 h	11
^{82}Sr–^{82}Rb (strontium-82–rubidium-82)	Cardiac perfusion imaging (PET)	25.5 days	75 s	29,000
^{68}Ge–^{68}Ga (germanium-82–gallium-82)	Neuroendocrine imaging (PET)	271 days	68 min	5,800

Transient equilibrium

Transient equilibrium is illustrated in Figure 3.2. In this example, the half-life of the parent nuclide is approximately 10 times that of the daughter. Following an elution that removes all of the available daughter, the amount of the daughter nuclide rapidly increases until the daughter activity slightly exceeds that of the parent at about four to five half-lives. Thereafter the daughter activity declines at the same rate as the parent.

The preceding example of transient equilibrium is based on a decay scheme in which 100% of the parent nuclide decays to the daughter nuclide. However, in the commonly used ^{99}Mo–^{99m}Tc generator, only 86% of the parent molybendum-99 decays to the daughter technetium-99m; the remainder decays directly to Technetium-99 (Figure 3.3). As a result, the activity of ^{99m}Tc is always less than the activity of ^{99}Mo (see Figure 3.3).

Secular equilibrium

For generators where the half-life of the parent is greater than 100 times that of the daughter nuclide, since we are interested in time-scales on the order of the daughter half-life, we just consider the parent nuclide to be stable.

Secular equilibrium, like transient equilibrium, is achieved rapidly following an elution that removes all of the available daughter nuclide. Thereafter the activity of the daughter nuclide is approximately equal to that of the parent. However, the decay curve of the parent appears to be flat since its half-life is so much longer than that of the daughter nuclide. An example of secular equilibrium can be seen with the ^{82}Sr–^{82}Rb generator (see Figure 3.4).

Cyclotrons

Cyclotrons are circular devices (Figure 3.5) in which charged particles such as protons and alpha

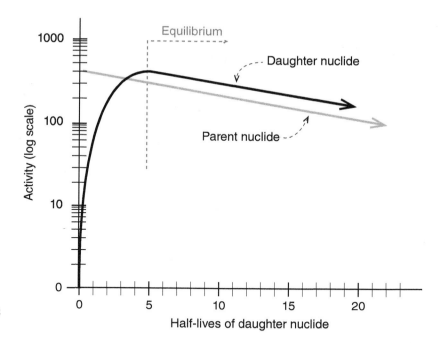

Figure 3.2 Transient equilibrium.

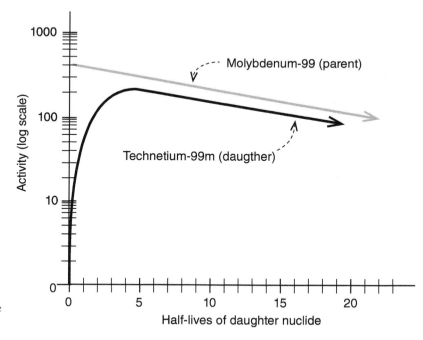

Figure 3.3 Transient equilibrium in a ^{99}Mo–^{99m}Tc generator.

particles are accelerated in a spiral path within a vacuum. The power supply provides a rapidly alternating voltage across the **dees** (the two halves of the circle). This produces a rapidly alternating electric field between the dees that accelerates the particles, which quickly acquire high kinetic ener-

gies. They spiral outward under the influence of the magnetic field until they have sufficient velocity and are deflected into a target.

A deflector is used to direct the particles out through a window of the cyclotron into a **target**. Some of the particles and kinetic energy from these particles are

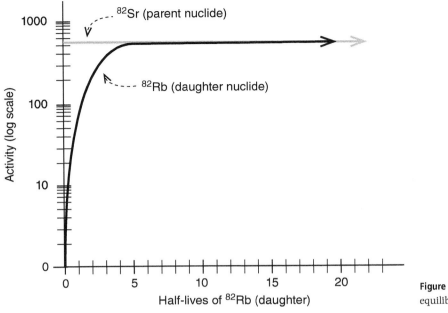

Figure 3.4 Secular equilibrium.

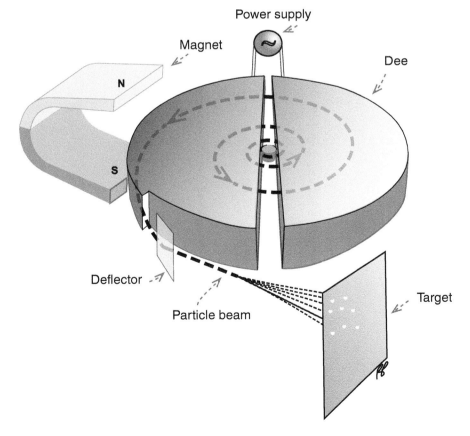

Figure 3.5 Cyclotron.

incorporated into the nuclei of the atoms of the target. These energized (excited) nuclei are unstable.

Indium-111 (^{111}In) is produced in a cyclotron. The accelerated (bombarding) particles are protons. The target atoms are cadmium-112 (^{112}Cd). When a proton enters the nucleus of a ^{112}Cd atom, the ^{112}Cd is transformed into ^{111}In by discharging two neutrons. This reaction can be written as:

Target atom (bombarding particle, emitted particles) product nuclide

Cadmium -112 (proton, two neutrons) Indium -111

or

$$^{112}\mathrm{Cd}\left(\mathrm{p,2n}\right)^{111}\mathrm{In}$$

Other examples of cyclotron reactions include ^{121}Sb(α,2n)^{123}I, ^{68}Zn(d,n)^{67}Ga, and ^{10}B(d,n)^{11}C, where the symbols α and d denote alpha particles and deuterons (proton plus neutron) respectively.

Reactors

Radionuclides for nuclear medicine are also produced in nuclear reactors. Some examples include ^{131}I, ^{133}Xe, and ^{99}Mo.

Reactor basics
A general schematic of a reactor is seen in Figure 3.6. A reactor is composed of **fuel rods** that contain large atoms (typically Uranium-235,

Uranium-238, or Plutonium-239) that are inherently unstable. These atoms undergo **fission**, (see Figure 1.14). Two or three neutrons and approximately 200 MeV of heat energy are emitted during this process. These neutrons leave the nucleus with moderately high **kinetic** energy and are referred to as **fast neutrons**. The neutrons are slowed with a **moderator** such as graphite, water, or heavy water. These "very slow" or **thermal neutrons**, and to a lesser extent the fast neutrons, in turn impact other fissionable atoms causing their fission, and so forth (Figure 3.7). If this **chain reaction** were to grow unchecked, the mass would explode. To maintain control, cadmium **control rods** are inserted to absorb the neutrons in the reactor. They can be further inserted or withdrawn to control the speed of the reaction. Medical nuclides are made in reactors by the processes of fission or neutron capture.

Kinetic energy

Kinetic means "motion." The form of energy attributable to the motion of an object is its kinetic energy. Kinetic energy is related to both the mass (m) and velocity (v) of the object, specifically $\frac{1}{2}\,mv^2$. A moving car has kinetic energy, a parked car does not. A speeding car contains a great deal of kinetic energy that can be dissipated rapidly as heat, noise, and the destruction of metal in a collision.

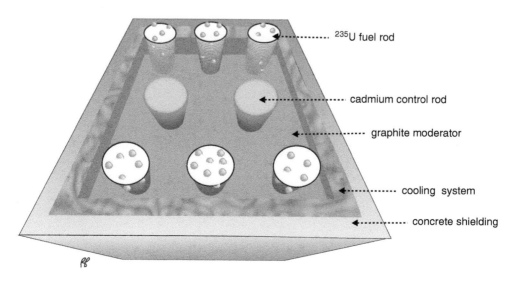

Figure 3.6 Schematic of a nuclear reactor.

Spontaneous fission of ^{235}U atom

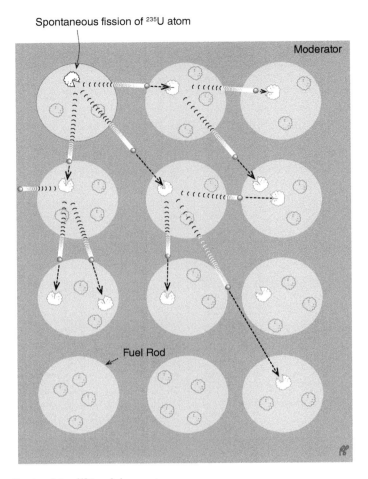

Figure 3.7 Chain reaction involving ^{235}U and slow neutrons.

Fission

In this process, the desired radionuclide is one of the **fission fragments** of a heavy element (Z > 92), either the fuel atom itself or the atoms of a **target** placed inside the reactor. The **by-product** is chemically separated from the other fission fragments. The fission reaction is denoted as

$$^{235}\text{Uranium}\,(\text{neutron,fission})\,\text{daughter}$$
$$\text{nuclide}$$

For example, the formation of iodine-131 and molybdenum-99 are written as

$$^{235}\text{U}\,(\text{n,f})^{131}\,\text{I}\,\text{and}\,^{235}\text{U}\,(\text{n,f})^{99}\,\text{Mo}$$

Neutron capture

In neutron capture the target atom captures a neutron. The new atom is radioactive and emits gamma photons or charged particles to produce the daughter nuclide (Figure 3.8). A gamma photon is emitted following capture of a thermal (slow) neutron. This reaction is written as

$$\text{Target}\,(\text{neutron,gamma})\,\text{daughter nuclide}$$

For example:

$$^{98}\text{Mo}\,(\text{n,}\gamma)\,\text{Mo}^{99}$$

When the target atom captures a fast neutron a proton can be emitted. This capture reaction is sometimes referred to as **transmutation** and is symbolized as

$$\text{Target}\,(\text{neutron,proton})\,\text{daughter nuclide}$$

For example:

$$^{32}\text{S}(\text{n},\text{p})^{32}\text{P}$$

A list of common medical nuclides and their methods of production, modes of decay, and decay products is provided in Appendix A.

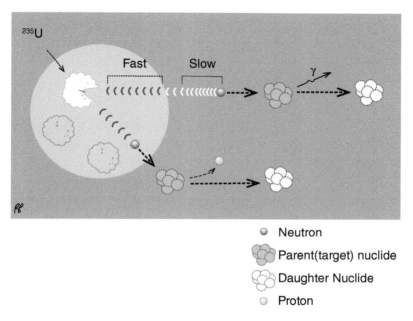

● Neutron

◉ Parent(target) nuclide

◎ Daughter Nuclide

○ Proton

Figure 3.8 Neutron capture by target nuclide placed in a reactor. Thermal (slow) neutron capture causes gamma emission (top), fast neutron capture results in proton emission (bottom).

Radionuclide production

There is often more than one way to make a radionuclide. For example, ^{111}In is most commonly made in a cyclotron using the ^{112}Cd(p,2n)^{111}In reaction but it can also be made from a cadmium-111 target using the ^{111}Cd(p,n)^{111}In reaction or from a silver-109 target in the reaction ^{109}Ag(α,2n)^{111}In. The tradeoffs involve the relative efficiencies of production for various cyclotron energies and the issues involved in separating and purifying the product. In general, bombardment of a target by charged particles in a cyclotron increases the charge to mass ratio and so nuclei in the product are likely to be charge-rich (neutron-poor) and thus decay via beta-plus decay or electron capture. This is the reason that most PET radionuclides, such as ^{18}F, are produced using a cyclotron. Conversely, bombarding a target with neutrons in a reactor tends to increase the mass of the target nuclei rendering them neutron-rich and thus likely to decay by beta-minus decay.

Questions

1. Which of the following statements are true about medical radionuclide generators:
   (a) The parent nuclide always has a shorter half-life than the daughter nuclide.
   (b) If the $T_{1/2}$ of the parent nuclide is 50 times greater than the $T_{1/2}$ of the daughter nuclide the equilibrium portion of the activity curve is basically flat and is categorized as "secular" equilibrium.
   (c) The parent nuclide is less tightly bound to the column than the daughter nuclide.
   (d) All of the above.
   (e) None of the above.

2. True or False: During an equilibrium state within a ^{99}Mo–^{99m}Tc generator the total activity of ^{99m}Tc is always less than the total activity of ^{99}Mo because 14% of ^{99}Mo decays directly to ^{99}Tc, bypassing the metastable state.

3. Which of the following is an example of a generator that reaches secular equilibrium?
   (a) ^{99}Mo–^{99m}Tc.
   (b) ^{82}Sr–^{82}Rb.

4. Associate each of the following terms (a) through (k) with the most appropriate of the three methods of nuclide production listed here (a term can apply to more than one method):
   (1) Reactor.
   (2) Cyclotron.
   (3) Generator.
       (a) Moderator.
       (b) Chain reaction.
       (c) Thermal neutron.
       (d) Dee.
       (e) Control rod.
       (f) Target.
       (g) Cow.
       (h) Pig.
       (i) Column.
       (j) Elution.
       (k) By-product.

5. Associate each of the following nuclear reactions (a) through (d) with the most appropriate of the three listed production methods.
   (1) Cyclotron.
   (2) Fission reaction (reactor).
   (3) Neutron capture (reactor).
       (a) ^{111}Cd(p,n)^{111}In.
       (b) ^{68}Zn(p,2n)67Ga.
       (c) 235U(n,f)99Mo.
       (d) 98Mo (n,γ)^{99}Mo.

6. ^{18}F is produced:
   (a) In a generator.
   (b) In a cyclotron.
   (c) From by-product material of nuclear fission.
   (d) By neutron bombardment in a nuclear reactor.

7. ^{99}Mo is produced (select all that apply):
   (a) In a generator.
   (b) In a cyclotron.
   (c) From by-product material of nuclear fission.
   (d) By neutron bombardment in a nuclear reactor.

8. ^{99m}Tc is produced:
   (a) In a generator.
   (b) In a cyclotron.
   (c) From by-product material of nuclear fission.
   (d) By neutron bombardment in a nuclear reactor.

9. The half-life of ^{99m}Tc is 6 hours and the half-life of ^{99}Mo is 66 hours. At 8 AM Monday morning, the Tc/Mo generator is eluted of all ^{99m}Tc and the yield is 86 mCi. Approximately how much total ^{99m}Tc will we be able to elute from the generator on Friday at 8 AM.
   (a) Essentially zero since more than 10 half-lives have elapsed.
   (b) 31 mCi.
   (c) 86 mCi.
   (d) 54 mCi.

Answers

1. (e) None of the above: (a) the parent half-life is always longer than the daughter half-life; (b) if the half-life of the parent is between 10 and 100 times greater than the half-life of the daughter, the activity curve is downward sloping and the equilibrium is termed "transient"; and (c) the daughter nuclide is less tightly bound, thereby it can be removed or eluted for use.

2. True.

3. (b) The half-life of the parent nuclide, ^{82}Sr, is more than 100 times that of the daughter nuclide, ^{82}Rb.

4. (a), (b), (c), (e), (f), (k) are terms for reactors; (d), (f) are terms for cyclotrons; (g), (h), (i), (j) are terms for generators.

5. (a) 1; (b) 1; (c) 2; (d) 3.

6. (b) In a cyclotron.

7. (c) and (d) .

8. (a) In a generator.

9. (b) 31 mCi.

$$A(t) = A(0)e^{-0.693t/T1/2}$$

Since only 86% of the ^{99}Mo decays to ^{99m}Tc the original amount of ^{99}Mo or $A(0) = 100$ mCi and $t = 96$ hours and $T_{1/2} = 66$ hours.

$$A(t) = 100 \text{ mCi} \times e^{-0.693 \times 96\,hours/66\,hours}$$
$$= 100 \text{ mCi} \times 0.36 = 36 \text{ mCi}$$

Since only 86% of ^{99}Mo decays to ^{99m}Tc

$$^{99m}\text{Tc} = 0.86 \times 36 \text{ mCi} = 31 \text{ mCi}$$

This calculation can be simplified by using the $A(0)$ for ^{99m}Tc combined with the $T_{1/2}$ of ^{99}Mo:

$$A(t) = 86 \text{ mCi} \times e^{-0.693 \times 96\,hours/66\,hours} = 31 \text{ mCi}$$

CHAPTER 4

Nonscintillation Detectors

Because we generally cannot sense the presence of radioactivity, electronic equipment has been developed to detect ionizing radiation (both particles and photons). This chapter explores the common types of nonscintillation radiation detectors used in a nuclear medicine department; the next chapter discusses scintillation detectors.

Gas-filled detectors

Theory of operation

Gas-filled detectors function by measuring the ionization that radiation produces within the gas. There are several types of detectors that operate on this general principle, but they differ greatly in the details of construction and in the manner in which the radiation-produced ionization is gauged. As might be expected, each type has one or more applications for which it is best suited.

Principles of measurement

Charge neutralization

Perhaps one of the simplest and oldest methods for quantifying the ionization produced in a gas detector is the visual observation of the filament of an electroscope. An example is the pocket dosimeter, illustrated later in this chapter in Figure 4.10, which contains a small gas-filled chamber within which a thin filament of wire is attached to a metal frame. When positively charged, the filament is repelled by the frame, which also carries a positive charge. The filament is observed to return to its resting position as the charge is neutralized by the radiation-produced ions. The greater the incoming radiation, the closer the filament moves toward the neutral position.

Charge flow

Measuring current: A related approach is to measure the flow of the charges that ionizing radiation produces in a gas-filled detector. The ions produced by the radiation are charged particles. The negative particle is either a free electron or an oxygen or nitrogen molecule that has absorbed a free electron. The positive particle is a molecule of gas that has lost an electron.

The gas-filled detector has both a positive and a negative electrode (Figure 4.1). As shown in a cross-section in Figure 4.2, the potential difference between them is maintained by a battery. The positive and negative ions produced in the gas by the radiation move in opposite directions, positive ions toward the negatively charged cathode where they acquire an electron and the negative ions toward the positively charged anode where they discharge an electron. This movement of ions (charges) is an electric current, which can be detected by a sensitive meter. The current between the electrodes is a measure of the amount of incoming radiation. The **ionization chamber**, about which more is said later in this chapter, is a practical instrument that functions in this way.

Counting pulses of current: The alternative to measuring the current is counting the individual pulses produced as each individual charged particle or photon enters the gas. The **Geiger counter** is an example of this type of detector. The rate at which counts occur in such detectors is a direct measure of the amount of incoming radiation.

The process of ionization, collection of the charges produced, and recording of the count takes place very quickly, but it is far from instantaneous. Time is

Essentials of Nuclear Medicine Physics, Instrumentation, and Radiation Biology, Fourth Edition.
Rachel A. Powsner, Matthew R. Palmer, and Edward R. Powsner.
© 2022 John Wiley & Sons Ltd. Published 2022 by John Wiley & Sons Ltd.

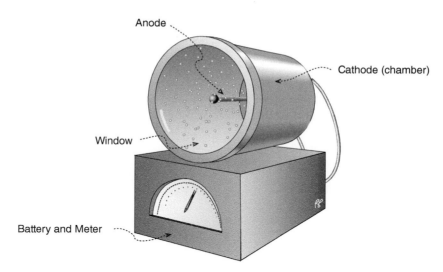

Figure 4.1 Simple gas-filled detector.

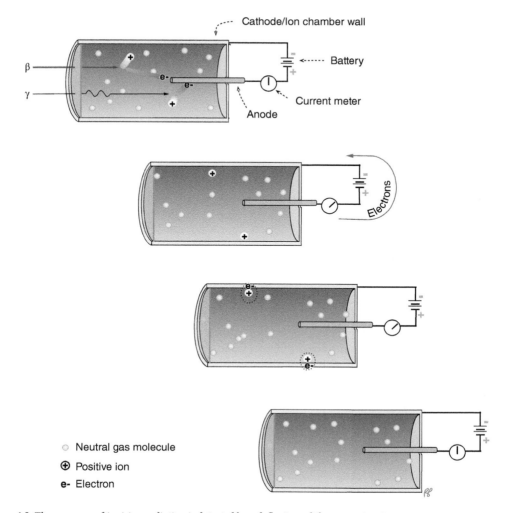

Figure 4.2 The presence of ionizing radiation is detected by a deflection of the current meter.

required for the ions to reach their respective electrodes and for the detector to return to its resting state. What transpires in this time depends on the construction of the detector, the kind of gases it contains, and the strength of the applied voltage. The last of these is almost directly proportional to the voltage applied to the electrodes. Although all three factors determine the characteristics of the detector, it is instructive to examine the role of the applied voltage in more detail.

Characteristics of the major voltage regions applied across a gas-filled detector

Low

In the gas-filled detector, the magnitude of the voltage between the electrodes determines the type of response to each charged particle or photon. When the voltage between the electrodes is relatively low, the field within the gas is weak and many of the ions

simply recombine, leaving only a small fraction to reach the electrodes. Little if any charge flows between the electrodes and the meter in the external circuit remains at zero.

At a somewhat higher voltage, referred to as the **ionization region** (Figure 4.3), most of the ions that are formed reach the electrodes. A further, small increase in the voltage does not increase the current once the voltage is sufficient to collect 100% of the ions formed. The brief pulse of current, generated by ionizing radiation entering the chamber, ceases until the next charged particle or photon enters the gas. This current is small and difficult to count as an individual event.

In this region, the current is relatively independent of small increases in voltage. It is, however, affected by the type of radiation. An alpha particle, because it carries two units of charge and is relatively massive, produces many ion pairs while traveling a short distance in the gas; a beta particle, which is

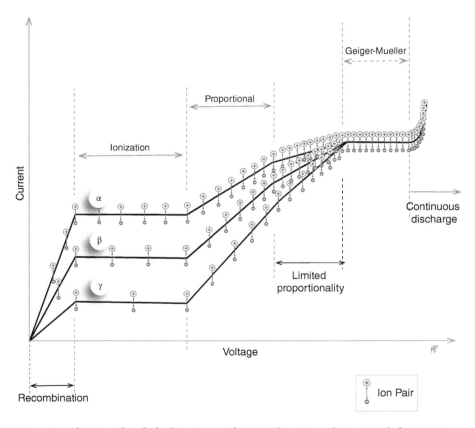

Figure 4.3 Current as a function of applied voltage in a gas detector. The regions of interest include ionization, proportional, and Geiger.

much lighter and carries only a single charge, produces fewer ion pairs per unit distance traveled; a photon, because it carries neither charge nor mass, creates even fewer ion pairs. In any case, practically all of the ion pairs that are created are collected on the electrodes because the applied voltage creates a strong enough electric field to prevent recombination.

In small detectors, some of the ionization from beta radiation and much or even most of the ionization from photon radiation may escape detection. In this situation, the current following irradiation by an alpha particle will be much larger than that caused by a beta particle of similar energy, and the current following both particles will be for both larger than that caused by photon radiation of similar energy.

Intermediate

With further increase in voltage, the detector passes into the next region of operation (see Figure 4.3).

In this so-called **proportional region,** a new phenomenon is observed—**gas amplification** (Figure 4.4). Accelerated more intensely toward the positive electrode at this higher voltage, the electrons produced by the radiation (called primary particles) travel so rapidly that they themselves are able to ionize some of the previously neutral gas molecules. This process, similar to that produced by the original radiation particle, can be imagined as a speeding electron knocking out a molecular electron (the new negative ion) and leaving behind a positively charged gas molecule (the new positive ion). The newly separated electrons (called **delta** or secondary particles) also accelerate toward the positive electrode and, in turn, ionize additional gas molecules. The pulse of charge started by the incoming radiation is greatly amplified by this brief chain reaction.

In this region, the current produced is proportional to the number of ion pairs produced by the incoming radiation. The current is higher for an

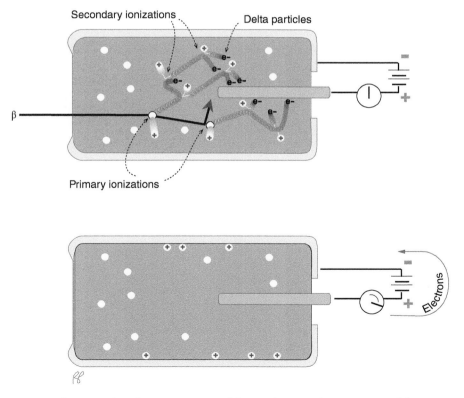

Figure 4.4 Proportional counter. The voltage causes gas amplification that gives electrons separated during primary ionization enough energy to cause secondary ionization.

alpha particle than for a beta, and currents for both are higher than for a photon. Because of gas amplification, the total number of ion pairs, primary plus secondary, is much higher than in the low-voltage ionization region. This resulting pulse of current is large enough to detect as an individual, countable event.

High

For detectors operating at still higher voltages, above the proportional region, the pulse of current is larger but becomes independent of the number of ions produced by the initial event. As the voltage is increased, a point is reached at which most of the gas within the detector is massively involved in the multiple, successive ionizations (Figure 4.5). Once all the gas is involved, no greater gas amplification is possible so that any further increases in voltage have little effect on the size of the pulse of current. This is the so-called **Geiger (or Geiger–Müller) region**. A detector operating in this region is called

a Geiger counter, or Geiger–Müller counter, after its early developers. In the Geiger region, not only is the size of the current pulse almost independent of small changes in voltage, but the size of the pulse is also independent of the amount of ionization produced by the incoming radiation. In other words, in the Geiger region the current produced by a charged particle or photon is large compared to that produced in the proportional region. The current is independent of fluctuations in voltage, and the size of each pulse of current is dependent on the characteristic of the detector itself rather than of the incoming particle or photon.

Voltages above the Geiger region are not used because, even in the absence of the radiation the counter is designed to detect, there is a spontaneous and **continuous ionization** of gas molecules that stops only when the voltage is lowered. This is similar to the visible ionizations seen in a neon sign (Figure 4.6). With such high voltages, the device is not useful as a radiation detector.

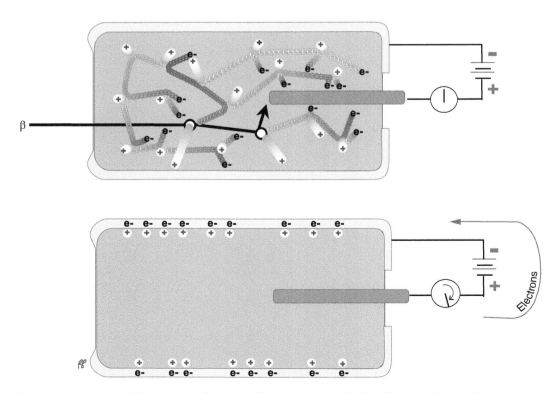

Figure 4.5 Geiger counter. The primary radiation rapidly triggers a cascade of further ionizations involving most of the gas.

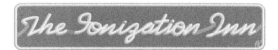

Figure 4.6 Continuous discharge. The voltage applied to a neon sign is high enough to generate spontaneous ionization that continues until the power is turned off.

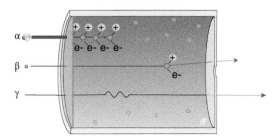

Figure 4.7 Ionization by alpha and beta particles and by photons in the gas-filled detector.

Sensitivity

Intrinsic

A gas-filled detector will respond to virtually every radiation event that causes ionization in the gas. To be detected, a particle or photon must be energetic enough to cross the detector face into the sensitive volume of gas, but must not be so energetic that it will pass right through the gas without causing any ionization. The first limitation is important for low-energy alpha or beta particles, which have only limited ability to penetrate the "window" of the detector, but once inside ionize strongly. The second is a consideration for high-energy photons, which penetrate easily but may pass through the detector causing little or no ionization (Figure 4.7). Sensitivity for charged particles (alpha or beta) can be increased by using thin, penetrable materials for the detector window such as a thin sheet of mica or, for greatest sensitivity, by actually placing the radioactive sample inside the sensitive volume. Sensitivity for moderately high-energy photons is improved by increasing the size of the sensitive volume or, equivalently, by "cramming" in more gas molecules under pressure, or by using a thicker wall for the chamber (some of the photons that would normally pass undetected through the chamber will instead interact with molecules of the inner surface of the

tube metal causing release of additional electrons into the chamber).

Typical gas-filled detectors are sensitive to alpha particles with energies greater than 3 to 4 MeV, beta radiation above 50 to 100 keV, and gamma radiation above 5 to 7 keV. The upper limit for gamma or X-ray radiation depends on the type and pressure of the gas and the type of material used for the window and walls of the detector.

Geometric

The larger the window and the closer the source, the more radiation will enter the detector. At long distances from compact sources, the amount of radiation reaching the detector decreases with the square of the distance. The controlling factor, aside from absorption of radiation in the intervening air, is the portion of the source seen by the window. As can be seen in Figure 4.8, this is the fraction of the sphere subtended (or seen) by the window.

Types of gas-filled detector

Ionization chambers

Structure and characteristics

Structure: The ionization chamber, in its simplest form, is a gas-filled can (the gas is usually air) with a radiation permeable end (the window), a central wire, a meter, and a battery (see Figure 4.1). The gas is most often at normal atmospheric pressure, but it may be filled under pressure, as discussed under Geiger counters below. A thin window at one end of the can admits radiation. A battery or power supply maintains the central wire (anode) at a positive potential relative to the surrounding walls of the can, which act as the negative electrode (cathode). The magnitude of the voltage is set relatively low to ensure operation in the ionization region, hence the name ionization chamber (see Figure 4.3). A sensitive meter to measure the current of ions completes the device.

Function: The ionization chamber is not ordinarily used to count discrete radiation events but rather to measure the average number of ionizations per minute occurring within the gas. If the events are sufficiently infrequent, the attached meter may be

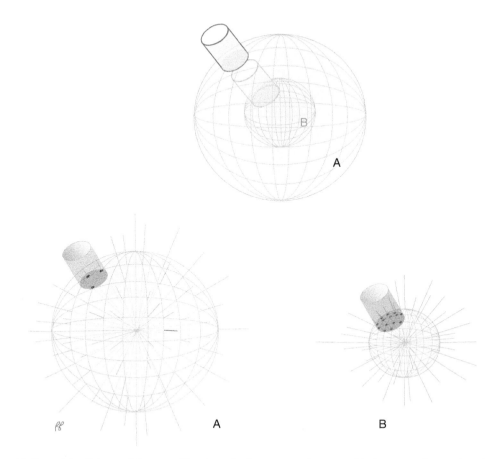

Figure 4.8 Geometric efficiency of detectors. The closer the detector is to the source (b), the greater the number of photons that will cross the detector window.

observed to move up a short distance as a particle or photon of radiation triggers the detector and falls back slowly in the interval before the next event.

Sensitivity: The lower limit of sensitivity for an ionization chamber is determined by the sensitivity of the meter used to measure the current. In terms of radiation exposure, sensitivity down to <1 mR for low- and moderate-energy photons (10 keV to 1 MeV) is available in standard survey meters and dosimeters.

Energy independence: In the ionization region of operation, the electrodes collect practically all of the ion pairs formed in the gas. Because the number of ionizations is almost directly proportional to the

energy of the incoming radiation, the current that results is a measure of the rate at which energy is being deposited within the gas by the ionizing radiation. The rate of ionization, the consequent current, and the radiation dose are all similarly dependent on the energy of the incoming particles or photons. As a result, at least for the ideal ionization chamber, the meter reading gives a reliable measure of the radiation dose rate. Note, however, that this reliability has its limits. As alluded to above, at very low energies the radiation may not even penetrate the ion chamber, and at very high energies the radiation may pass completely through the device without having many ionizing interactions with the gas.

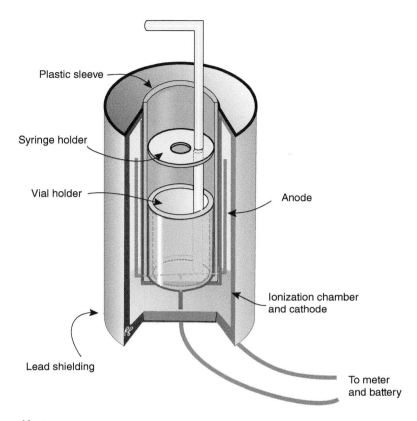

Plastic sleeve

Syringe holder

Vial holder

Anode

Ionization chamber
and cathode

Lead shielding

To meter
and battery

Figure 4.9 Dose calibrator.

Applications

Dose calibrator: The dose calibrator is most frequently used in the nuclear medicine department
as a table-top ionization chamber to confirm that
the correct amount of activity has been dispensed
before a dose of radiopharmaceutical is administered (Figure 4.9). The dose calibrator consists of
an ionization chamber surrounding an open well.
The walls of the well are permeable to photons.
The current produced in the circuitry is
proportional to the number of primary ionizations
in the chamber. The amount of current is registered as radioactivity in MBq or mCi. The dose
calibrator can only report the activity, not the type
of radiation or radiopharmaceutical.

The accuracy of the reading is affected by such
factors as the type of dose container, its proper placement in the dose calibrator well, and the calibration
and regular recalibration of the instrument itself.
Because of the importance of administering the correct amount of activity to patients, there are strictly

enforced rules for the use and calibration of the dose
calibrator. These are discussed in Chapter 14.

Survey meter: When the ionization chamber is used
as a survey meter, the current reading is usually
interpreted as the average intensity of radiation in
roentgens (R) per hour. For example, a survey meter
might register a 30 mR/h exposure rate at one
meter from a person who was treated with 370 MBq
(10 mCi) of ^{131}I. The roentgen is defined in terms of
ionization produced in air and it is no coincidence
that the ionization chamber can be used for the
measurement of radiation intensity in roentgens.

Roentgen (R)

A measurement of gamma or X-ray radiation
exposure in air, not tissue. One roentgen is the
quantity of radiation that will produce 2.58×10^{-4}
coulombs (C) of charge (or 2×10^9 ion pairs) per
kilogram of dry air under standard conditions.

Pocket dosimeters: A small ionization chamber is the heart of the classic pocket dosimeter. For this application, a small, straight filament, insulated from the walls of the chamber, is mounted within the ionization chamber (Figure 4.10). To prepare the chamber for use, a positive charge is placed on the filament by a charger that briefly connects the positive terminal of a battery to the filament. When charged, the positive filament is repelled by the positively charged frame. When radiation penetrates the walls of the chamber, the gas is ionized and the ions are attracted to the frame and fiber or walls of the chamber, which partially neutralizes their charge. The filament is less strongly repelled by the frame and begins to move toward a neutral position. The position of the filament can be viewed through a lens against a scale on the end of the chamber

calibrated in roentgens or rads per hour. Properly insulated from the case of the chamber, the positive charge can remain on the filament for hours.

Pocket dosimeters of this type are relatively inexpensive and can be used to measure exposures to photons in the range of zero to several hundred mR. A separate charging device is required.

Proportional counters

Structure and characteristics

Chamber and filling gas: In its construction, the proportional counter is very similar to an ionization chamber. The filling gas is more likely to be argon or an argon–methane mixture than air, but the essential difference between them is the higher voltage and

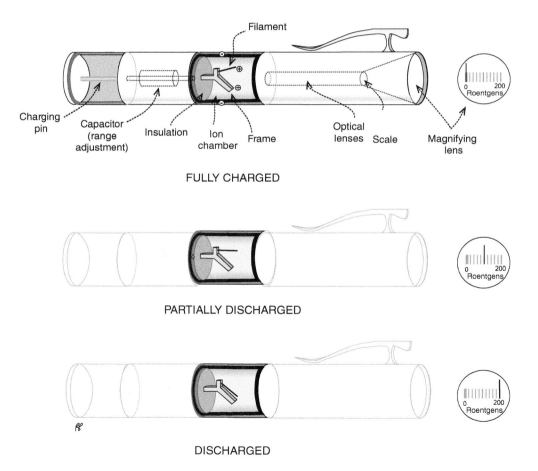

FULLY CHARGED

PARTIALLY DISCHARGED

DISCHARGED

Figure 4.10 Pocket dosimeter. Ions produced in the gas neutralize the charge on the filament and frame and the filament returns toward its neutral position. Source: Courtesy of Federal Emergency Management Agency. Adapted from drawing of the FEMA dosimeter.

the resulting gas amplification. For this reason, the incoming radiation causes a pulse of current large enough to be registered as an individual count.

Applications as survey meter: The proportional counter is particularly suitable when it is important to distinguish among various types of radiation. Because the size of the pulse from a proportional counter is proportional to the initial ionization, alpha particles, which ionize more heavily than beta particles, produce larger pulses, and this difference can be used to distinguish between them.

Counting low-energy particles may require very close proximity of the detector to the sample. Proportional counters can be built for this type of counting with no window or only a very thin, somewhat leaky membrane between the sample and the gas of the chamber. In the windowless type, the sample is placed directly within the gas-filled chamber. A continuous flow of gas through the detector compensates for any loss of gas as the samples are inserted or, in the case of the thin window, for any gas that leaks through the membrane. Gas-flow counting is relatively exacting and, for many purposes, has been replaced by the less exacting liquid scintillation counting (see Chapter 5).

Geiger counters

Structure and characteristics

The tube and the filling gas: The Geiger counter is an ionization chamber that operates at a relatively high applied voltage (Figure 4.11). The chamber is usually filled with argon containing traces of other gases such as halogen or methane, although a detector will function with a filling as simple as dry air. The sensitive end of the probe is generally a mica window protected by an external metal mesh. In some applications, the thin window of the ionization chamber is covered by an aluminum cap. Photons striking the cap knock out secondary electrons that in turn ionize the gas within the chamber. The walls of the chamber may also function similarly.

The gas in the chamber may be filled to atmospheric pressure or it may be pressurized to increase sensitivity. At higher pressure, usually a few times normal atmospheric pressure, the number of gas molecules "crammed" into the chamber is greater. This raises the probability that incoming radiation will encounter and ionize a gas molecule within the chamber. Pressurization is particularly useful for photon radiation for which the energy is high enough, and therefore its range in gas long enough, to allow it to pass completely through an unpressurized chamber without encountering and ionizing a gas molecule. The Geiger counter cannot distinguish between types of radiation because each interaction of the radiation with the gas causes maximum ionization.

Quenching: The gas multiplication, which characterizes the Geiger region, causes a single incoming radiation event to give a large current pulse, but gas amplification carries the disadvantage that the discharge, once started by the radiation, is likely to sustain itself indefinitely. The discharge continues because as the positive ions reach the cathode (wall

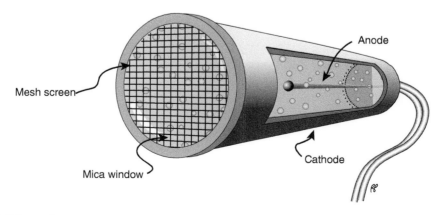

Figure 4.11 Geiger probe.

of the chamber) and acquire a free electron they also acquire excess energy. This energy is discharged by emitting photons or dislodging another electron which in turn can cause further avalanches (Figure 4.12 top). While the discharge continues, the detector is not affected by any further incoming radiation; it is effectively paralyzed (this **dead time** lasts 100–500 μs for Geiger counters). The discharge must be quenched before the tube can count again. The two common methods of **quenching** are to quickly drop the applied voltage or to add a quenching material to the filling gas. The quenching material is usually a halogen diatomic molecule composed of two identical atoms such as Br_2 (two bromide atoms). The latter serves to quench the discharge by absorbing the positive charge from the filler gas atom making it inert so it doesn't

travel to the cathode. Instead, the newly charged quenching atom strikes the cathode, acquiring an electron and excess energy. However, instead of releasing energy in a photon and/or dislodging an additional electron it can absorb the excess energy by splitting into two atoms which then quickly recombine (Figure 4.12 bottom).

Applications: The Geiger counter has long been the most widely used of the gas-filled detectors. Its principal uses are the monitoring of areas such as nuclear medicine laboratories for radiation and the detection of contamination. When used as a **radiation monitor** to detect individual photons or their rate (usually referred to as counts or count rate, respectively), the Geiger counter is relatively independent of the energy of the photon. This is

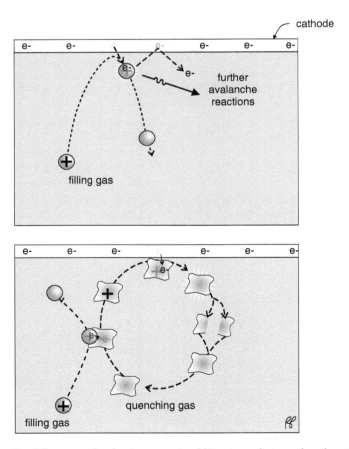

Figure 4.12 Quenching. Top: Filler atoms absorb extra energy in addition to an electron when they strike the cathode, this energy can be discharged by causing the emission of photons or additional electrons adding to the avalanche response. Bottom: Halogenic diatomic molecules quench the reaction by absorbing the positive charge from filler atoms, when they strike the cathode discharge the excess energy by splitting into two atoms which then recombine.

true provided that the photon is sufficiently energetic to enter the counting chamber but not so energetic that it passes through it without interacting. When used as a **survey meter** to measure the exposure rate, usually as mR/h, the meter reading is strongly affected by the energy of the photons. For low-energy photons, typically those below 100 keV, the actual exposure rate is only a fraction of the reading displayed on the meter. The reason for this is that the counter detects individual photons, not their energy, whereas the exposure rate depends both on the photon and the energy of the photon. The usual meter is calibrated for a photon of moderate or even high energy such as that of ^{137}Cs or ^{60}Co. It must be recalibrated if the energy of the photon is expected to be very different from that used for the factory calibration.

Sensitivity: The Geiger counter can be expected to respond to any individual particle or photon whose energy is high enough to permit it to penetrate into the chamber but low enough so that it does not, or is unlikely to, pass through without ionizing any gas molecules. From this, it is apparent that geometric considerations—the size and shape of the detector and its distance from the source—can be the most important factors limiting sensitivity.

For monitoring radiation of low intensity, sensitivity is further limited by the background count. The count rate of the monitored radiation must be sufficient to increase the total significantly above background. For radiation of high intensity, sensitivity may be limited by the so-called dead time of the counter, which, as described above, is the time before one discharge has been quenched and the tube is able to count another event.

Semiconductor detectors

Introduction
Semiconductors are crystalline materials with fewer loosely bound outer shell electrons than a metallic material. As a result, the flow of electrical charge in these materials is less than that of a metal such as copper, hence the name semiconductors. **Semiconductor detectors** can be thought of as functionally equivalent to a gas detector but with all the advantages of a solid material. Like their gaseous

counterparts, the more loosely bound outer shell electrons of the molecules of these solids can be "dislodged" by ionizing radiation or light photons. Instead of positively charged gas molecules, positive "holes" are created within the crystalline structure as a positively charged atom is left behind when an electron migrates. In a manner similar to their gaseous counterparts, for which the ion pairs of electron and positively charged gas molecules migrate within the gas chamber, the electrons and the positive "holes" migrate within the semiconductor. These charged entities, the electrons and "holes", are attracted to an anode and cathode attached to opposite sides of the detector, this will be discussed later in more detail.

The primary advantage of using solid materials instead of gas for detectors is their much higher density. The higher the density of a material the more likely the interaction of the incoming radiation with atoms of the material. In addition, the electrons in the semiconductor are less tightly bound to their atoms than the electrons in the atoms of gas molecules. It takes only 2 to 3 eV to "release" an electron in a semiconductor material compared to approximately 35 eV to release an electron in air. This means that for any incoming radiation there is a much greater yield of charges (positive holes and negative electrons) in the semiconductors than in air (or other gases) of a similar volume. As a consequence, a relatively smaller volume of solid material is needed, which allows the production of much smaller detectors.

Semiconductor materials
The most common semiconductor material is silicon (Si), others are germanium (Ge), cadmium telluride (CdTe), cadmium zinc telluride (CdZnTe or CZT), and zinc telluride (ZnTe). Silicon and germanium are examples of semiconductor materials which are only efficient for detecting lower energy photons such as light photons; they have a low stopping power for the higher energy gamma and X-ray photons used in medical imaging. As a result, they must be coupled to scintillators (discussed in the next chapter) which "convert" the energy from incoming gamma and X-ray photons into light photons which can then be detected by these semiconductors. Cadmium zinc telluride (CZT), however, has a greater stopping power for higher energy photons and therefore can be used independently for gamma and X-ray detection. Because of

the high cost of manufacturing semiconductor materials, they were initially only used in specialty applications such as intraoperative probes, however, they are becoming more widely used in imaging systems.

The remainder of the discussion will focus on the more commonly used silicon-based semiconductors although many of the concepts apply to other semiconductor materials as well.

Doped silicon for semiconductors

In a silicon crystal, each atom is covalently bound (shares its four outer shell electrons) with four adjacent atoms. As a result, each atom ends up with a stable configuration of eight outer shell electrons (Figure 4.13a).

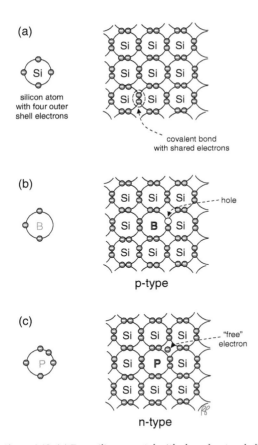

Figure 4.13 (a) Pure silicon crystal with shared outer shell electrons. (b) Positive-type semiconductor: boron "doping" results in a missing electron or positive "hole". (c) Negative-type semiconductor: phosphorus "doping" results in a surplus free electron.

The responsiveness of the crystal to photon impacts can be improved by replacing some of the silicon atoms with atoms with three (such as boron) or five (phosphorus) outer shell electrons. This process is called "**doping**".

When a boron atom, which only has three outer shell electrons, is substituted for a silicon atom one of the four surrounding covalent bonds is incomplete; there is a "hole" where the 8th electron should reside (Figure 4.13b). This hole is considered to be positively charged as it "attracts" electrons. When an electron in a nearby atom jumps into this hole, it leaves behind another hole; in this sense, the first hole has "moved" to a new position. This crystal is said to a **p-type** (positive type) semiconductor.

When a phosphorus atom, which has five outer shell electrons, is substituted for a silicon atom four of its five electrons contribute to covalent bonding; the residual 5th electron is therefore relatively free to dissociate from the crystalline structure (Figure 4.13c). This crystal is said to be an **n-type** (negative type) of semiconductor.

Single photon avalanche detector (SPAD)

Single photon avalanche detectors (SPAD) are composed of layers of doped silicon arranged such that the response of the detector to a single photon is greatly enhanced much like the previously described avalanche response in gas detectors.

P-N junctions and the depletion zone: Within a single photon avalanche detector there are adjacent p- and n-type semiconductors. At the junction of the p- and n-type semiconductors (**P-N junctions**) the free electrons from the n-type diffuse into the p-type and the holes in the p-type diffuse into the n-type. They leave behind positively or negatively charged fixed (non-moveable) atoms adjacent to the junction (the boron atom, losing a hole becomes negatively charged and the phosphorus atom, losing an electron becomes positively charged). The number of fixed positively and negatively charged atoms eventually increases to the point where their cumulative charge blocks the movement of the free electrons and holes. This zone is called the "**depletion**" zone as it has become depleted of free electrons and holes (Figure 4.14) and there is no current flow.

In a simple single photon avalanche detector, the p-type semiconductor is attached to an anode

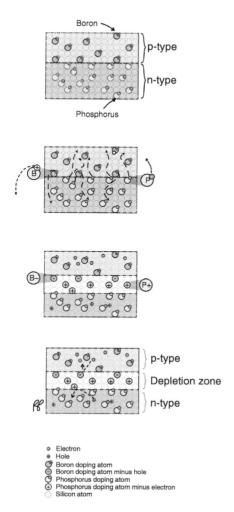

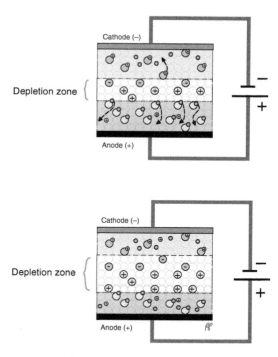

Figure 4.15 The depletion zone is widened by the application of a high voltage across the p- and n-type semiconductors.

Figure 4.14 Depletion zone is created after the free electrons and positive holes diffuse out of the junction between p-type and n-type semiconductors

Geiger–Müller range voltage across the SPAD causes this free electron to accelerate at high speed towards the anode. Due to its high kinetic energy, it strikes the atoms in the crystal multiple times releasing many electron hole pairs, these liberated electrons in turn are also subject to rapid acceleration by the high voltage causing further impacts and release of more electron hole pairs. The resulting avalanche of free electrons creates a current within the SPAD which travels through the anode and is detected by the electronics in the silicon photomultiplier.

Silicon photomultipliers (SiPM)

Silicon photomultipliers (SiPM) are composed of numerous SPADs and are the semiconductor version of the vacuum tube photomultiplier tube which will be discussed in the next chapter. Each silicon photomultiplier measures only several millimeters in length and width and is composed of 100–10,000 individual cells. Each cell contains a SPAD connected to a resistor and a battery (Figure 4.17). Between photon impacts there is no current in the SPAD and therefore there is no current in the cell circuit; the SPAD functions like a

(positively charged) and the n-type to a cathode (negatively charged). A high voltage in the Geiger–Müller range (see Figure 4.3) is applied by an external battery between the anode and cathode. Because of this some of the holes in the p-type material are drawn towards the cathode and some of the electrons in the n-type material are drawn towards the anode; the depletion region is therefore widened (Figure 4.15).

SPAD response to incoming photons: It is in this nearly current free depletion zone that the incoming photon interacts with the crystal, liberating a free electron and a positive hole (Figure 4.16). The

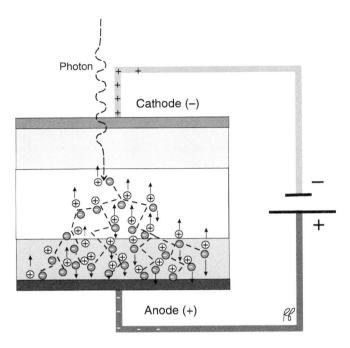

Figure 4.16 An incoming photon impacts an atom in the depletion zone causing release of a free electron and positive hole, this electron in turn, is accelerated causing an avalanche of free electrons and holes.

switch in the "off "position. When there is an impact in the depletion zone of the SPAD current flows in the SPAD and the circuit and the SPAD functions like a switch in the "on" position. The current from the cell is detected by the SiPM.

However, the current also flows through the resistor in the cell circuit which, because resistors reduce current flow, causes a drop in the voltage throughout the circuit and as a result there is a drop in the voltage across the SPAD. The drop of voltage across the SPAD slows the speed of the electrons within the detector and the avalanche of electrons halts. The SPAD no longer conducts current and the cell turns "off" until another photon impacts the detector.

Each SiPM receives constant input from the 100-10,000 cells it contains, the number of simultaneous "on" signals can range from 0 to the maximum number of cells (10,000 for example). So, although each individual cell has only a discrete output of "on" or "off", the overall SiPM output has a nearly continuous range or analog output (Figure 4.18).

The silicon photomultipliers have the advantage of not being affected by magnetic fields (as will be discussed in PET/MRI in Chapter 11) and are also much smaller than the vacuum tubes.

Photographic and luminescent detectors

There are several types of radiosensitive materials that are typically used to measure the cumulative exposure received by personnel working with radioactivity. These materials are encased in plastic and worn by the user in either badge or ring form. Unlike the pen dosimeter, which can be read by the user, these badges must be sent to an outside laboratory for interpretation.

Photographic detectors

The **film badge** depicted in Figure 4.19 is one such detector. It is simply a plastic holder containing film that is radiosensitive. Strips of materials of different densities (such as aluminum, cadmium, and lead) are placed within the badge in the space in front of the film. These strips attenuate the incoming radiation and reduce the degree of exposure of the film located immediately behind the strip. As discussed in Chapter 2, the amount of attenuation is dependent on the type of radiation (alpha, beta, gamma, or X-ray), the energy of the radiation, and the density of the absorber. By comparing the amount of exposure of film behind each strip (including a fourth

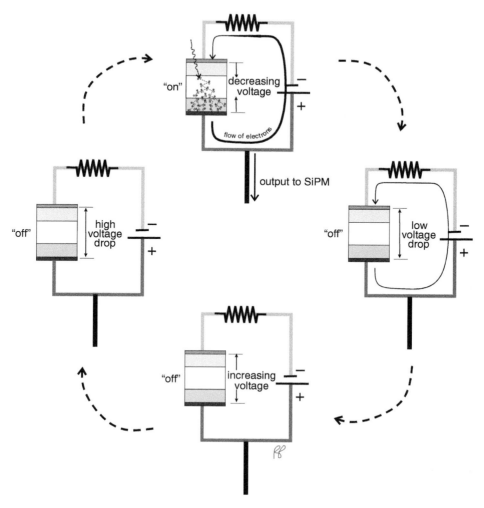

Figure 4.17 Each cell within the silicon photomultiplier is composed of a single photon avalanche detector connected to a resistor and battery.

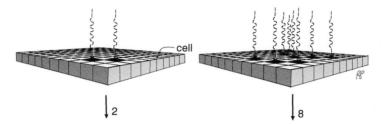

Figure 4.18 The large number of cells within a silicon photomultiplier results in a nearly continuous (analogue) output signal.

uncovered area), some estimate as to the type and energy of the radiation can be determined.

Thermoluminescent and optically luminescent detectors

Crystalline materials that emit light when exposed to energy (in the form of light, heat, radiation, etc.) are called **luminescent**. Luminescent crystals that can absorb energy from gamma rays, X-rays, and alpha and beta particles and then emit the energy as light are used in nuclear medicine for counting, imaging (see scintillation crystals in the next chapter), and for recording cumulative radiation exposure.

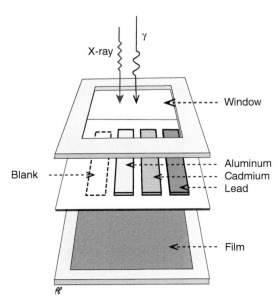

Figure 4.19 Film badge. The strips of metal absorbers assist in estimating the type and energy of radiation exposure.

Radioactive particles and photons striking theses crystals (Figure 4.20a) cause electrons (and the positively charged holes) to be released from the atoms of the crystal (Figure 4.20b). These "excited" electrons contain excess energy. The excited electrons return to a stable state as they recombine with the positive holes and in the process release their excess energy as light (Figure 4.20c and d).

Crystals that emit light as soon as they are exposed to radiation are useful for imaging, but not for recording cumulative radiation exposure.

Fortunately some luminescent crystals absorb energy from radiation, but do not emit all of the absorbed light immediately. A portion of the absorbed energy remains in the crystal until it is exposed to another external energy source such as heat or laser light. Usually the absorptive properties of these crystals are improved by contaminating or "doping" the crystals with small amounts of other minerals (Figure 4.21).

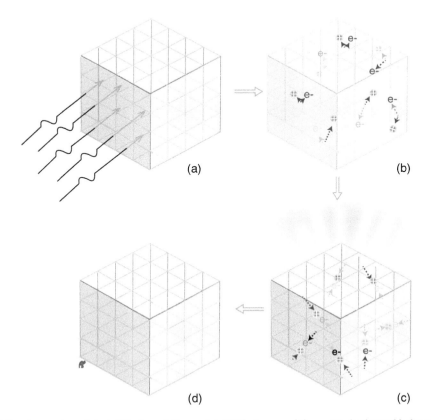

Figure 4.20 Luminescent crystals: (a) Photons strike crystal. (b) Electrons and the positively charged holes are released and then recombine (c) causing emission of light photons. (d) Crystal returns to stable state.

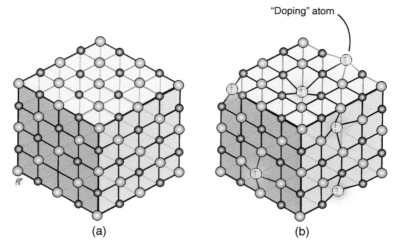

"Doping" atom

(a) (b)

Figure 4.21 Luminescent crystals without (a) and with "doping" (b). Atoms used for doping are depicted as cross-hatched spheres.

The added atoms alter the crystalline structure such that the electrons and holes released by radiation exposure are prevented from returning to a stable state; the electrons and holes are "trapped" until external energy is applied to the "doped" crystal. This applied external energy alters the crystalline structure enough for the electrons and holes to escape their "traps" and return to a stable state. As they return to their stable state they release the excess energy that was deposited by the initial radiation exposure (Figure 4.22).

Thermoluminescent detectors

Examples of crystalline substances that are commonly used to make thermoluminescent badges are calcium fluoride doped with manganese (CaF_2:Mn) and lithium fluoride doped with magnesium and titanium (LiF:Mg,Ti). When these badges are sent (usually after a period of one or more months) to an outside laboratory for reading they are carefully exposed to heat (the "thermo" portion of "thermoluminescent"). The application of energy in the form of heat causes the release of the trapped electrons (and positive holes). As the electrons and holes return to their stable state their excess "stored" energy is released as light. The amount of released light is proportional to the amount of energy stored in the crystal during its repeated exposures to radiation. Since, during the process of heating, the atomic configuration returns to a stable state these badges can only be read once

(however, once read, they are restored to their original state and can be reused).

Optically luminescent detectors

An example of a common crystalline substance that is used for these detectors is aluminum oxide doped with carbon (Al_2O_3:C) Instead of heat, laser light (thence the term "optical") is applied to these detector materials to release the electrons and positive holes from their "traps" in the doped crystal. As with thermoluminescent materials the quantity of light emitted from the crystals as the electrons recombine with positive holes is proportional to the amount of cumulative radiation exposure of the crystal. Because only a portion of the electrons and positive holes are released during each exposure to laser light these detectors can be re-read several times.

Badge dosimeters made from thermoluminescent crystals or optically luminescent crystals (in a powder form enclosed within plastic) also contain small squares of different types of attenuating materials which are placed in front of the crystals much as strips of these materials are placed in front of the film in photographic film badges (see Figure 4.19). By comparing the amount of light emitted from the portion of the crystalline material behind each attenuator some characterization of the type (alpha, beta, and gamma) and energy of the initial radiation exposure can be estimated.

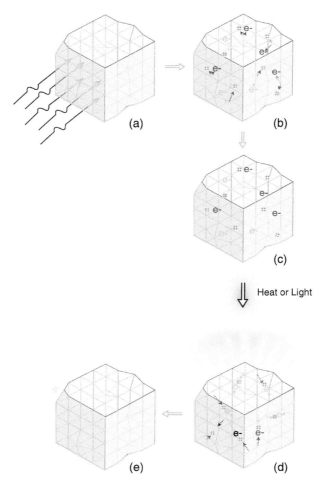

Figure 4.22 Thermoluminescent and optically luminescent crystals. (a) Photons strike crystals. (b) Electrons and positively charged holes are released and remain trapped (c) until energy in the form of heat or laser light is applied after which they recombine (d) and the crystal returns to a stable state (e).

Questions

1. Rank the following major voltage regions for gas detectors from highest applied voltage to lowest applied voltage:
   (1) Ionization region.
   (2) Proportional region.
   (3) Geiger (Geiger–Müller) region.

2. True or false: Gas-filled detectors are highly efficient for detection of high-energy gamma photons and X-rays as well as low energy beta particles.

3. Which of the following radiation detectors are classified as ionization chambers?
   (1) Pen dosimeter.
   (2) Geiger counter.
   (3) Dose calibrator.

4. True or false: Because of the near-maximal ionization of the gas molecules in a Geiger counter in response to each radiation interacting with a gas molecule in the detector, Geiger counters cannot be used to distinguish between types or energies of radiation.

5. True or false: The film badge, unlike the pen dosimeter, can provide some information about the type and energy of the radiation an individual has received.

6. Which of the following are true about a dose calibrator?
   (1) It functions in the proportional region of voltages for gas chambers.

(2) It is a type of ionization chamber.

(3) It can be used to measure the activity of radionuclides because the current produced in the circuitry is proportional to the number of primary ionizations produced in the chamber by the nuclide.

7. True or false: The roentgen is a measure of radiation exposure in tissue.

8. Pocket dosimeters are useful because:
   (1) They do not need charging.
   (2) They can differentiate different types of radiation.
   (c) They can be used for immediate readings of radiation exposure.

9. True or false: Quenching gases are added to reduce the dead time between counts in gas amplification chambers such as the Geiger counter.

10. Which of the following are true about semiconductor materials?

(1) For incoming radiation of the same energy more ion pairs are created in a semiconductor than in air.

(2) Semiconductors have more loosely bound outer-shell electrons than metals.

(3) They are relatively expensive to produce.

11. Which of the following semiconductor materials has the greatest stopping power for higher energy photons and therefore does not need to be coupled to a scintillator in order to detect gamma photons and X-rays?
    (1) Cadmium zinc telluride (CZT).
    (2) Silicon (Si).
    (3) Germanium (Ge).

12. Which of the following materials can be used for measuring accumulated exposure for individuals working with radioactivity?
    (1) Gas detectors.
    (2) Film.
    (3) Optically luminescent detectors.
    (4) Geiger counters.
    (5) Thermoluminescent detectors.

Answers

1. High: Geiger, intermediate: proportional, low: ionization.

2. False. High energy photons and X-rays will often pass through the detector without interacting with a gas molecule and low-energy betas may not pass through the detection window.

3. (1), (3). All of the above are gas detectors, but only the pen dosimeter and the dose calibrator can be classified as ionization chambers. The Geiger counter functions at a higher voltage range, the Geiger–Müller range, than the ionization chambers.

4. True

5. True

6. (2), (3).

7. False: It is a measure of radiation exposure in air only.

8. (3).

9. True.

10. (1) and (3). Option (2) is not correct as semiconductors have fewer loosely bound outer-shell electrons than metals.

11. (1). Choices (2) and (3) are incorrect as they are only efficient for detecting light photons which are low-energy photons.

12. (2), (3), (5).

CHAPTER 5

Scintillation Detectors

This chapter focuses on the properties of scintillation detectors, in particular the most commonly used scintillation material, the sodium iodide crystal. A discussion of how the crystal converts gamma or X-ray photon energy into light photon energy is followed by a discussion of other components of the detector that convert and amplify this light photon output into a detectable electric current. The resulting sodium iodide energy spectrum is covered as well as the characteristics, and common nonimaging applications, of scintillation detectors.

Structure

Scintillation crystals

Scintillation is another term for luminescence, but has been specifically applied to a subset of luminescent crystals that emit light when exposed to particles or photons from radiation. Scintillation crystals are translucent slabs in which gamma rays are converted to light. The most widely used crystals are made of sodium iodide (NaI); they are fragile and can easily be cracked. Because sodium iodide crystals absorb moisture from the atmosphere, they must be sealed in an air-tight aluminum container.

Except at very low temperatures, pure sodium iodide crystals don't scintillate unless they are doped with small amounts (a fraction of a percent) of stable thallium (Tl). The thallium atoms dispersed in the crystal are said to "activate" the scintillation and alter their response to the gamma ray photons (Figure 5.1).

The process of converting gamma rays to light is complex, but it can be summarized as absorption of the gamma ray energy by the crystal, leaving its electrons in an excited state. The gamma photon transfers its energy in one or more Compton or photoelectric interactions in the crystal. Each of these energetic electrons produced by the gamma ray interactions in turn distributes its energy among electrons in the crystal leaving them in an excited state. As these return to their original state, some of their energy is released as **light photons** (Figure 5.2). For each keV of gamma ray energy absorbed by the crystal, approximately 40 light photons are emitted. In a typical detector arrangement, photomultiplier tubes (discussed below) are optically coupled to the scintillation crystals to detect these light photons. The design of the crystal affects its performance. The thickness of the sodium iodide crystal ranges from less than a centimeter to several centimeters. Thicker crystals, by absorbing more of the original and the scattered gamma rays, have a relatively high sensitivity in which almost all of the gamma ray energy reaching the crystal is absorbed (Figure 5.3). Thinner crystals have lower sensitivity because more photons escape. For photons in the 140 keV range (^{99m}Tc), typical thicknesses range from 0.6 to 1.2 cm.

After the crystal absorbs energy from a gamma ray impact the excited electrons within the crystal do not return to their original state at exactly the same time, but over the course of a few nanoseconds to milliseconds, depending on the scintillator. As a result, the light photons are also emitted by the crystal over a very short span of time instead of as a single simultaneous burst. Although we cannot perceive it, if one were to plot the amount of light released following a single gamma ray impact it would appear as a curve instead of a sharp spike.

Photomultiplier tubes

The **photomultiplier tube** (PMT) is a vacuum tube with a **photocathode** on the end adjacent to the

Essentials of Nuclear Medicine Physics, Instrumentation, and Radiation Biology, Fourth Edition.
Rachel A. Powsner, Matthew R. Palmer, and Edward R. Powsner.
© 2022 John Wiley & Sons Ltd. Published 2022 by John Wiley & Sons Ltd.

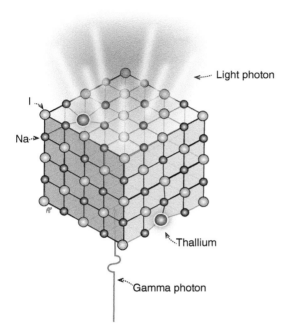

I

Na

Light photon

Thallium

Gamma photon

Figure 5.1 Scintillation crystal. The sodium iodide crystal "doped" with a thallium impurity is used to convert gamma photons into light photons.

crystal. A photocathode is a light-sensitive material, usually a type of semiconductor. The PMT is coupled with a light-conductive transparent gel to the surface of the crystal (Figure 5.4). The transparent gel has the same refractive index as the crystal and the PMT window. The light striking the photocathode causes it to emit electrons, referred to as photoelectrons. On average, four to six light photons strike the photocathode for each photoelectron produced.

The number of electrons produced at the photocathode is greatly increased by the multiplying action within the tube (Figure 5.5). As soon as they are produced, the electrons cascade along the multiplier portion of the tube successively striking each of the tube's **dynodes**. These are metal electrodes, each held at a progressively higher voltages. As an electron strikes a dynode, it knocks out two to four new electrons, each of which joins the progressively larger pulse of electrons cascading toward the anode at the end of the tube. In other words, for each electron entering a cascade of just three such dynodes, there will be between 2^3 and 4^3 electrons leaving; cascading against 10 dynodes will yield between 2^{10} and 4^{10} electrons.

Amplifiers

The current from the photomultiplier must be further amplified before it can be processed and counted. Despite the multiplication within the photomultiplier tube, the number of electrons yielded by the chain of events that begins with absorption of a single gamma ray in the crystal is still small and must be further increased or amplified. This small current is increased by the amplifier as much as a thousand-fold (see Figure 5.5).

Pulse-height analyzer

The amplifiers are designed to ensure that the amplitude of each pulse is proportional to the energy absorbed in the crystal from the gamma radiation. The amplitude of each electrical pulse from the amplifiers is measured in the electrical circuits of the **pulse-height analyzer**. A tally is kept showing the number of pulses of each height. A plot of the number of pulses against their height—that is, their energy—is called a **pulse-height spectrum**.

The pulse-height analyzer is often used to "select" only pulses (conventionally called **Z-pulses**) that correspond to a range of the acceptable energies. This range is called the **energy window**. A window setting of 20% for the 140 keV photopeak of ^{99m}Tc means that Z-pulses corresponding to a 28 keV range centered on 140 keV (126 to 154 keV) will be accepted and counted (Figure 5.6).

Sodium iodide detector energy spectrum

The shape of the pulse-height spectrum is dependent on the photon energies and the characteristics of the crystal detector. We shall now review some of the general features of the spectrum, and examine the components of the spectrum of a NaI crystal, the most commonly used crystal.

Calibrating the energy spectrum

The energy scale (horizontal axis in Figure 5.6) can be calibrated in absolute terms by using a radionuclide whose photon energy is well known, and usually one with a simple decay scheme. The most prominent peak, seen as a high point in the spectrum, is then assigned the energy value corresponding to the known energy of the principal gamma ray of the radionuclide under observation.

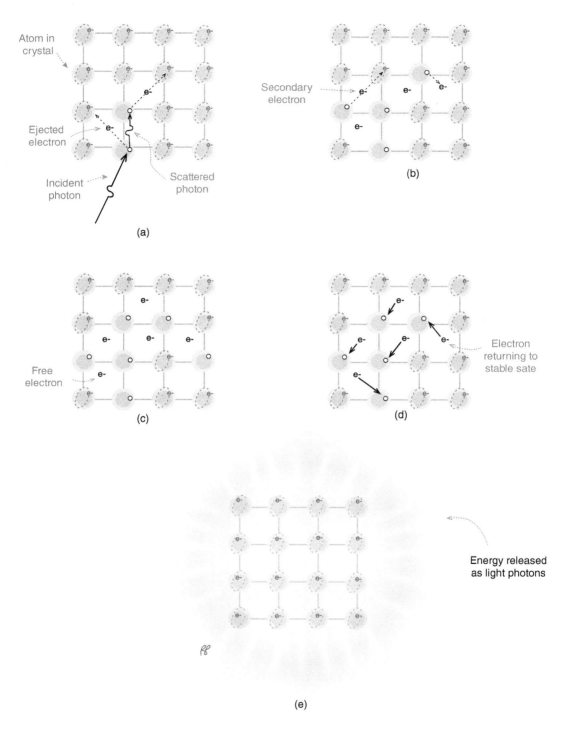

Figure 5.2 Light photons. (a) Gamma rays eject electrons from the crystal through Compton scattering and the photoelectric effect. (b, c) The ejected electrons in turn produce a large number of secondary electrons. (d, e) During de-excitation (oversimplified in this drawing) energy is released in visible light.

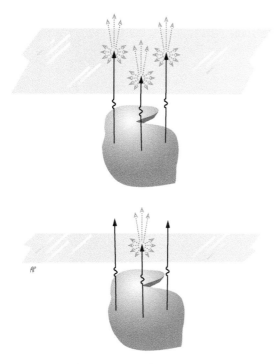

Figure 5.3 Thick crystals stop a larger fraction of the photons.

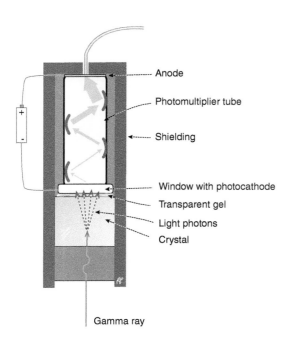

Figure 5.4 Sodium iodide crystal scintillation detector.

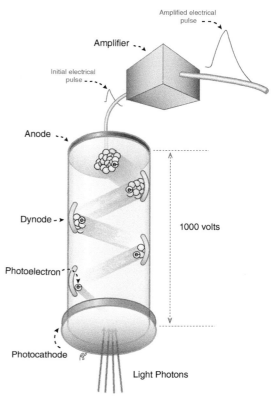

Figure 5.5 Photomultiplier tube and its amplifier.

Photopeak

When a gamma photon deposits all of its energy in the crystal, the amplifier output is a single electrical pulse whose amplitude is, as discussed above, proportional to the energy of the original gamma photon. Ideally this conversion of gamma energy to electrical pulse would be identical for each photon, and a plot of these pulses would appear as a single narrow "spike." However, due mainly to the statistical variation in the number of visible light photons produced upon interaction of the gamma ray in the scintillator, the plot of electrical pulses corresponding to the photon energy is a blurred version of the original spike (Figure 5.7).

Photopeaks in the spectrum correspond to the principal energies of gamma rays from the radioactive source. Figure 5.8 shows a typical spectrum, one from a sample of ^{99m}Tc. The relatively sharp, prominent peak at 140 keV is called the photopeak. It is produced by the prominent gamma photon from the decay of ^{99m}Tc. The horizontal axis of the pulse-height spectrum represents energy, typically in keV or MeV.

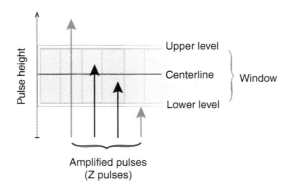

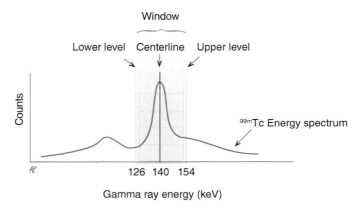

Figure 5.6 Pulse-height analyzer. The incoming pulse (Z-pulse) is proportional to the energy of the initial gamma ray photon. The pulse-height analyzer accepts only those that fall within the window (depicted as black arrows in top of illustration).

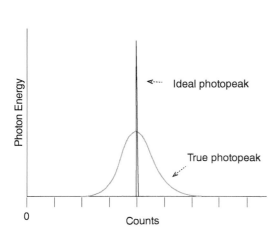

Figure 5.7 Blurring of photopeak due in part to statistical variation in the number of light photons produced when a gamma ray interacts with the crystal.

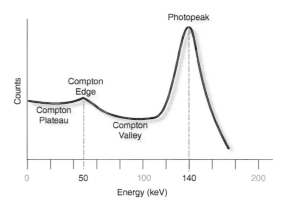

Figure 5.8 Compton peak (edge). (Adapted from Harris CC, Hamblen DP, Francis JE. Oak Ridge National Laboratory basic principles of scintillation counting for medical investigators. In: Ross DA, ed. *Medical Gamma-ray Spectrometry*. Oak Ridge, TN: US Atomic Energy Commission, Division of Technical Information, 1959.)

The vertical axis represents the number of photons detected at each point on the energy scale.

Other peaks in the energy spectrum of the source

Several other important peaks—Compton, iodine escape, annihilation, and coincidence—are briefly discussed below.

Compton peak (or Compton edge)

Compton scattering was introduced in Chapter 2. If both the **Compton electron** and deflected photon are detected, their total energy will equal that of the incident photon, and the event will register in the photopeak. However, the scattered photon often escapes detection, so that the event leaves only the energy of the Compton electron in the crystal. These Compton electrons, whose energies are always less than that of the incident photon, register to the left of the photopeak.

The Compton electrons can have any energy from nearly zero up to a characteristic maximum called the **Compton peak** or **edge**. The value of the maximum energy can be calculated as follows:

$$E_{\text{maximum Compton electron}} = \frac{E^2_{\text{incident photon}}}{\left(E_{\text{incident photon}} + 256 \text{ keV}\right)}$$

For example, the maximum Compton electron energy for a ^{99m}Tc 140 keV photon is 50 keV.

The **Compton plateau** refers to electron energies that are less than the Compton peak; the **Compton valley** reflects the sum energy of multiple Compton electrons generated by a single photon (see Figure 5.8).

Iodine escape peak

The photoelectric effect indirectly contributes to the existence of a small peak below the photopeak. When an incoming photon is absorbed as a result of a photoelectric interaction in the sodium iodide crystal, a K-shell electron is usually ejected. Because the K-shell vacancy is then filled by an L-shell electron (see Chapter 3) a 28-keV X-ray (the difference in binding energies between the L and K shells of iodine) is emitted. If this x-ray escapes detection, the total energy absorbed from the original photon is diminished by 28 keV, and a new, small peak is created 28 keV below the photopeak (Figure 5.9). This is called the **iodine escape peak**. It can only be seen as separate

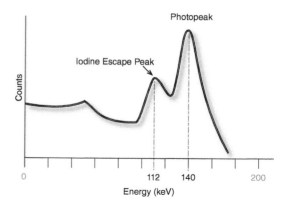

Figure 5.9 Iodine escape peak. (Adapted from Harris CC, Hamblen DP, Francis JE. Oak Ridge National Laboratory basic principles of scintillation counting for medical investigators. In: Ross DA, ed. *Medical Gamma-ray Spectrometry*. Oak Ridge, TN: US Atomic Energy Commission, Division of Technical Information, 1959.)

from the photopeak at relatively low energies where the spread of the photopeak is relatively small; at higher photopeak energies, the iodine escape peak is obscured by the spread of the photopeak.

Annihilation peak

If an entering photon is energetic enough (>1.02 MeV), it may be absorbed near the nucleus of an atom, creating a positron and an electron. This process is called **pair production**. The positron (β^+) will undergo annihilation with an electron, producing two 511-keV electrons. When one of these 511-keV photon escapes the detector, the energy detected from the original photon (which would have been 2.76 MeV in Figure 5.10 prior to the escape) will be reduced by 511 keV; if both photons escape, the energy will be reduced by 1.02 MeV. The resulting peaks are called the **single escape** and **double escape annihilation peaks**.

Coincidence peak

Some nuclides emit two or more photons. Most often, each of these produces its own characteristic photopeak in the spectrum. However, if two photons impact the crystal simultaneously, the detector will record only a single event with an energy equal to the sum of the two photon energies. This result is the so-called **coincidence peak** (Figure 5.11).

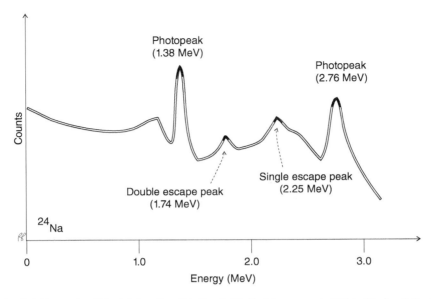

Figure 5.10 Annihilation peaks. (Adapted from Ross DA, Harris CC. *The Measurement of Clinical Radioactivity*. Oak Ridge, TN: Oak Ridge National Laboratory. (ORNL-4153), 1968.)

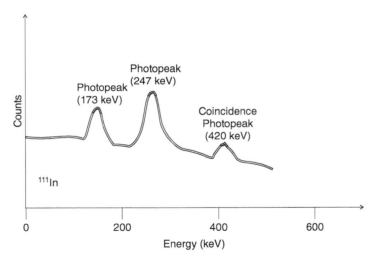

Figure 5.11 Coincidence peak for ^{111}In equals the sum of the individual photopeaks.

Effect of surrounding matter on the energy spectrum

So far we have considered the appearance of the energy spectrum for a point source in air. However, the daily practice of nuclear medicine rarely involves imaging point sources in air with unshielded NaI(Tl) crystals. The lead used to shield the crystal and the water and tissue surrounding the radioactive source alter the shape of the energy spectrum.

Backscatter peak

When lead shielding surrounds the crystal, photons may exit the crystal without detection only to be scattered 180° off the lead back into the crystal. These photons account for the **backscatter peak**. Their energy is equal to

$$E_{backscattered\ photon} = \frac{E_{incident\ photon}}{\left(1 + E_{incident\ photon} / 256\ keV\right)}$$

Backscatter peaks are only evident when the incident energy is great enough to contribute a significant degree of Compton scattering in lead (approximately 200 keV).

Characteristic lead X-ray peak

A photoelectric interaction in the lead shield will result in ejection of a K-shell electron along with the prompt emission of an X-ray. This X-ray energy is 72 keV and is equal to the difference between the binding energies of the L and K shells of lead. The emitted X-ray can be detected by the crystal and contributes to the **characteristic lead X-ray peak** at 72 keV.

Additional Compton scattering from medium surrounding source

Many of the photons emitted by a source will undergo Compton scattering in surrounding water or tissue. As a consequence, there will be fewer counts in the photopeak. The Compton photons may be seen by the detector and add to the counts below the photopeak. The effects of water on the energy spectrum of Cr-51 can be seen in Figure 5.12.

Characteristics of scintillation detectors

Energy resolution

Because the peaks of an energy spectrum are not sharp spikes but are statistically broadened, the detector may not be able to separate peaks produced by photons of similar energy. The distance between the closest peaks that the detector can distinguish determines the energy resolution of the detector.

Decay time

Although scintillation detectors absorb incoming radiation virtually instantaneously, the emission of visible light takes place over an extended period of time. This brief interval is referred to as the **decay time** of the crystal and is 230 nanoseconds for NaI(Tl). If a second gamma photon enters the crystal during this time it will add to the total output of the light pulse in a process referred to as **pulse pile-up**. These events cannot be distinguished as separate detection events and so the energy measured by the analyzer will be the sum of the two gamma energies.

Efficiency

The fundamental meaning of efficiency is the amount observed as a fraction of the amount expected. The **overall efficiency** of a detector can be considered in terms of **geometric** and **intrinsic efficiency**.

Overall efficiency

The ratio of the number of counts actually registered by the detector to the number of decays generated by a source in a given period of time is the

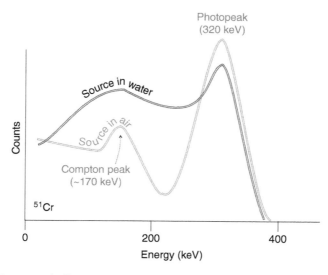

Figure 5.12 The effect of water on the ^{51}Cr energy spectrum. (Adapted from Harris CC, Hamblen DP, Francis JE. Oak Ridge National Laboratory basic principles of scintillation counting for medical investigators. In: Ross DA, ed. *Medical Gamma-ray Spectrometry*. Oak Ridge, TN: US Atomic Energy Commission, Division of Technical Information, 1959.)

overall efficiency. For a well detector, this is simply the number of counts recorded divided by the number of decays in the specimen. For a camera, it is the ratio of the number of counts within the image of the target organ, the so-called region of interest (ROI), to the number of decays of the radionuclide present in the organ. Overall efficiency can be measured, or at least reasonably approximated, by counting a sample container filled with a known quantity of radioactivity.

Using this method, the efficiency is given by the ratio of the number of counts recorded (if using a well detector) or seen in the ROI (if using a camera) to the number of actual decays. Except for attenuation within the sample or its container, the number of decays in the specimen will be 10^6 decays per megabecquerel (MBq) or 3.7×10^4 decays per microcurie (μCi).

As a practical matter, the efficiency of modern detectors is not a consideration in the daily work of the nuclear medicine department. Not only are relatively high count rates available from patients and specimens, but most quantitative work is based on the comparison of the sample (such as a urine sample) to a standard (such as the standard used for a Schillings test) count rate using the same device. Because the efficiency is the same for both standard and sample, the exact value of the efficiency is inconsequential. The detector efficiency is more important when measuring the radioactivity in a wipe test. **Wipe tests** are performed by wiping a small absorbent pad over a countertop or other surface and measuring the pad for any radioactive contamination. Here it is necessary to determine whether the activity measured on an absolute scale is below a prescribed limit, for example, less than 37 Bq/cm^2 (1 nCi/cm^2).

Geometric efficiency

The size and shape of the detector relative to the organ being imaged determines how much of the radiation emanating from the organ is actually "seen" by the face of the detector. Because radiation emanates in all directions, a detector receives only a fraction of the total. The fraction of radiation striking, or "seen" by, the face of the detector obviously will be less for a smaller crystal than larger ones and will further decrease the farther away the detector is placed from the source.

Geometric efficiency is the ratio of the number of photons striking the face of the detector to the number of photons emitted by the target organ, assuming no significant losses in the air between patient and detector. Because the measurement of the number of photons actually striking the face of the detector may be difficult, it is usually satisfactory to infer the geometric efficiency from the physical measurement of the area of the detector face and the distance between it and the target.

Intrinsic efficiency

Intrinsic efficiency, a component of overall efficiency, is the ratio of the number of counts recorded by the system to the number of photons striking the face of the detector. The **intrinsic efficiency** can be calculated most easily if a known source emitting a known number of photons is placed directly against the face of the detector. In this arrangement, any effect of geometric factors is usually small enough to be ignored.

Types of scintillation-based detectors

Some commonly used scintillation-based detectors are described below. All contain a sodium iodide crystal coupled to a single photomultiplier tube. The output of the photomultiplier tube is then routed through the amplifier, and pulse-height analyzer, as described above.

Thyroid probe

The **thyroid probe** (Figure 5.13) is a crystal scintillation detector for measuring the radioactivity in a patient's thyroid gland. The detector is supported on a stand by an adjustable arm that permits placement of the detector against the patient's neck. A cylindrical or slightly conical extension of the shielding around the crystal limits the field of view to the region of the thyroid gland. For measuring ^{123}I or ^{99m}Tc uptake in the gland, the sodium iodide scintillation crystal need be only one-half centimeter thick. Thicker crystals, up to 2-cm thick, are more efficient for higher energy radionuclides, such as ^{131}I.

Well counter

The **well counter** (Figure 5.14) is a shielded crystal with a hole, the "well", drilled in the center to hold a specimen in a test tube or vial. In this

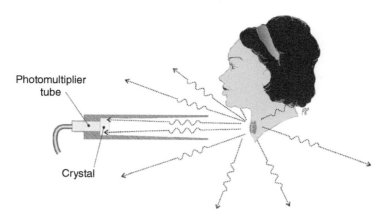

Figure 5.13 Thyroid probe. Shielded crystal scintillation detector as used for measuring thyroid uptake.

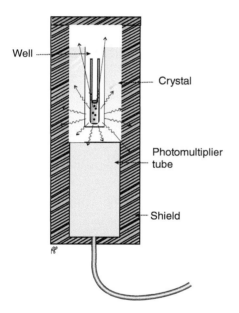

Figure 5.14 Well counter. Crystal scintillation detector constructed with an internal well for counting samples in vitro.

arrangement, the specimen is surrounded by the crystal so that only a small fraction of the radiation escapes through the opening of the well. The size and thickness of the crystal are selected for efficient capture of photons. For radionuclides with low-energy emissions, typical crystals are cylinders of

2 to 3 cm. Two or three times larger crystals are more efficient for higher energies such as those of ^{131}I.

Liquid scintillation counters

Alpha particles and lower energy beta particles that cannot travel far enough to reach a detector or are blocked by the walls or windows of previously described detection equipment can be placed in close proximity to scintillation molecules by immersing the sample in a liquid solvent containing these molecules. The radioactive sample (such as a wipe test) is immersed in this liquid and, as with solid scintillation crystals, light photons are emitted following an impact by the incident particles. The light photons are detected, converted to photoelectrons, and the signal is amplified by photomultiplier tubes.

Dosimeters and area monitors

Scintillation detectors are available for dosimeters and handheld survey meters for the purpose of monitoring or searching for a source. Others are placed more permanently for area monitoring. In one commercial design, a series of detectors are arranged in a door-like frame through which personnel must pass before leaving a restricted area of the laboratory. The device is often equipped with an audible alarm to signal when the radiation is above an acceptable level.

Questions

1. Connect the following events with the corresponding components of a scintillation detector:
   (a) Photoelectrons are released in response to light photons.
   (b) Light photons are released in response to gamma photons.
   (c) The output of the PMT is amplified to a detectable level of current.
   (d) The multiplying action of successive steps yields a very large number of electrons in response to each photoelectron.
   (1) Photomultiplier tube (PMT).
   (2) Amplifier.
   (3) Crystal.
   (4) Photocathode surface of PMT.

2. Name the following features that can be seen in the energy spectrum obtained from a sodium iodide crystal detector:
   (a) Can be seen at 28 keV below photopeak.
   (b) Energy of photon source.
   (c) Can be seen at 511 and 1020 keV below photopeak of high-energy photon.
   (d) Peak near 420 keV emitted by a ^{111}In source.
   (e) Maximum Compton electron energy.
   (f) 72 keV.
   (1) Photopeak.
   (2) Compton peak or edge.
   (3) Annihilation escape peaks.
   (4) Iodine escape peak.
   (5) Coincidence peak.
   (6) Characteristic lead X-ray peak.
   (7) Backscatter peak.

3. True or false: A detector that can distinguish separate photopeaks at 200 and 205 keV has a better energy resolution than a detector that can only distinguish photopeaks as close as 200 and 250 keV.

4. Match each of the listed terms (1)–(3) below to one of the following definitions:
   (a) Electrical output from amplifiers connected to the PMTs in response to photon interaction in the crystal.
   (b) Range of acceptable photon energies.
   (c) Used to select Z pulses within the upper and lower limits of the energy window.
   (1) Pulse height analyzer (PHA).
   (2) Energy window.
   (3) Z pulse.

5. For an I-123 imaging study in a gamma camera a single 15% energy window is set symmetrically on the 159 keV photopeak. The lower and upper energy windows are:
   (a) 0 keV and 159 keV.
   (b) 159 keV and 183 keV.
   (c) 143 keV and 175 keV.
   (d) 147 keV and 171 keV.
   (e) 135 keV and 159 keV.

6. Scintillation crystals convert:
   (a) Gamma ray energy into a current.
   (b) Visible light into ultraviolet light.
   (c) Gamma ray energy into visible light.
   (d) Electron energy into potential energy.
   (e) Voltage into current.

7. Liquid scintillation counters are used for detecting which of the following types of radiation (choose all that are correct).
   (a) High-energy gamma photons.
   (b) Low-energy gamma photons.
   (c) High-energy beta particles.
   (d) Alpha particles.
   (e) Low-energy beta particles.

Answers

1. (a) 4. (b) 3. (c) 2. (d) 1.
2. (a) 4. (b) 1. (c) 3. (d) 5. (e) 2. (f) 6.
3. True.
4. (a) 3. (b) 2. (c) 1.

5. (d).
6. (c).
7. (d), (e).

CHAPTER 6

Imaging Instrumentation

Theory and structure

The daily workload in a nuclear medicine department consists of "functional" imaging of organs including the thyroid, brain, heart, liver, and kidney. This is accomplished using a large scintillation device. In the 1950s, Harold Anger developed the basic design of the modern nuclear medicine camera. The **Anger camera**, was a significant improvement over its predecessor, the rectilinear scanner. The components of the Anger camera are depicted in Figure 6.1.

Components of the imaging system

The following components of the imaging system are described in the order they are encountered by the gamma ray photons emitted from the patient's body.

Collimators

A **collimator** restricts the photons or X-ray from the source so that each point in the image corresponds to a unique point in the source. Collimators are composed of thousands of precisely aligned **holes** (channels), which are formed by either casting hot lead (most common method of production) or folding lead foil. They are usually depicted in cross section (Figure 6.2). Nuclides emit gamma ray photons in all directions. The collimator allows only those photons traveling directly along the long axis of each hole to reach the crystal. Photons emitted in any other direction are absorbed by the **septa** between the holes (Figure 6.3). Without a collimator in front of the crystal, the image would be indistinct (Figure 6.4).

There are several types of collimators designed to channel photons of different energies. By appropriate choice of collimator, it is possible to magnify or minify images and to select between imaging quality and imaging speed.

Parallel-hole collimators

Low-energy all-purpose collimators (LEAP): These collimators have relatively large holes which allow the passage of many of the photons emanating from the patient. As such they have relatively high sensitivity at the expense of spatial resolution.

Because the holes are larger photons arising from a larger region of the source are accepted. As a result, image resolution is decreased (Figure 6.5 top image). The sensitivity of one such collimator has been calculated at approximately 500,000 cpm for a 1-μCi source, and the resolution is 1.0 cm at 10 cm from the surface of the collimator (Nuclear Fields Precision Microcast Collimators, Nuclear Fields B.V., The Netherlands; 140-keV ^{99m}Tc source). These collimators are useful for imaging low-energy photons such as those from ^{201}Tl for which thick septa are not necessary. In addition, because of their moderately high sensitivity (resulting from thinner septa and bigger holes) they are advantageous for images of short duration such as the sequential one-per-second images for a renal flow study. These collimators are sometimes called GAP or general all-purpose collimators.

High-resolution collimators: These collimators allow collection of higher resolution images than the LEAP collimators. They have more holes that are both smaller in diameter and longer in length. The calculated sensitivity of a representative high-resolution collimator is approximately 185,000 cpm for a 0.037-MBq (1-μCi) source, and its nominal resolution is 0.65 cm at 10 cm from the face of the collimator (Nuclear Fields B.V.).

Essentials of Nuclear Medicine Physics, Instrumentation, and Radiation Biology, Fourth Edition.
Rachel A. Powsner, Matthew R. Palmer, and Edward R. Powsner.
© 2022 John Wiley & Sons Ltd. Published 2022 by John Wiley & Sons Ltd.

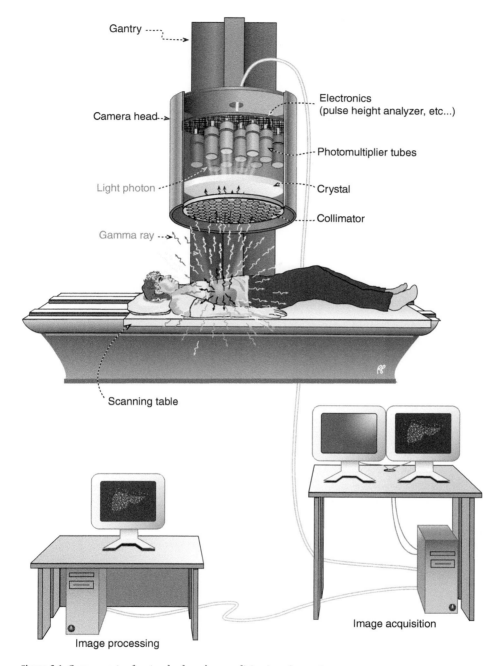

Figure 6.1 Components of a standard nuclear medicine imaging system.

To compare the performance of a LEAP with a high-resolution collimator, let us look at the photons from two radioactive points in a liver. The photons from each of the points are emitted in all directions, but the detector can "see" only those photons that pass through the holes of the collimator.

The relatively large hole in the LEAP collimator will also admit photons scattered at relatively large angles from the direct line between liver and the crystal. This lowers the resolution because the angled photons have the effect of merging the images of two closely adjacent points (Figure 6.5 top).

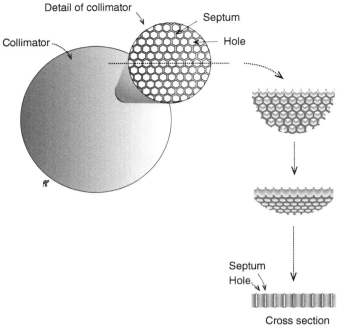

Detail of collimator

Septum

Hole

Collimator

Septum

Hole

Cross section

Figure 6.2 Collimator detail.

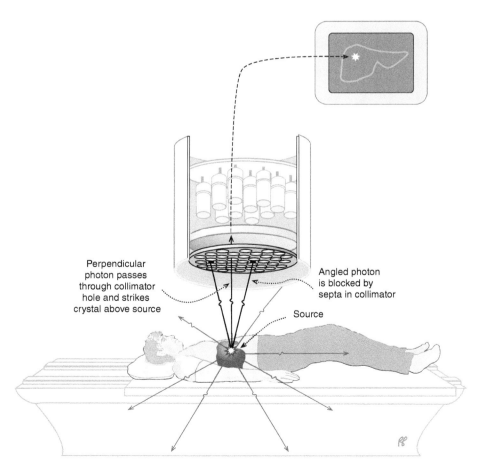

Perpendicular photon passes through collimator hole and strikes crystal above source

Angled photon is blocked by septa in collimator

Source

Figure 6.3 A collimator selects photons perpendicular to the plane of the collimator face.

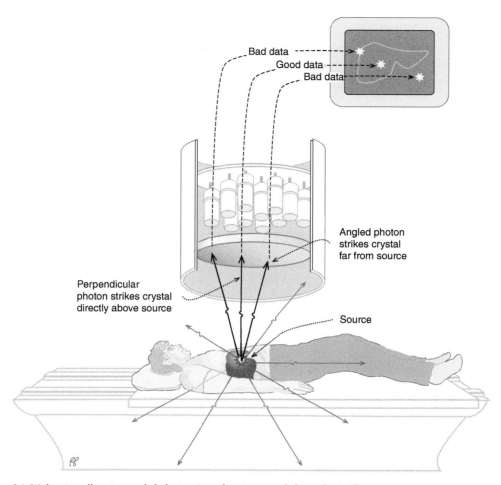

Figure 6.4 Without a collimator, angled photons introduce improperly located scintillations.

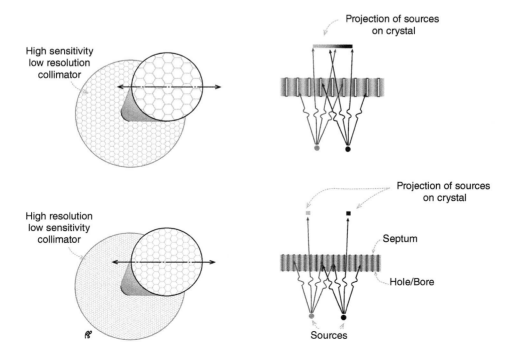

Figure 6.5 For the same bore length, the smaller the diameter the higher the resolution.

At the same time, the larger holes and correspondingly thinner septa give the LEAP a higher sensitivity by admitting a higher percentage of the photons. The high-resolution collimator, on the other hand, admits photons from a smaller fraction of the organ, because more of its face is blocked by septa. In a reciprocal way, the narrower (see Figure 6.5 bottom) and/or longer (Figure 6.6) bore of its holes better collimate those photons that do enter the collimator. As a result, relatively closely spaced details in the source are more likely to appear clearly separated in the image. Resolution is sometimes expressed as the angle of acceptance. Only photons falling within the angle of acceptance (defined by the length and diameter of the hole) can reach the crystal (Figure 6.7).

High- and medium-energy collimators: Low-energy collimators are not adequate for the higher-energy photons of nuclides such as ^{67}gallium (it emits 394-keV, 300-keV, and 185-keV photons, in addition to its

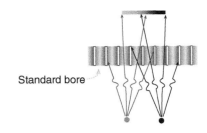

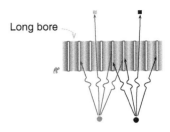

Figure 6.6 For the same hole diameter, the longer the bore the higher the resolution.

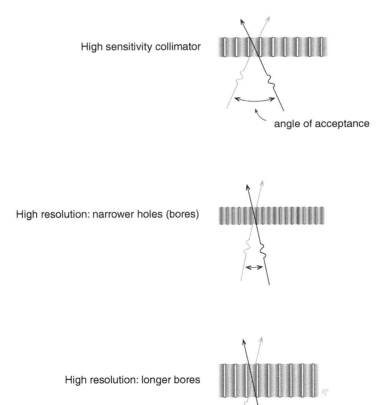

Figure 6.7 Angle of acceptance. The narrower the angle of acceptance of a collimator the better the resolution of the image.

low-energy 93-keV photon), ^{131}iodine (364 keV), and ^{111}indium (245 and 173 keV). The photons of these nuclides can penetrate the thinner septa of both the LEAP and the high-resolution collimators, resulting in poorer resolution. High-energy collimators with thicker septa (Figure 6.8) to reduce septal penetration are used, but thicker septa also mean smaller holes and, consequently, lower sensitivity. High-energy collimators are useful for ^{131}iodine.

Medium-energy collimators have characteristics between those of low- and high-energy collimators.

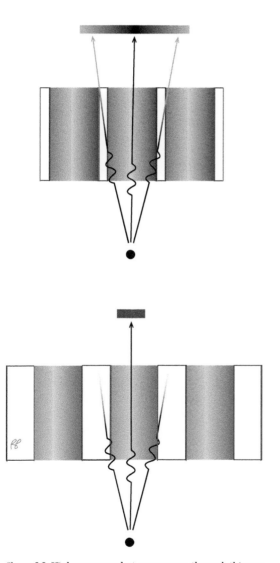

Figure 6.8 Higher energy photons can pass through thinner collimator septa (top). Thicker septa (bottom image) are used to block high- and medium-energy photons.

They can be used to image photons emitted by ^{67}gallium and ^{111}indium. The terms high-, medium-, and low-energy are not rigidly defined, and usage may vary from institution to institution.

Sensitivity

Sensitivity refers to the ability of the imaging camera to detect the photons generated by the nuclides. A low sensitivity system detects a smaller fraction of the generated photons; a high sensitivity system detects more of them. Sensitivity of a gamma camera is specified as the count rate recorded by the detector for a small amount of activity placed 10 cm from the collimator. The units are counts per minute per mCi or kBq.

Spatial resolution

Spatial resolution refers to the ability of the camera to distinguish between adjacent points in the organ. The higher the spatial resolution the closer the points that can be distinguished, in other words, the finer the detail that can be seen. Spatial resolution is characterized by the **point-spread function (PSF)** or the **line-spread function (LSF)** which are the images obtained when a point or line sources of activity are placed in the field of view (Figure 6.9). PSF and LSF are specified in terms of their full-width at half maximum (**FWHM**) and full-width at one-tenth maximum (**FWTM**) in mm. Those are the width of the distributions measured at 50% and 10% of the peak intensity respectively (middle and bottom images in Figure 6.10).

Sensitivity and spatial resolution play off against each other: increasing the spatial resolution by using a high-resolution collimator decreases the system sensitivity—fewer counts would be recorded for a given imaging session but would be localized with a higher accuracy. Conversely, a general purpose collimator employed for the same imaging task would allow more counts to be acquired but result in a blurrier image. The choice of which one to favor and therefore which collimators to choose therefore depends on the objectives of the imaging tasks.

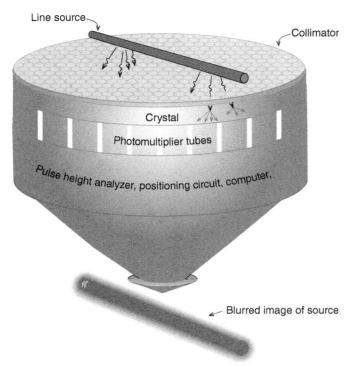

Figure 6.9 Blurring of a line source.

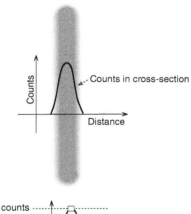

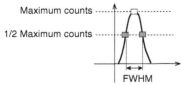

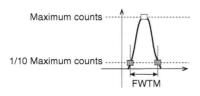

Figure 6.10 Full-width at half-maximum and full-width at tenth-maximum.

Modulation transfer function

The LSF can be expressed in the frequency domain by applying a Fourier transform which will be discussed in Chapter 12. As we will discuss at that time images can be represented as a collection of waves in frequency space. The **modulation transfer function** plots show the ability of the camera to reproduce these waves at each of the spatial frequencies. Each camera system has a unique frequency response. This is analogous to stereo systems; some reproduce more of the treble (higher frequency waves), others reproduce more of the bass (lower frequency waves), and the better the system the more of both bass and treble it can reproduce.

In nuclear medicine systems the higher frequencies are necessary to reproduce the sharp edges and fine details of an image; the lower and middle frequencies produce the remainder of the image. Figure 6.11 contains plots of the modulation transfer functions of two hypothetical camera systems. System A accepts a greater proportion of lower frequencies, system B accepts a greater proportion of higher frequencies.

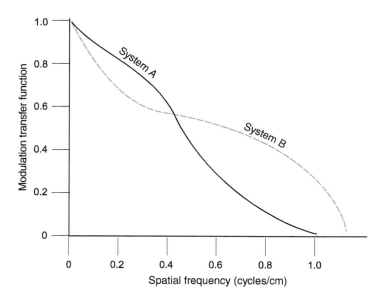

Figure 6.11 Modulation transfer function.

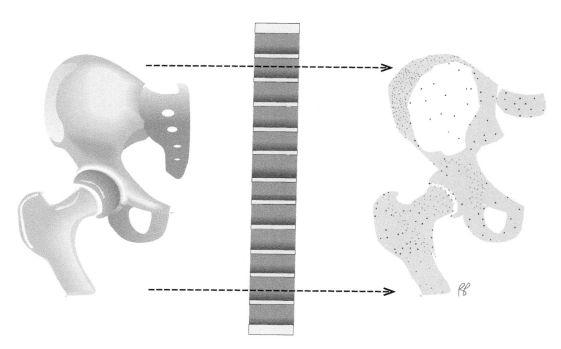

Figure 6.12 Parallel-hole collimator.

Nonparallel-hole collimators: Nonparallel-hole collimators provide a wider or a narrower field of view. The cone-like pattern of holes allows these collimators to enlarge or reduce the size of the image.

Converging and diverging collimators: A parallel-hole collimator and its image are shown in Figure 6.12. At least for this simple example, the organ and the image are the same size. In a converging collimator, however, the holes are not parallel but are angled inward, toward the organ, as shown in Figure 6.13. Consequently, the organ appears larger at the face of the crystal.

Diverging collimators achieve a wider field of view by angling the holes the opposite way, outward toward the organ. This is used most often on a camera with a small crystal, such as a portable camera. Using a diverging collimator, a large organ such as the lung can be captured on the face of a smaller crystal (Figure 6.14).

Pinhole collimators: These have a single hole—the pinhole—usually 2 to 4 mm in diameter. Like a camera lens, the image is projected upside down and reversed right to left at the crystal (Figure 6.15). It is usually corrected electronically on the viewing screen. A pinhole collimator generates magnified images of a small organ like the thyroid or a joint.

Fan beam collimators: These are a cross between a converging and a parallel-hole collimator. They are designed for use on cameras with rectangular heads

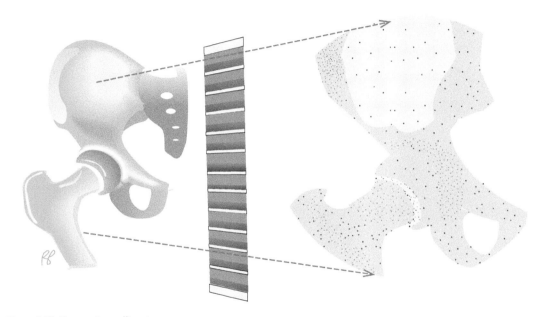

Figure 6.13 Converging collimator.

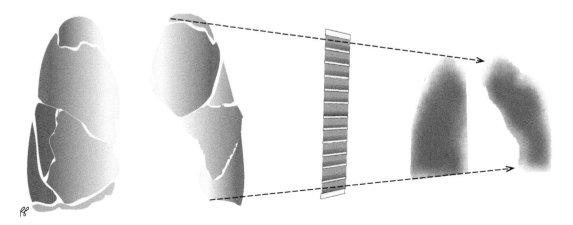

Figure 6.14 Diverging collimator.

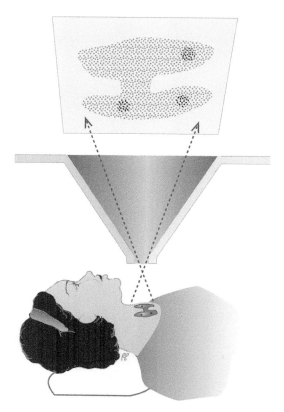

Figure 6.15 Pinhole collimator.

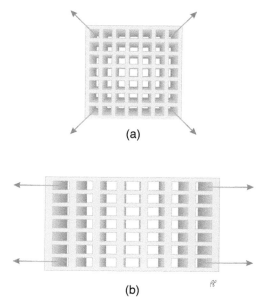

(a)

(b)

Figure 6.16 (a) In a converging collimator, holes converge toward the patient in both directions and uniformly enlarge an image. (b) In a fan beam collimator, holes converge in one direction but are parallel in the other. Arrows demonstrate the paths of photons coming from the patient.

when imaging smaller organs such as the brain and heart. When viewed from one direction (along the short dimension of the rectangle), the holes are parallel. When viewed from the other direction (along the long dimension of the rectangle), the holes converge (Figure 6.16). This arrangement allows the data from the patient to be spread to better fill the surface of the crystal.

Camera head

The camera head contains the crystal, photomultiplier tubes, and associated electronics (see Figure 6.1). The **head housing** envelopes and shields these internal components. Typically, it includes a thin layer of lead. A **gantry** supports the heavy camera head.

Crystals, photomultiplier tubes, and amplifiers: The crystal for an imaging camera is a large slab of thallium-"doped" NaI crystal similar to that used for the scintillation probes described in Chapter 5. It should be noted that the thickness of a crystal

affects its resolution as well as its sensitivity. Although thicker crystals have higher sensitivity, the resolution is lower because gamma rays may be scattered and absorbed farther from the point at which they entered the crystal (Figure 6.17).

Sixty or more photomultiplier tubes (described in Chapter 5) may be attached to the back surface of the crystal using light conductive jelly. The amplifier is also discussed there.

Positioning algorithm: The amount of light received by a photomultiplier tube (PMT) is related to the proximity of the tube to the site of interaction of the gamma ray in the crystal. The photomultiplier tube closest to the site of interaction receives the greatest number of photons and generates the greatest output pulse; the tube farthest from the nuclide source receives the fewest light photons and generates the smallest pulse. Although an image can be composed solely of the points corresponding to the photomultiplier tube with the highest output at each photon interaction, the number of resolvable points is then limited to the total number of PMT tubes (up to 128 per camera).

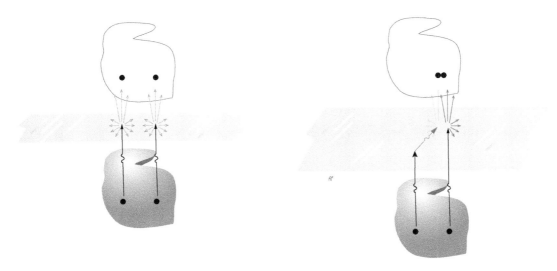

Figure 6.17 Scattering of photons in a thicker crystal reduces resolution.

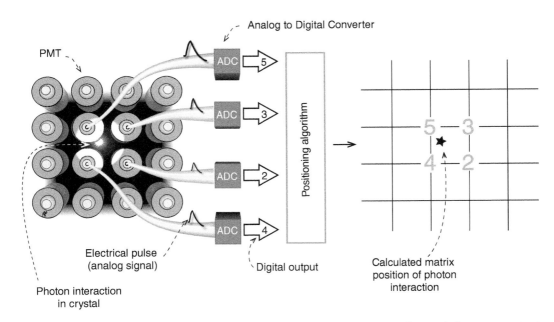

Figure 6.18 The positioning algorithm improves image resolution. The closer the PMT to the site of photon interaction in the crystal the greater the analog signal output (current pulse). This signal is converted to a digital value by the ADCs and this digital value is used to calculate the corresponding matrix position of the photon interaction in the image stored on the computer.

The **positioning algorithm** improves resolution by combining the signals from adjacent tubes (Figure 6.18). The electrical pulse generated by each PMT is first digitized by an analog to digital converter (ADC). These digital values are then transmitted to the positioning algorithm which is a part of the computer processing equipment in the camera head. Since the computer/positioning algorithm "knows" the location of each PMT tube on the surface of the crystal it can estimate the site of the gamma ray interaction in the crystal by "weighing-in" the digital value of the amount of light each PMT receives.

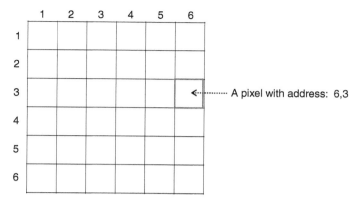

Figure 6.19 Pixel address: column number, row number.

Pulse-height analyzer: The function of the pulse-height analyzer is discussed in the preceding chapter (see Figure 5.6). Following each gamma photon interaction in the crystal, the sum of digital output from all of the PMTs is proportional to the energy of the gamma photon striking the crystal. This summed output is called the **Z-pulse**. The pulse-height analyzer accepts only those Z-pulses that correspond to the gamma energy of interest. Each accepted Z-pulse and its location (as determined by the positioning algorithm) is stored in the computer.

Persistence scope

In the past, the **persistence scope** was made with a phosphor that faded very slowly to provide a slowly changing view of the x,y location of the Z-pulses that are accepted (each of which corresponds to the location of a gamma ray). At present, the same result is achieved with much greater flexibility by storing the image in computer memory and using it to update the image on the screen slowly or rapidly. This allows the person who is acquiring the scan to adjust the position of the patient prior to recording the final image on film or computer.

Computers

Nuclear medicine computers are used for the acquisition, storage, and processing of data. The image data are stored in digital form (**digitized**) as follows: For each Z-pulse that is accepted by the pulse-height analyzer, one count is added to the storage location that corresponds to its x,y location determined by the positioning circuit. The data

storage can be visualized as a **matrix**, a kind of two-dimensional checkerboard. Each matrix position corresponds to a **pixel**, which has a unique "address" composed of the column and row of its location (Figure 6.19). Data are digitized by assigning a matrix position to every accepted photon (Figure 6.20). Matrices are defined by the number of subdivisions along each axis. The operator can select from several matrix configurations of successively finer divisions; 64 × 64, 128 × 128, 256 × 256, and 512 × 512, or more. These numbers refer to the number of columns and rows in these square matrices. Notice that the outside physical dimensions of all matrices are the same size; what varies is the pixel size and hence the total number of pixels. A 64 × 64 matrix has 4096 pixels; a 128 × 128 matrix has 16,384 pixels; and so on.

The greater the number of pixels the smaller is each pixel for a given field of view, and the better preserved is the resolution of the image (Figure 6.21). The camera and computer system cannot reliably distinguish between two points that are separated by less than 1 pixel. In Figure 6.22, three "hot spots" are seen in the kidney parenchyma. With a coarser matrix (larger pixel size) depicted in the upper portion of the figure, two of the three spots are within a single pixel. In the finer matrix pictured below, all three points are distinct as there are now several "cold" pixels between the "hot" pixels.

The size of a pixel is inversely related to the dimensions of a matrix for a given field of view. For a 32-cm camera field of view mapped onto a 64 × 64 computer matrix, each pixel will measure 0.5 cm on a side. For the same camera, each pixel of

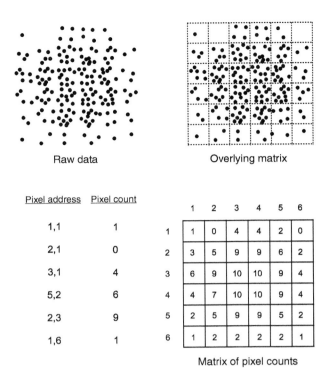

Raw data

Overlying matrix

Pixel address	Pixel count
1,1	1
2,1	0
3,1	4
5,2	6
2,3	9
1,6	1

	1	2	3	4	5	6
1	1	0	4	4	2	0
2	3	5	9	9	6	2
3	6	9	10	10	9	4
4	4	7	10	10	9	4
5	2	5	9	9	5	2
6	1	2	2	2	2	1

Matrix of pixel counts

Figure 6.20 Storing image data in a matrix.

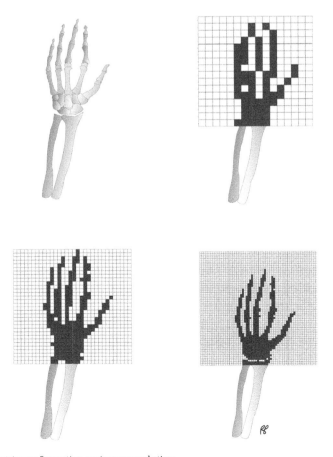

Figure 6.21 Effect of matrix configuration on image resolution.

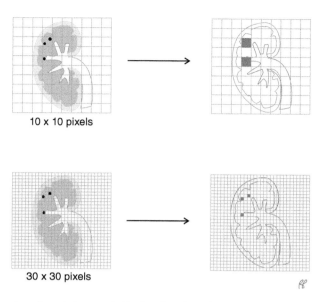

10 x 10 pixels

30 x 30 pixels

Figure 6.22 A matrix cannot resolve points separated by less than 1 pixel.

a 128×128 matrix will measure 0.25 cm on a side. Similarly, a matrix of 256×256 will divide the field of view into pixels measuring 0.125 cm on a side. This means that points that are closer to each other than 0.5 cm, 0.25 cm, and 0.125 cm, respectively, cannot be separately distinguished.

Of course, the maximum resolution of the image is limited by the resolution of the camera and collimator. Once the data is stored in a matrix, images can be displayed on the computer screen or film.

Planar imaging

Image acquisition

The gamma photons emitted by the patient may be acquired in various forms: static, dynamic, gated, or tomographic images.

Static images

Static imaging is used to collect images of different regions of the body or differently angled (oblique) views of a particular region of interest. For example, a bone scan is composed of static images of 12 different regions of the body (three head views, left arm, right arm, anterior chest, posterior chest, and so on) or anterior and posterior whole body images with additional static views of select regions of the skeleton. The whole body images seen in Figure 6.23 were obtained by moving the gantry at a steady rate

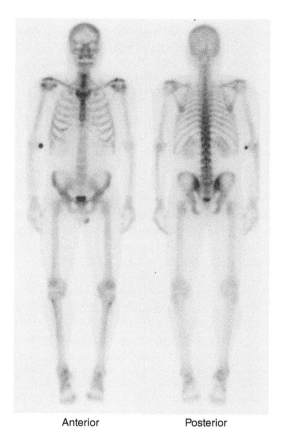

Anterior   Posterior

Figure 6.23 Bone scan.

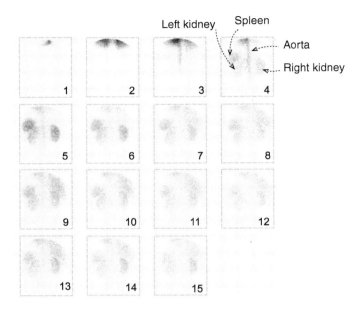

Figure 6.24 Sixty-second renal flow study.

of 12 cm/min while acquiring the imaging data. Liver scans are generally composed of six angled views of the liver and spleen; thyroid scans may have three or four angled views of the thyroid. In all of the above cases there is very little change in the distribution of nuclide in the organ of interest during the time the images are being acquired.

Dynamic images

If the distribution of nuclide in the organ is changing rapidly and it is important to record this change, multiple rapid images of a particular region of interest are acquired. This type of image acquisition is called **dynamic imaging**. It is used, for example, to collect sequential one-second images (called **frames**) of the vascular flow of nuclide through the kidney. In the example shown in Figure 6.24, these 60 frames are summed or **compressed** into 15 frames of four seconds each by adding every four frames together.

In Figure 6.25, sequential anterior abdominal images demonstrate an active bleeding site originating in the colon at the splenic flexure. Radiolabeled blood progresses through the descending colon to the rectum. The images were first acquired as 96 frames of 30 seconds-duration. These images were then "compressed" into 16 images of three minutes each. Dynamic imaging can be thought of as a type of video recording to "catch" images of fast action; static images are similar to photographs.

Gated images

Gated images are a variation of dynamic images: Continuous images are obtained of a moving organ (generally the heart) and data are coordinated with the rate of movement (using electrocardiographic leads to keep track of the R–R interval for heart imaging). Gating is used to divide the emission data from the radioactive blood pool in a Gated Blood Pool Study (GBPS) or Multigated Acquisition (MUGA) into "frames" so that wall motion can be evaluated and a left ventricular ejection fraction can be calculated. During gated imaging, each cardiac cycle (the interval between R waves on the electrocardiogram) is divided into frames (Figure 6.26). The output of the electrocardiogram (EKG attached to the patient) is connected to the nuclear medicine camera/computer. Each R wave will "trigger" the collection of a set of frames. In this simplified example, the camera/computer is programmed to collect eight frames of 0.125 seconds each. This assumes that each heart beat is of one second's duration. Images of the cardiac blood pool collected from approximately 600 cardiac cycles are summed to create a single composite gated cycle image.

Bleeding site

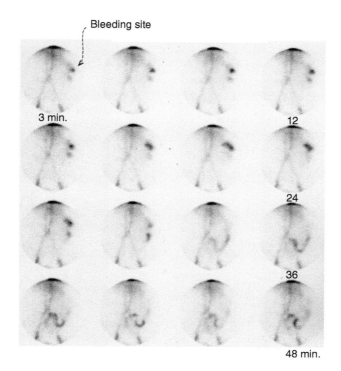

Figure 6.25 Gastrointestinal bleeding scan.

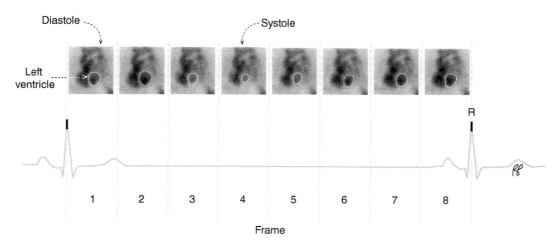

Figure 6.26 Gated blood pool study.

Questions

1. True or false: A parallel hole collimator providing both high sensitivity and high resolution is difficult to design principally because the requirements for sensitivity conflict with those for resolution.

2. Starting with a standard low energy all-purpose collimator, what will happen to the images if you alter the collimator design by (select all that apply):
   (a) Lengthening the bores?
   (b) Increasing the number of holes while decreasing the size of each hole?
   (c) Decreasing the width of the holes and thickening the septa?
   (d) Widening the holes and making the septa thinner?
      (i)   Higher resolution, lower sensitivity.
      (ii) Less septal penetration by higher energy photons.
      (iii) Lower resolution, higher sensitivity.

3. True or false: In the converging-hole collimator, the holes angle inward toward the organ to be imaged. In consequence, the organ appears larger at the face of the crystal.

4. How many pixels of data can be stored in a 64 × 64 image matrix? Choose one.
   (a) 128.
   (b) 256.
   (c) 512.
   (d) 1024.
   (e) 2048.
   (f) 4096.

5. The usual gamma camera head contains all of the following elements except:
   (a) Crystal.
   (b) Photomultiplier tubes.
   (c) Collimator.
   (d) Positioning circuit.
   (e) Pulse-height analyzer.
   (f) Focusing assembly.

6. Match the part of the imaging system with its function:
   (a) Positioning algorithm.
   (b) Photomultiplier tube.
   (c) Crystal.
   (d) Collimator.
   (e) Gantry.
   (f) Pulse height analyzer.
      (i)   Converts photon energy to light energy.
      (ii) Supports the camera head(s).
      (iii) Converts light energy to a small electrical pulse.
      (iv) Improves image resolution by factoring in the output of each PMT to better localize the position of the photon interaction in the imaging field.
      (v)   Accepts summed PMT output (Z-pulses) that correspond to the photon energy of the source.
      (vi) Restricts photon entry to the crystal so that each point in the image corresponds to a unique point in the source.

7. What is the pixel size for an image acquired with a field of view size of 32 cm × 32 cm and a matrix size of 128 × 128?

Answers

1. True. For example, high sensitivity design calls for large holes with thin septa while high resolution calls for small holes and thick septa.
2. (a) (i). (b) (i). (c) (i) and (ii). (d) (iii).
3. True.
4. (f) (4096). In a square matrix, 64 × 64 = 4096.
5. (f) (Focusing assembly). This is an undefined term.
6. (a) (iv). (b) (iii). (c) (i) (d) (vi). (e) (ii). (f) (v).
7. 2.5 × 2.5 mm (320 mm/128 = 2.5 mm).

CHAPTER 7

Single-photon Emission Computed Tomography (SPECT)

Single-photon emission computed tomography (SPECT) cameras acquire multiple planar views of the radioactivity in an organ. The data are then processed mathematically to create cross-sectional views of the organ. SPECT utilizes the single photons emitted by gamma-emitting radionuclides such as ^{99m}Tc, ^{111}In, and ^{123}I. This is in contrast to positron emission tomography (PET), which utilizes the paired 511-keV photons arising from positron annihilation. PET is the subject of Chapter 8.

Equipment

Types of camera

The simplest camera design for SPECT imaging is similar to that of a planar camera but with two additional features. First, the SPECT camera is constructed so that the head can rotate about the patient to acquire multiple views (Figure 7.1). Second, it is equipped with a computer that integrates the multiple images to produce the cross-sectional views of the organ.

To increase overall efficiency, most SPECT cameras are manufactured with more than one head—two being the most common. The heads are mechanically rotated around the patient to obtain the multiple projection views. In addition a number of dedicated cardiac SPECT cameras are available for use and will be discussed briefly at the end of this chapter.

Angle of rotation of heads

Single-headed cameras must rotate a full 360° to obtain all necessary views of most organs. In contrast, each head of a double-headed camera need

rotate only half as far, 180°, and a triple-headed camera only 120° to obtain the same views. The cost of the additional heads must be balanced against the benefits of increased speed of acquisition.

Two-headed cameras: fixed and adjustable

Two-headed cameras can have a fixed, parallel configuration or fixed, perpendicular configuration or adjustable heads (Figure 7.2). Fixed, parallel heads (opposing heads) can be used for simultaneous anterior and posterior planar imaging or can be rotated as a unit for SPECT acquisition. Fixed, perpendicular heads, in an L-shaped unit, are used almost exclusively for cardiac or brain SPECT imaging.

Adjustable heads allow positioning of the heads in different angular configurations. The moveable head can be moved closer to or farther along the ring from the other head so that the two heads are parallel (opposing), perpendicular (L-shaped), or separated by an intermediate angle. Thus the adjustable two-headed camera can be used for planar imaging and for large and small organ tomography.

> ### Tomography
>
> *Tomos* is the Greek word for "cut" or "section". "Tomography" is a name originally used for conventional X-rays that were modified to bring only a single plane through the patient into focus.

Acquisition

The numerous, sequential planar views acquired during tomographic acquisition are called **projection**

Essentials of Nuclear Medicine Physics, Instrumentation, and Radiation Biology, Fourth Edition.
Rachel A. Powsner, Matthew R. Palmer, and Edward R. Powsner.
© 2022 John Wiley & Sons Ltd. Published 2022 by John Wiley & Sons Ltd.

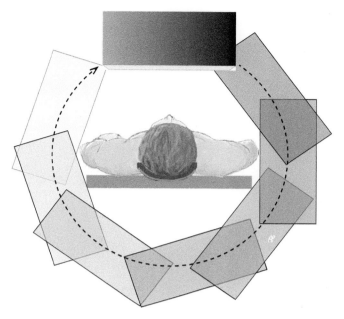

Figure 7.1 SPECT camera.

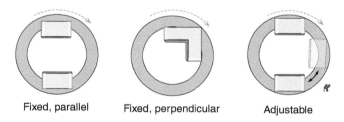

Fixed, parallel　　Fixed, perpendicular　　Adjustable

Figure 7.2 Two-headed SPECT camera configurations.

views. They are little more than an intermediate step toward creating slices. Figure 7.3 shows an entire set of projection views that can be used to construct tomographic images of the liver and spleen. Because of the large number, 64 in this case, compared to the five typically used for a conventional liver–spleen scan (Figure 7.4), these projection views are most useful when displayed as a moderately rapid sequential presentation, the so-called **cine** view. The term cine is used because of its resemblance to movies.

Arc of acquisition

Tomographic projection views are most often acquired over an arc of 360° or 180°. The 360° arc of rotation of the camera heads is regularly used for most organs. The 180° arc is used for organs that are positioned on one side of the body, such as the heart.

Views of the heart are obtained in a 180° arc extending from the right anterior oblique position to the left posterior oblique position. The data from this 180° is considered adequate, because photons exiting the body from the right posterior and lateral chest travel through more tissue and suffer greater attenuation than those exiting through the left side (Figure 7.5).

Number of projection tomographic views

Over a full 360° arc, 64 or 128 tomographic projections are usually collected; similarly, 32 or 64 views are generally obtained over a 180° arc.

Collection times

For a given dose of radiopharmaceutical, better images are generated using the higher count statistics from longer acquisitions. However, patient comfort and cooperation limit imaging times.

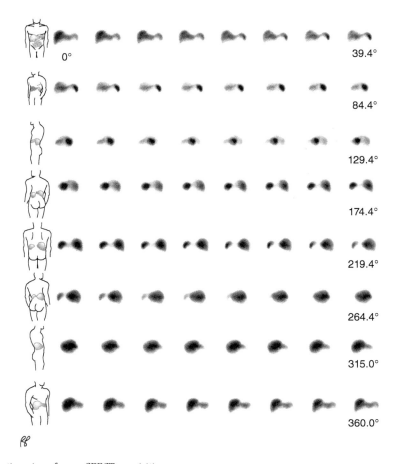

Figure 7.3 Projection views from a SPECT acquisition.

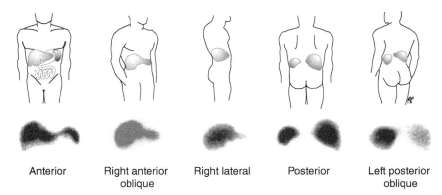

Anterior   Right anterior   Right lateral   Posterior   Left posterior
                   oblique   oblique

Figure 7.4 Five-view planar liver–spleen scan.

Acquisition times of 20 to 40 seconds per projection view are standard.

Step-and-shoot vs. continuous acquisition

The standard method for collection of tomographic projection views is called **step-and-shoot acquisition**. In this technique, each projection view is acquired in entirety at each angular **stop** (position). There is a short pause of a few seconds between views to allow for the automatic rotation of the camera head to the next stop. The camera makes a single rotation around the patient. In the

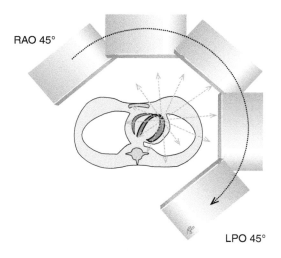

RAO 45°

LPO 45°

Figure 7.5 180° cardiac SPECT.

example depicted in Figure 7.6, projection views of 20 seconds' duration were obtained every 5.6° for a total of 64 views. The camera paused for two seconds after acquiring each view as the head moved into position for the next view. The total acquisition time was 1408 seconds. Since 126 seconds of this total were "consumed" by pauses, there was a total of imaging time of 1282 seconds.

In **continuous acquisition**, data are collected over one or several sequential 360° rotations. There are no pauses; rotation is continuous. In the example depicted in Figure 7.7, the camera rotated a full 360° every 140.8 seconds. Ten such rotations provided 1408 seconds of imaging time (compared to the 1282 seconds from the step-and-shoot acquisition).

Circular, elliptical, and body contouring orbits

Scans on older systems were acquired with a **circular orbit**. The camera head rotated at a fixed distance from the center of the body. Since the body is more nearly elliptical than circular in cross section, the camera did not come as close to the organ as possible over a significant portion of its rotation. Because image resolution is better if the camera is as close to an organ as possible, **elliptical**, and more recently **body contouring** orbits allow the camera heads to more closely follow the contour of the body and therefore remain closer to the organ being imaged (Figure 7.8). The body contouring orbits are enabled by electronic sensors placed on the collimators. As the gantry rotates, the detector

radii are dynamically adjusted to get close to the body while avoiding collisions.

Patient motion and sinograms

Significant patient motion can cause artifacts or blurring in an image. To detect patient motion, the cine display and/or the **sinogram** (see below) should be reviewed prior to releasing the patient. Small amounts of patient motion can be corrected by automated correction algorithms which shift the projection views to align the organ of interest. Repeat acquisition is recommended if these algorithms are not successful.

A **sinogram** image is a stack of slices of the acquired projection views from 0° to maximum angle of rotation, either 180° or 360°. Each row of the sinogram image consists of data acquired at a different angle of rotation, but all of the rows in the sinogram come from the same axial (y) position. In other words, there is a separate sinogram image for each slice location along the y-axis (the long axis) of the patient. Figure 7.9a is an illustration of the construction of a sinogram representing a thin slice of the heart obtained from sample projection views from a 180° arc around the patient, Figure 7.9b is the complete sinogram containing all of the projection views. Figure 7.10 shows sinograms taken at the level of the heart, the gallbladder, and the bowel. Figure 7.11 shows discontinuities seen in the sinogram of a patient who moved in the direction of x-axis (side to side motion) and the y-axis (motion along the long axis) of his body during the acquisition of his images. It is not always possible to distinguish the direction of motion from examination of the sinogram, but the cine images provide this information. Figure 7.12 is an example demonstrating artifacts created by patient motion in the direction of the y-axis. Correcting motion in the x-axis (created by side to side rotation or shifting in the axial plane) is more difficult than correcting motion in the direction of the y-axis (the long axis of the patient).

Dedicated cardiac SPECT cameras

A camera designed specifically for imaging the heart as opposed to any organ or the whole body can have a sensitivity advantage by focusing relatively large detectors at the relatively small space in the body containing the heart. In addition, since the

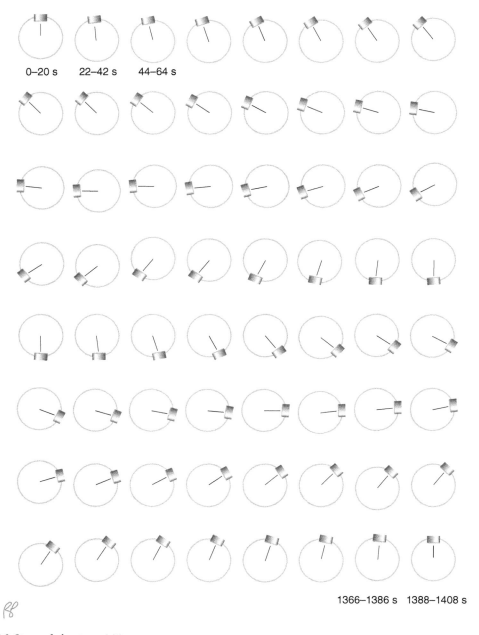

0–20 s   22–42 s   44–64 s

1366–1386 s   1388–1408 s

Figure 7.6 Step-and-shoot acquisition.

application is limited, designers can simplify or optimize the gantry arrangement to reduce costs and improve patient comfort. Conventionally, cardiac imaging is performed on a general purpose two-headed SPECT camera with the heads oriented at (or close to) 90 degrees; the gantry rotates approximately 90 degrees to acquire the 180 degrees of cardiac SPECT data (shown in Figure 7.5).

Dedicated cardiac cameras employ a similar strategy to sample photons over a limited arc with the patient upright, semi-reclined or supine. Some of these camera designs are relatively minor variations on the general-purpose camera where multiple heads move to fill an arc of just over 180 degrees (Figure 7.13a). Others employ apparently stationary heads but have moving internal detector

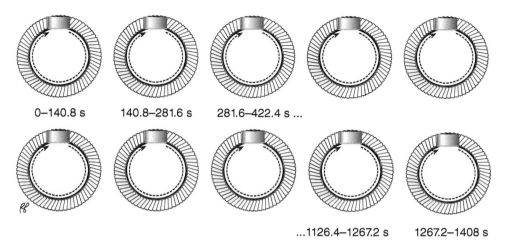

0–140.8 s   140.8–281.6 s   281.6–422.4 s ...

...1126.4–1267.2 s   1267.2–1408 s

Figure 7.7 Continuous acquisition.

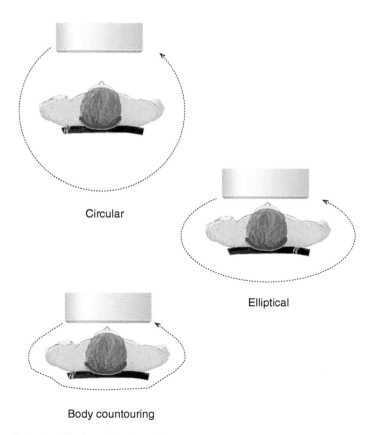

Circular

Elliptical

Body countouring

Figure 7.8 Circular, elliptical, and body contouring orbits.

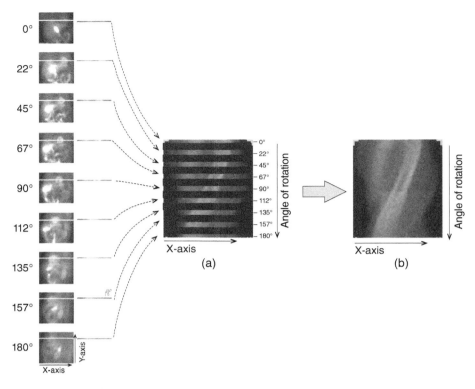

Figure 7.9 (a) Slices through the level of the heart from selected projection views are stacked to create a sonogram, a sample of projection views are shown. (b) Complete sinogram containing slices from all projection views.

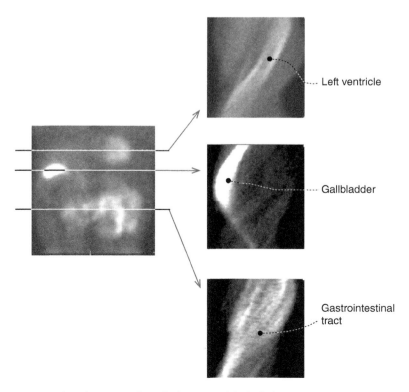

Figure 7.10 Sinograms at selected positions along the long axis of the body (y-axis).

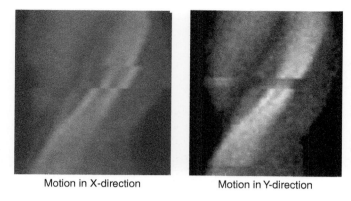

Motion in X-direction   Motion in Y-direction

Figure 7.11 Effects of patient motion in the X- and Y-directions on sinograms of a slice of the heart.

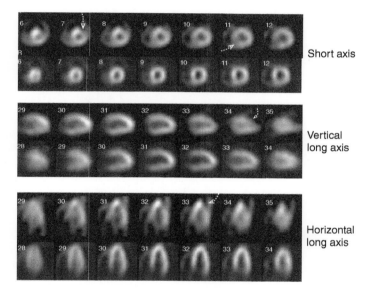

Short axis

Vertical
long axis

Horizontal
long axis

Figure 7.12 First, third, fifth rows: artifacts created by patient motion (arrows). Second, fourth, and sixth rows: motion corrected images.

assemblies (Figure 7.13b) and others employ completely stationary heads which sample the photons via multiple pinhole collimators (Figure 7.13c).

Quantitation of lesion activity in SPECT studies

An estimate of the amount of radionuclide activity in a lesion can be helpful in differentiating benign from malignant lesions and for tracking disease progression or response to treatment. A semi-quantitative estimate of this activity is the **standardized uptake value (SUV)**, which has been used in PET imaging for many years. More recently, due to

improvements in SPECT image reconstruction, particularly with better quality attenuation correction maps derived from CT data and better algorithms for reducing the contribution of scattered photons, SUV calculations for SPECT data have become available on some of the newer scanners.

The formula for calculation of SUV for SPECT and PET are identical:

$$SUV = \left(\frac{\text{concentration of activity in the}}{\text{volume of interest in Bq / ml}} \right) \times \frac{(\text{mass of the patient in g})}{(\text{injected activity in Bq})}$$

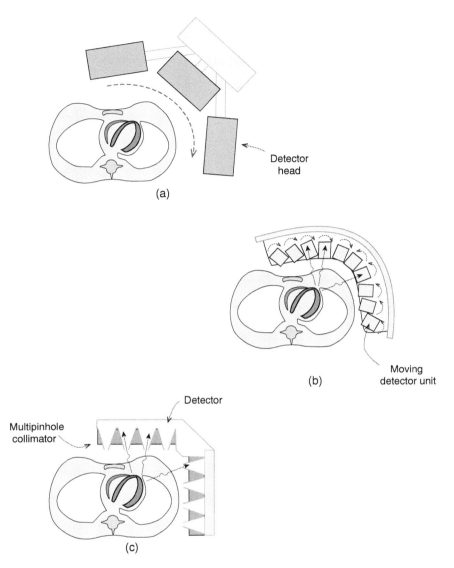

Figure 7.13 Newer cardiac SPECT cameras. (a) Multiple heads. (b) Stationary head with internal moving detector units. (c) Stationary head with pinhole collimators.

SPECT scanners, just like PET scanners, intrinsically measure counts per second and converting that to Bq/ml requires multiplication by a calibration factor. This calibration factor is often termed the well-counter calibration factor since it is analogous to the efficiency factor that describes the fraction of counts recorded by a well-counter per disintegration in the radionuclide being counted. The calibration factor for each scanner must be determined from a simple phantom experiment in which a known activity is dispersed uniformly in a known volume—hence Bq/ml. The scanner then acquires and reconstructs images and regions of interest (ROI) are placed in a number of locations within the uniform distribution and counts in the ROIs are averaged. The calibration factor is the ratio of the known activity concentration to the averaged ROI count value. This number can then be used to estimate the amount of activity within ROIs in the patient images.

Further discussion of SUV values can be found near the end of Chapter 8.

Questions

1. Match the following phrases to the terms listed below:
   (1) Individual images acquired at each stop of the SPECT camera as it rotates around the patient.
   (2) "Movie" of all of the projection views.
   (3) Reconstructed horizontal slices of the patient data.
   (4) A stack of slices from each acquired projection views, each slice taken at the same level of the y-axis (along the length of the body).

Terms:
   (a) Cine views.
   (b) Projection views.
   (c) Sinogram.
   (d) Transverse slices.

2. True or false: Elliptical and body contouring orbits for SPECT image acquisition improve image resolution compared to circular orbits because the camera remains closer to the patient as the heads rotate around the patient.

3. True or false: Examination of cine images or sinogram images prior to discharging the patient from the nuclear medicine lab is no longer necessary since motion correction software can compensate for almost any patient motion.

4. True or false: A 360 degree arc of acquisition is usually used for acquiring SPECT images of the heart and a 180 degree arc is used for acquisition of most other organs.

Answers

1. (1) b. (2) a. (3) d. (4) c.
2. True.
3. False, software algorithms can only correct a small amount of motion.
4. False: the heart is eccentrically located in the chest and therefore a 180 degree arc of rotation from the right anterior oblique projection to the left posterior oblique projection is used for cardiac SPECT imaging, for all other SPECT imaging a 360 degree arc of rotation is used.

CHAPTER 8

Positron Emission Tomography (PET)

Positron emission tomography (PET) cameras are designed to detect the paired 511-keV photons generated from the annihilation event of a positron and electron. Following emission, any positron travels only a short distance before colliding with electrons in surrounding matter. As discussed in Chapter 2, the paired 511-keV annihilation photons travel in opposite directions (180° apart) along a line (Figure 8.1).

Following the acquisition of the images of positron emissions, the data are reconstructed in a manner similar to that used for SPECT, with the exception that attenuation correction is always performed using a radionuclide transmission scan or, more commonly, CT data. PET has a number of advantages compared to SPECT. Most important are its greater sensitivity and resolution and the existence of positron emitting isotopes for elements of low atomic number elements for which no suitable gamma emitters are available. The principal disadvantage of PET is the added cost of the equipment and the short half-life of some of the most useful positron emitters.

Advantages of PET imaging

Sensitivity

As pointed out earlier, a collimator reduces a camera's sensitivity because the collimator's septa cover part of the camera crystal's face. A collimator is not required for PET since PET cameras use the detection of the simultaneous and oppositely directed 511-keV photons of positron annihilation to locate the direction from which the photons originated. This is referred to as "**annihilation coincidence detection.**" For SPECT, the origins of the single photons can only be located if the camera is equipped with a collimator to absorb any photons not traveling perpendicular to the face of the crystal. Therefore, a PET camera, needing no collimator, is inherently more sensitive (by at least a factor of 100) compared to a SPECT camera and has a higher count rate for similar quantities of radioactivity.

Resolution

Coincidence detection

If two detectors located on opposite sides of the annihilation reaction register coincident photon impacts, the annihilation reaction itself occurred along an imaginary line, called a **line of response (LOR)**, drawn between these detectors (Figure 8.2). A **coincidence circuit** registers these as simultaneous events.

Events that arise from a single positron annihilation that follow the emission of a positron are referred to as **true coincidence events** (Figure 8.2). The impact of an unpaired photon, called a **singles event**, is rejected. A singles event is registered when an unpaired photon from a non-annihilation gamma ray impacts a detector (Figure 8.3a). A singles event is also registered when only one of a pair of annihilation photons impacts a detector; the other photon can leave the plane of detection (Figure 8.3b) or it can be absorbed or scattered by the surrounding medium (Figure 8.3c).

Unfortunately, by chance, photons generated simultaneously from separate sites in the body may

Essentials of Nuclear Medicine Physics, Instrumentation, and Radiation Biology, Fourth Edition.
Rachel A. Powsner, Matthew R. Palmer, and Edward R. Powsner.
© 2022 John Wiley & Sons Ltd. Published 2022 by John Wiley & Sons Ltd.

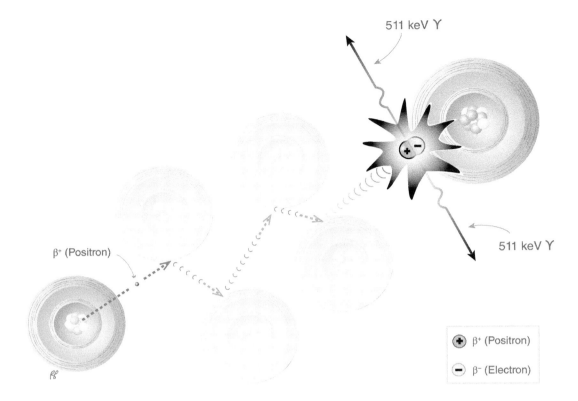

Figure 8.1 Annihilation reaction.

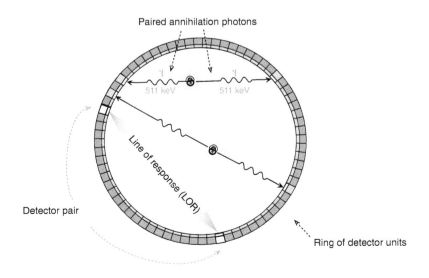

Figure 8.2 Line of response and examples of coincident events.

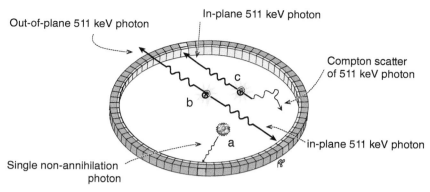

Figure 8.3 Singles events.

reach the crystal at the same time. These separate events are incorrectly perceived as though resulting from annihilation of a single positron emission occurring along a line between the two detectors. These photons can arise from annihilation events (Figure 8.4a), when one of each pair of two annihilation events registers as a simultaneous event (their respective partners are out-of-plane events), or from simultaneous detection of non-annihilation photons (Figure 8.4b). Other mistakes in identification may also occur. For example, when scattering of one of the 511-keV photons alters its path, the location of the annihilation event may incorrectly be presumed to be on a line connecting the detectors (Figure 8.4c). These are referred to as **random events** (a sort of false positive happening). The probability of random events increases significantly with increasing radioactivity within the field of view of the scanner, and thus are of most concern at high count rates. Scatter and random events are undesirable because they contribute to an increase in image background counts and consequently cause a reduction in image contrast.

Time of flight

To improve resolution, some systems also measure **time of flight** under the assumption that the location of the annihilation can be localized along the line of flight of the coincident photons by measuring the time of arrival of each of the photons at the opposing crystals. Unless the event occurs in the exact center of the detection ring, one of the photons will arrive before the other. The time difference will be proportional to the difference in distances traveled by the two photons and can be used to calculate the position of the event along the line con-

necting the detectors (Figure 8.5). Unfortunately, due to current electronic timing limitations, the calculated position of the annihilation event is not precise (Figure 8.6). However, knowing the approximate location of the annihilation event helps constrain the reconstruction algorithm and does provide information which is used to improve the quality of the image.

Radiopharmaceuticals

One of the greatest advantages of PET imaging is the large number of low atomic number elements for which positron emitters exist (Table 8.1). This permits incorporation of positron emitters into many biologically active compounds, including isotopic forms of oxygen, carbon, nitrogen, and fluorine. Very specific physiologic properties of an organ can therefore be imaged; for example, the oxygen consumption and the glucose metabolism of the brain can be independently imaged using $[^{15}O]_2$ and ^{18}F-fluorodeoxyglucose. Other radiopharmaceuticals that can be used in PET are listed in Table 8.2.

PET camera components

A common PET detector consists of rings of crystals (Figure 8.7). The rings may or may not be separated by septa. The individual detector contains one or more large segmented crystals or a collection of small crystals. A standard **detector unit** or **block** consists of a group of small crystals watched by PMTs, one such arrangement consists of 36 small crystals arranged in a 6 × 6 matrix, coupled to four PMTs. More recently semiconductor materials are replacing PMT tubes (see Chapter 4 for an in-depth discussion of semiconductors).

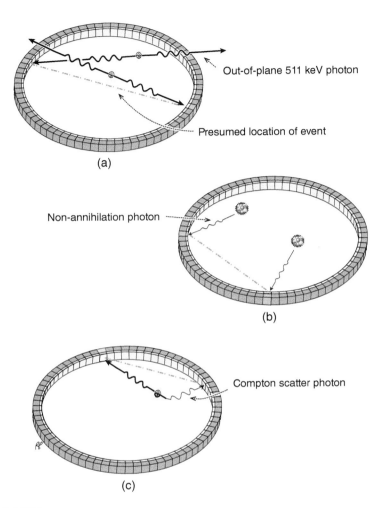

(a)

Out-of-plane 511 keV photon

Presumed location of event

Non-annihilation photon

(b)

Compton scatter photon

(c)

Figure 8.4 Random events.

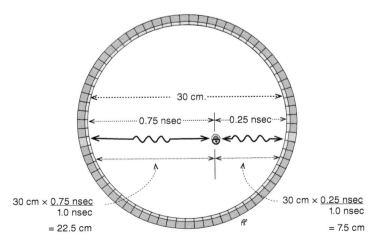

30 cm.

0.75 nsec   0.25 nsec

30 cm × $\dfrac{0.75\ \text{nsec}}{1.0\ \text{nsec}}$

= 22.5 cm

30 cm × $\dfrac{0.25\ \text{nsec}}{1.0\ \text{nsec}}$

= 7.5 cm

Figure 8.5 Time-of-flight PET systems.

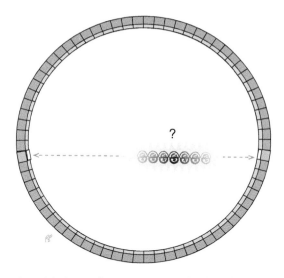

Figure 8.6 Current limitation in time-of-flight technology.

Table 8.1 Common positron-emitting nuclides [1]

Nuclide	Half-life (min)	Positron yield (%)	Maximum energy (MeV)	Method of production
^{11}C	20.4	99.8	0.960	Cyclotron
^{13}N	9.96	99.8	1.200	Cyclotron
^{15}O	2.04	99.9	1.720	Cyclotron
^{18}F	110	96.7	0.634	Cyclotron
^{64}Cu	642	17.9	0.653	Cyclotron
^{68}Ga	67.7	88.9	1.900	Generator
^{82}Rb	1.26	95.4	3.380	Generator

Table 8.2 Some of the available PET radiopharmaceuticals

Radiopharmaceutical	Physiologic imaging application
$H_2[^{15}O]$	Myocardial blood flow
$[^{11}C]$-choline	Prostate tumor imaging
$[^{13}N]$ ammonia	Myocardial blood flow
^{18}F-florbetaben, florbetapir, flutemetamol	Brain imaging for amyloid deposits
^{18}F-flortaucipir	Brain imaging for tau proteins
^{18}F-fluciclovine	Prostate tumor imaging
$[^{18}F]$-sodium flouride	Bone imaging
$[^{18}F]$-fluorodeoxyglucose	Tumor localization
^{68}Ga dotatate	Neuroendocrine tumor localization
$[^{82}Rb]$ chloride	Myocardial blood flow

Crystals

The basic crystal function of converting gamma photon energy into light photon energy is discussed in Chapter 5. Thallium-doped sodium iodide (NaI(Tl)) crystals were originally used for PET systems; however, NaI has a relatively low density and is less effective at stopping the high-energy 511-keV photons. To compensate for the lower density, thicker crystals were employed for 511-keV imaging than those used for detecting the lower-energy single photon emissions (3.8 cm as opposed to 0.6 to 1.2 cm).

Crystals with higher densities and higher atomic numbers (Z), such as bismuth germinate oxide (BGO), leutetium orthosilicate (LSO), and gadolinium orthosilicate (GSO), were developed for use with 511-keV imaging due to their greater stopping power for annihilation photons. This is because the likelihood of any photon interaction per unit volume increases linearly with density and the probability of photoelectric interactions increases rapidly with increasing Z (proportional to Z^3) (see Figure 2.1 in Chapter 2). In detector design, photoelectric interactions are favored over Compton interactions since most of the energy from the photon is transmitted to the photo-electron and this electron, being a charged particle, will deposit most of this energy in the material close to the location of the initial interaction (see Chapter 2). If, on the other hand, the initial interaction involving a 511 keV photon and the detector crystal is a Compton scatter event, only a small amount of the energy is transferred to an electron and deposited locally and much of the energy of the scattered photon may escape the crystal.

LSO and GSO have the advantage of a shorter **decay time** than BGO or NaI(Tl) for PET imaging. Decay time is the time required for the radiation-excited atoms in the crystal lattice to return to the ground (unexcited) state with the emission of light photons (see Figure 5.2 and associated text). During this time, a second gamma photon entering the crystal cannot be detected. A shorter decay time is desirable for rapid imaging.

A higher **light yield** is desirable because the greater the crystal light photon output per keV of absorbed gamma energy the greater the energy resolution and better spatial resolution. Improved energy resolution improves the ability to distinguish the lower energy scatter photons from the

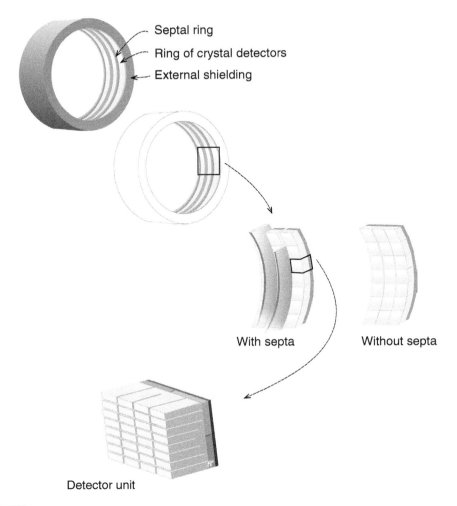

Septal ring
Ring of crystal detectors
External shielding

With septa   Without septa

Detector unit

Figure 8.7 PET camera.

high energy annihilation photons. The larger number of light photons makes it easier to identify which crystal has been struck by the annihilation photon thereby improving spatial resolution. As outlined in Table 8.3, the choice of crystal material involves a compromise among the factors of cost, density, decay time, and light yield. Currently, LSO and a similar composite: LYSO (leutetium–yttrium orthosilicate) are the predominant crystals used in the manufacture of PET systems.

Photomultipliers

Silicon photomultipliers (SiPM) are discussed in Chapter 4 and vacuum photomultiplier tubes (PMTs) in Chapter 5. Photomultipliers convert the light photon energy into an electrical signal. SiPMs

are rapidly replacing PMTs in PET scanners due to their compact size, their better temporal resolution, and increased sensitivity. They are used in PET/MRI systems (see Chapter 11) due to their insensitivity to magnetic fields. They are, however, more temperature sensitive than PMT tubes.

Unlike single photon imaging systems, where many PMT tubes are attached to a single large crystal, positron cameras are designed with many crystal subdivisions watched by a few SiPMs (or PMT tubes). The slits between crystal subdivisions channel the light photons toward the SiPMs. Localization of the site of impact is achieved by measuring the light detected in each SiPM; the closer the SiPM is to the site of impact the stronger the signal generated by the SiPM (Figure 8.8).

Table 8.3 Properties of crystals used for PET imaging

Crystal	Density (g/cm³)	Decay time (ns)	Light yield relative to NaI (%)
NaI(Tl)* (sodium iodide)	3.67	230	100
BGO (bismuth germanate oxide)	7.13	300	014
LSO (leutetium orthosilicate)	7.40	040	075

* 3.8 cm thick (compared to 0.6 to 1.2 cm thick for single photon emission cameras).
Source: Data from Early PJ. Positron emission tomography (PET). In: Early PJ, Sodee DB. *Principles and Practice of Nuclear Medicine.* St. Louis: CV Mosby, 1995:319; and Ficke DC, Hood JT, TerPogossian MM. A spheroid positron emission tomograph for brain imaging: A feasibility study. *J Nucl Med* 1996;37:1219–25.

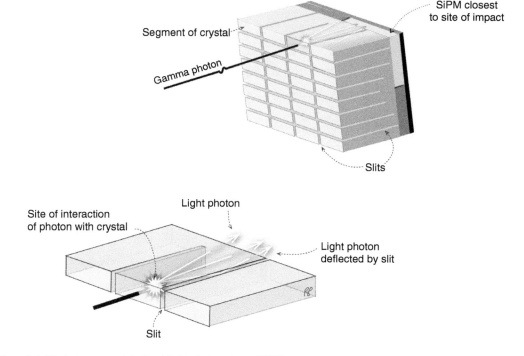

Figure 8.8 Slits between crystals direct light photons toward PMTs.

Pulse-height analyzers, timing discriminators, and coincidence circuits

The signals from the SiPM or PMT tubes are amplified (see Figure 5.5 and associated text). The system electronics must then determine which signals came from paired 511 keV coincident photons arising from an annihilation event occurring along a line of response between a pair of opposing detectors. This is accomplished primarily by measuring the size of each signal, which is proportional to the energy of the photon reaching the crystal, and by recording the time of detection of the signal. The pulse height analyzer (Figure 5.6) determines whether the signal is the correct amplitude (pulse height) to have come from a 511 keV photon interaction within the crystal. The **timing discriminator** records the time the signal was generated. The **coincidence circuit** then examines signals of adequate amplitude coming from opposing detectors and determines if the timing of the signals occurred within the **coincidence time window.** Typically, this coincidence timing window is set between 5–15 nanoseconds depending on the decay time of the selected crystal material. As illustrated

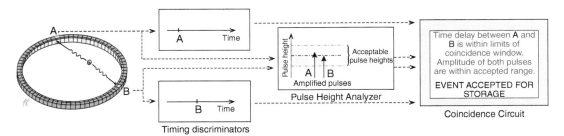

Figure 8.9 A coincident event is accepted after processing by the pulse height analyzers, timing discriminators, and coincidence circuits.

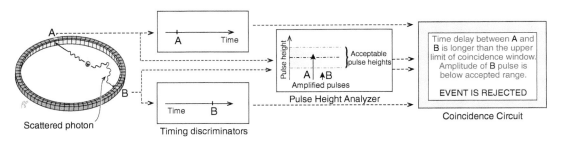

Figure 8.10 One of a pair of annihilation photons is scattered and their data is rejected.

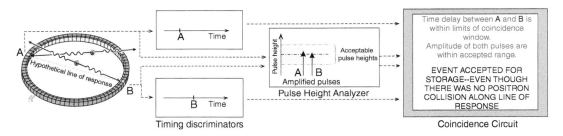

Figure 8.11 Random events can "pass" as true coincidence events.

in Figure 8.9, two 511 keV coincident photons coming from an annihilation event along the line of response between paired detectors will yield adequately sized pulses and a timing delay that is less than the upper limit of the coincidence window. A coincident event between the detector pairs will be recorded by the computer. In contrast, paired annihilation photons in which one or both of the photons have been subjected to scatter or absorption by surrounding tissue will usually be discarded by the coincident circuit, as seen in Figure 8.10. This is because scattered photons have lower photon energies and because in the process of scattering the photon is often delayed on its path to the crystal. Random events are more difficult to separate from

coincident events since they occur as the result of two 511 keV (or other high energy) photons arising from events occurring away from the line of response, but reaching the opposing detectors within the coincidence time window (Figure 8.11). Some systems estimate random event rates arithmetically using a product of the coincidence time window and measured singles rates. Other approaches are available, but are beyond the scope of this text.

Septa

Septal rings can be used to improve resolution by reducing the amount of scatter from photons originating outside the plane of one ring of

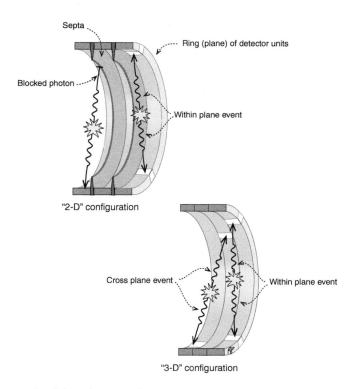

Figure 8.12 Two-dimensional and three-dimensional PET imaging.

crystals. The sensitivity of the scanner is reduced, however, because a significant fraction of true coincidence events are rejected. Removal of the septa will increase sensitivity and decrease resolution. Scans obtained with the septa in place are called **two-dimensional scans**; without septa the scans are called **three-dimensional scans**. In the "**2-D**" illustration in Figure 8.12, the septa block out-of-plane photons, allowing only within-plane coincidence events to be recorded. The "**3-D**" configuration permits coincident registration of cross-plane events, those in which the two 511-keV photons are detected in different rings. Septa reduce the number of random coincidence events.

Factors affecting resolution in PET imaging

Positron range in tissue
Positrons travel a short distance in tissue before undergoing annihilation with an electron. Therefore, the camera detects photons originating from an annihilation event at a distance from the true source of the beta particle emission (Figure 8.13a). For lower energy beta emitters (such as ^{18}F), this range is fairly small (1.2 mm in water); for higher energy beta emitters (such as ^{82}Rb), the distance traveled prior to detection can be quite large (12.4 mm in water) [2]. The minimum possible resolving power of any system for a positron nuclide is therefore limited to the average range of the positrons in the tissue.

Photon emissions occurring at other than 180°
Another factor causing degradation in resolution is the fact that 511-keV annihilation photons do not always travel in paths separated by exactly 180°. This is true because the positron–electron combination will often be in motion during the process of annihilation, thereby altering the angle of ejection of the 511-keV photons. The detectors, however, assume a standard 180° emission path of the photons and therefore the localization of the positron emission is miscalculated in these cases (Figure 8.13b).

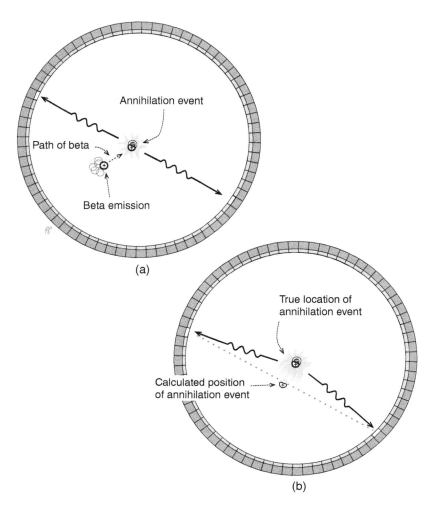

Figure 8.13 Factors limiting resolution in PET imaging. (a) The positron travels in tissue before becoming annihilated. (b) The combined positron/electron pair can travel during annihilation creating opposing photons at angles other than 180 degrees.

Parallax error

Resolution decreases toward the periphery of a ring of PET detectors. This is because some of the photons arising from peripheral annihilation events cross the ring of detectors at an oblique angle and can interact with one of several detectors along a relatively long path. When a photon interacts within a detector it is assumed the annihilation event occurred along a line of response originating at the front of the detector since the depth of interaction in the crystal is not recorded. The illustrations in Figure 8.14a and b show two different possible lines of response (involving two different pairs of detectors) from a single annihilation event occurring near the edge of the ring of detectors.

This effect is sometimes referred to as a **parallax error** or **depth of interaction effect**.

The larger the size of the ring of detectors, relative to the size of the body being imaged, the less the effect, since the annihilation events will be more centrally located and the photons will cross the detector at a less oblique angle. This is illustrated in Figure 8.14c, the opposing photons from an annihilation event each cross two detectors in the smaller ring, and only one in the larger ring.

Attenuation in PET imaging

Because of the relatively high energy of the positron-annihilation photon and because of the use of

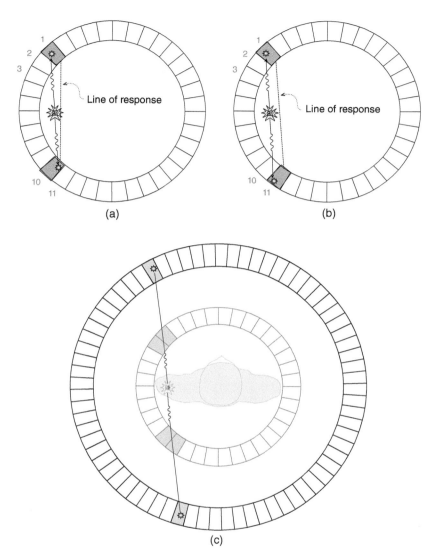

Line of response

(a)

Line of response

(b)

(c)

Figure 8.14 (a and b). Parallax error affects resolution near periphery of field. (c) Larger ring size reduces error.

coincidence detection, attenuation correction is simpler and more accurate in PET than it is in SPECT. The attenuation coefficient for a 511-keV photon of PET is more nearly uniform across the various kinds of body tissues, e.g., fat, muscle, and bone of the than it is for the lower energy photons encountered in SPECT. Also, the sum of the likelihoods of absorption for the two photons of the 511-keV pair will be the same regardless of the location of the annihilation event along the line of response. Figure 8.15 illustrates the paths of paired annihilation photons originating at different positions along the line. For example, for every position along this

line-of-response, the length of the path traversed by the photon traveling to the right increases the farther the annihilation has occurred from the point at which the photon exits. This increase is exactly offset by the decrease in the length of the path traversed by the left-traveling photon of the pair. In other words, adding the length of the path to the right to that for its pair-mate traveling to the left, one can see that the total amount of tissue traversed and therefore the total likelihood of absorption for the two photons of a pair will be the same no matter where along the line of response the annihilation occurred. If either photon of a pair is absorbed by

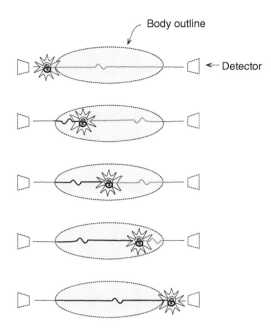

Figure 8.15 Attenuation is constant across a line connecting two detectors.

surrounding tissue, the annihilation will not register as a coincident event, and will not be counted.

Attenuation correction

The attenuation in PET imaging, i.e., loss of counts due to absorption of photons before they arrive at the detector is compensated for arithmetically by using data from transmission scans. Although, in the past, transmission scans for standalone PET scanners were created by using a rotating positron or high energy photon source, PET/CT scanners utilize the CT scan images for this purpose but because of the marked difference between X-ray photon energies and annihilation photon energies scaling factors are needed to correct the linear attenuation coefficients. Attenuation correction for both SPECT/CT and PET/CT will be discussed further in Chapter 12.

Standard uptake values

Determination of the amount of an injected radionuclide that is taken up by a tumor or organ is used in ^{18}F-fluoro-deoxy-glucose (FDG) scans to aid in the differentiation of benign from malignant masses and to follow tumor progression and/or post treatment regression. Because accurate measurement of uptake is confounded by, among other things, the variable and often poorly known extent of photon absorption in the surrounding tissues, a semi-quantitative

measure, the **standard uptake value (SUV)** is commonly used as an estimate of the actual uptake.

Calculation of the SUV requires a PET estimate of the concentration of activity in the tumor or organ in mCi/ml or mBq /ml, the mass of the patient in grams, and the amount of the injected activity in mCi or mBq.

$$SUV = (\text{concentration of activity in the tumor in mBq / ml}) \times (\text{mass of the patient in g}) / \text{injected activity in mBq}$$

The units of SUV are therefore g/ml, but since tissue is almost completely water, and one milliliter of water weighs one gram, SUVs are given without units.

The procedure for determining the calibration factor for converting the counts/second in the image to a measurement of the concentration of activity in mBq/ml is outlined at the end of Chapter 7.

SUV measurements are overestimated by the above formula in patients who are overweight because fat does not concentrate FDG as much as the rest of the tissue of the body. The contribution of the patient's weight towards the SUV is reduced if the patient's body surface area (BSA) is used in the calculation instead of his mass. This is because the formula for the calculation of the BSA incorporates the patient's height as well as his weight. There are several formulas that can be used to estimate BSA, one example is [3]:

$$\text{Body surface area} = (\text{weight in kg})^{0.425} \times (\text{height in cm})^{0.725} \times 0.007184$$

The formula for SUV based on body surface area, becomes:

$$SUV_{BSA} = (\text{concentration of activity in the region of interest in mBq/ml}) \times (\text{body surface area in m}^2) / (\text{injected activity in mBq})$$

References

1. NuDat 2.8. Nuclear Data Center, Brookhaven National Laboratory, www.nndc.bnl.gov/nudat2/
2. Llewellen, T, Karp, J, Pet Systems, Pages 179–194, in Wernick, M.N. and Aarsvold, Jn Emission Tomography, The fundamentals of PET and SPECT, Elsevier, Inc. 2004, page 180.
3. DuBois D, DuBois EF. A formula to estimate the approximate surface area if height and weight be known. Arch Int Med 1916; 17:863–71.

Questions

1. Match the following phrases with the choices listed below the phrases.
   (a) Two 511 keV photons arising from a single annihilation event striking opposing detectors simultaneously.
   (b) Two 511 keV photons arising from separate annihilation events striking opposing detectors simultaneously.
   (c) One 511 keV photon from a single annihilation event strikes a detector, the other is absorbed by surrounding tissue.

   Choices: singles event, random event, true coincidence event.

2. Which of the following characteristics are desirable for the crystalline materials used to detect 511 keV photons:
   (a) High density.
   (b) Short decay time.
   (c) High light yield.
   (d) All of the above.

3. True or false: Coincidence circuitry can more readily differentiate singles events from true coincidence events than random events from true coincidence events.

4. Which of the following factors tend to reduce resolution in PET imaging:
   (a) The positrons can travel a significant distance prior to annihilation.
   (b) Septa in 3-D imaging decrease the number of detected true coincidence events.
   (c) 511 keV photon emissions are not always exactly 180° apart following an annihilation reaction.
   (d) Proximity of source to edge of ring of detectors.

5. Which of the following are true about current "time of flight" annihilation detection technology on PET scanners:
   (a) Precise localization of the position of an annihilation event along a line of response is possible.
   (b) Approximate localization of an annihilation event along a line of response can be used to improve image quality.

6. True or false: Standard uptake values (SUV) measurements based on body surface area may be more accurate than those based on weight alone in obese patients because adipose tissue does not concentrate FDG as much as the rest of the tissue in the body.

Answers

1. (a) True coincidence event. (b) Random vevent.
   (c) Singles evevnt.
2. (d.)
3. True.
4. (a) and (c) and (d). (b) is incorrect because septa have nothing to do with 3-D scanning.
5. (b).
6. True.

CHAPTER 9

X-ray Computed Tomography (CT)

Computed tomography (CT) is a three-dimensional imaging modality based on X-ray imaging. In a CT scanner, multiple planar X-ray images are acquired and then processed mathematically to create three dimensional and cross-sectional images through the body, much like the image reconstruction of SPECT images discussed in Chapter 7. Relative to nuclear imaging, CT scanners are capable of low-noise, high-resolution, detailed anatomical images and are therefore highly complementary. As a result, the hybrid imaging techniques of PET/CT and SPECT/CT are widely utilized for nuclear medicine imaging and so an understanding of X-rays and CT scanners is essential for the nuclear medicine professional.

In this chapter, we will briefly introduce X-ray tubes and how they produce X-rays. We will then discuss the general configuration of a CT scanner.

X-ray production

Wilhelm Roentgen is usually credited with discovering X-rays. Although they had been observed earlier, Roentgen was the first to describe their basic properties in 1895 and in 1901, he was awarded the first Nobel Prize in physics. When he first observed them, the nature of the radiations was unknown and their properties surprising, if not actually mysterious. This is reflected in his use of the "X" in naming them "**X-ray**".

A modern **X-ray tube** (Figure 9.1) is an evacuated glass or ceramic tube with a window for the exiting X-rays. Within the vacuum tube, electrons are "boiled off" an electrically heated filament wire, the **cathode**, and are accelerated to high speed toward the positively-charged tungsten target, the **anode**, by the high potential difference (or voltage) maintained between filament and target (Figure 9.2). The vast majority of these electrons interact with outer shell electrons of the tungsten target and their kinetic energy is lost as heat. A small percent of the electrons bombarding the target, approximately 0.2% of them, cause the emission of an X-ray by either characteristic radiation or bremsstrahlung (see Chapter 2).

Medical imaging utilizes both characteristic and bremsstrahlung X-rays. Although characteristic X-rays have discrete, or specific, energies, bremsstrahlung interactions produce a full range of X-ray energies, from 0 keV to a maximum which is equal to the **maximum** or **peak voltage** applied between the filament and target. The energy of each bremsstrahlung X-ray is dependent upon the proximity of the moving electron and the nucleus of a nearby atom involved in the bremsstrahlung interaction. The closer the electron comes to the nucleus the greater the deceleration of the electron and the greater the energy of the X-ray produced by this interaction (for illustrations related to brehmsstrahlung emissions see Figures 2.13–2.15). The larger the peak applied voltage (expressed in kilovolts and abbreviated **kVp**) between the filament and the target in the X-ray tube the higher the maximum bremsstrahlung X-ray energy and the greater the number of X-rays created. An energy spectrum of a typical X-ray beam is shown by the dashed line in Figure 9.3.

The lowest energy X-rays in the X-ray beam add to the radiation dose to the patient, particularly to the skin, but are not penetrating enough to reach the detectors and contribute to the image quality. The glass of the vacuum tube blocks some of the

Essentials of Nuclear Medicine Physics, Instrumentation, and Radiation Biology, Fourth Edition.
Rachel A. Powsner, Matthew R. Palmer, and Edward R. Powsner.
© 2022 John Wiley & Sons Ltd. Published 2022 by John Wiley & Sons Ltd.

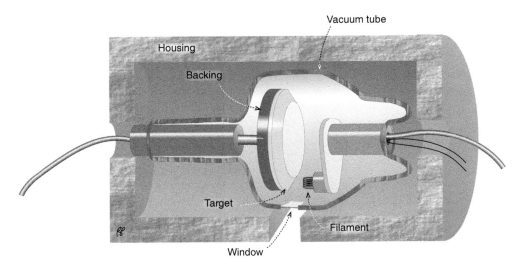

Figure 9.1 Basic components of an X-ray tube.

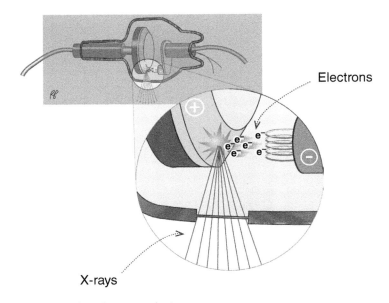

Figure 9.2 X-rays are generated when electrons strike the tungsten target.

lowest energy X-rays and others are attenuated by a **filter** (usually aluminum) placed in front of the tube window (Figure 9.4). Thus, both the applied voltage between the filament and target and the attenuation by the filter affect the range of energies of the X-rays delivered to the patient (solid line in Figure 9.3). In addition, the amount of electricity or current (expressed in milliamperes or **mA**) used to heat the filament to boil off the electrons and the duration of this current (in seconds) affect the total number of X-rays emitted. The last two quantities are often combined as a product and referred to as **mAs** (milliamperes-seconds). Finally, the X-ray beam is narrowed or **collimated** by lead shutters (Figure 9.4) to avoid radiating tissues other than those being imaged.

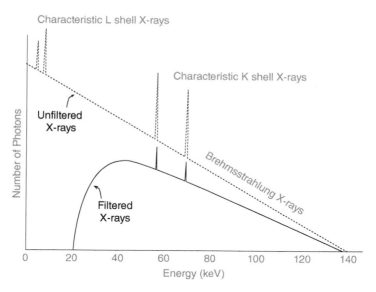

Figure 9.3 X-ray spectrum

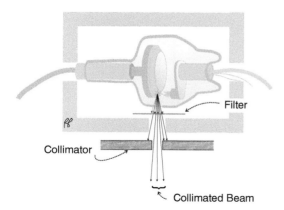

Figure 9.4 The filter attenuates the lower energy X-rays (depicted as short lines with larger arrows) and a collimator narrows the X-ray beam.

In general, the greater the kVP and mAs the better the image quality, but the greater the radiation dose delivered to the patient. When setting kVp and mAs parameters, particularly in CT imaging, a balance can be achieved between obtaining image quality needed for clinical diagnosis and keeping the radiation dose to the patient as low as possible.

An unavoidable accompaniment of bombardment of the target is the generation of **heat**. The tungsten, itself, is dense enough to stop the electrons and capable of withstanding the heating. The heat

is dissipated from the tungsten by a copper backing and by rapid rotation of the target, which spreads the heat over a larger area and allows a brief rest period for any one spot to "cool down" before serving again as the focus point of the electron beam. Further methods of cooling include limiting the duration of the bombardment, and external air or oil cooling.

The contents of the X-ray tube are in a vacuum so that there are no gas particles to impede the flow of the electrons.

X-ray imaging

Images created by projecting X-rays at the body, also called X-rays by convention, are in essence shadows. They can be thought of as "inverse shadows", the denser tissues such as bone, which block much of the X-rays, appear as white on the film or digital detectors, and lungs, which are mainly composed of air, appear to be very dark in the image.

Computed tomography

Overview

An X-ray of a patient using a stationary X-ray source and detector is called a planar image. Chest X-rays are probably the most common example of a planar X-ray image. If, on the other hand, the X-ray data is recorded over the full 360° path encircling the patient this data can also be "back-projected" to create transaxial slices. The X-ray source and detectors in most current scanners are arranged in one of two configurations. Either the X-ray source rotates within a stationary complete ring of detectors (called **rotate–stationary** systems) as illustrated in Figures 9.5 and 9.6 or, more commonly, the X-ray source and an opposing arc of detectors rotate in synchrony around the patient (called **rotate–rotate** systems) as seen in Figure 9.7. At the current time rotate-stationary configurations are too expensive to manufacture for multislice detectors (see below) and therefore rotate-rotate systems are the predominant configuration. The process of acquisition and reconstruction of X-ray data is called **computed (trans)axial tomography (CAT)** or simply **computed tomography (CT)** scanning.

The X-ray source is moved in increments around the patient. At each position the X-ray tube is turned on and the patient is exposed to a fan-shaped beam of X-rays (Figure 9.7).

The X-rays that are not attenuated by the patient's body are registered by the detectors on the opposite side of the patient. The detectors are composed of **ceramic scintillators** which like the NaI(Tl) crystal discussed in Chapter 5 emit light in response to X-rays. Because the scintillator detectors used in CT scanners must respond to the large rapidly changing flow of X-rays generated by the CT X-ray source, the chemical composition of the materials in the ceramic are more complex than the NaI(Tl) crystal. In particular, these scintillators must have very rapid decay times; both the initial light output in response to the X-ray excitation must be rapid, and the residual light within the scintillator present after the initial response, called the **afterglow**, must dissipate rapidly.

The ceramic scintillators are backed by **photodiodes** which generate electrical pulses/current

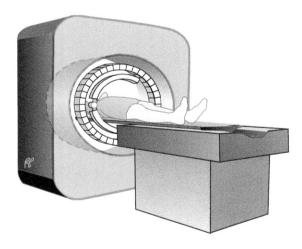

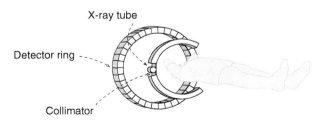

Figure 9.5 Basic components of one type of CT scanner containing a stationary detector ring and rotating inner X-ray tube.

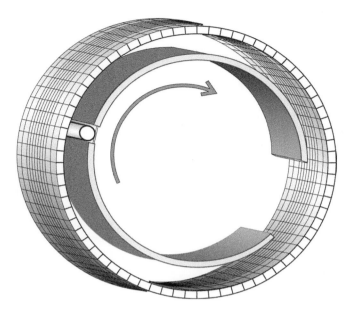

Figure 9.6 Rotate–stationary configuration. A rotating source and collimator generate a fan-shaped X-ray beam which is directed towards a stationary ring of detectors.

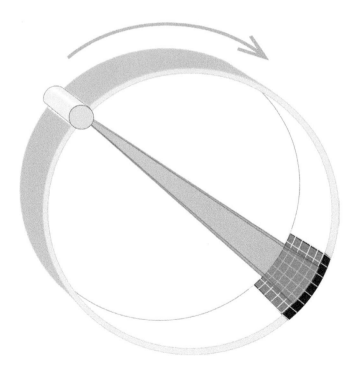

Figure 9.7 Rotate–rotate configuration. Opposing source and detector rotate synchronously.

in response to the light photons. The photodiodes are semiconductors that function similarly to photomultiplier tubes (PMTs) by converting light photon energy into current. Semiconductors and PMTs are discussed in Chapters 4 and 5 respectively.

Multislice detector configuration

Older CT scanners were equipped with a single row of detectors. Most CT scanners are now manufactured with multiple detector rows arranged side by side along the z-axis of the scanner (Figure 9.8a) and are called multidetector or more commonly, multislice CT scanners. Having multiple detector rows allows for faster scanning times as a larger area of the patient can be imaged during a single rotation of the X-ray tube. The total number of detector rows used during scanning is determined by the collimated width of the beam (Figure 9.8b).

Within each row the detectors are of uniform size. On most new scanners, the innermost rows of detectors contain smaller detectors than the outermost rows. Single detector rows can be used to collect a "slice" of data or one or more adjacent rows of detectors can be "grouped" together and collected as a slice. The number of slices in a scanners designation (such as 64-slice CT) refers to the number of simultaneous data slices, sometimes called data channels, that can be collected and not to the total number of detector rows. A 4-slice or 16-slice scanner can have, for example, 16 or 32 detector rows. If the smallest detectors are each assigned to a slice or channel then the images will have the finest detail or greatest resolution, but the scan acquisition time will be longer. If adjacent rows are grouped together there will be lower image resolution but the acquisition time will be faster. Figure 9.9 shows a hypothetical four slice scanner with a detector array composed of 12 rows; the innermost eight rows are 0.5 mm wide and the outermost rows are 1 mm wide. By grouping increasing number of detector rows (and widening the collimated beam) slices of 0.5, 1, and 2 mm width are collected.

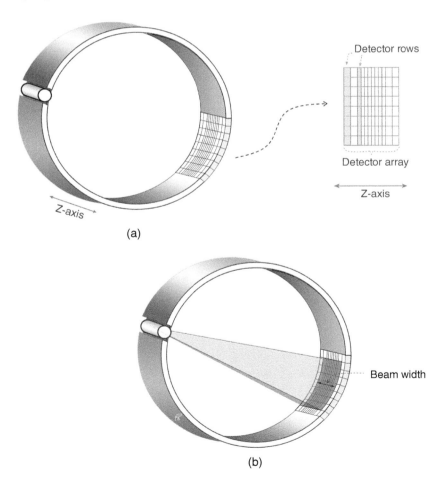

(a)

(b)

Figure 9.8 Multislice CT detector array composed of multiple rows of detectors placed side by side along the z-axis.

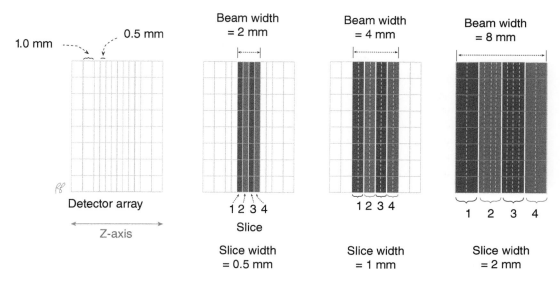

Figure 9.9 Grouping detector rows allows acquisition of slices of varying widths.

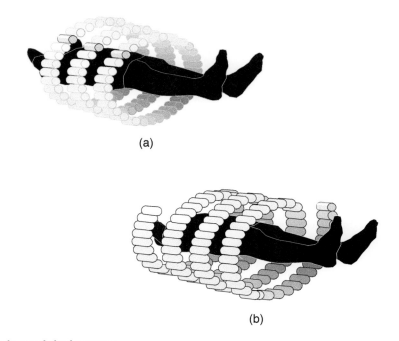

Figure 9.10 Axial versus helical scanning.

Axial and helical scanning

Older CT scanners acquired individual axial slices. The patient bed (pallet) was advanced in small increments. After each increment the bed was stopped and an axial slice was acquired (Figure 9.10a).

Newer CT scanners acquire continuously as the bed advances continuously so that the path of the X-ray source is much like the peel of a tubular apple or a helix, therefore this is referred to as a helical scan (Figure 9.10b). Some authors use the name **spiral** instead of helical to refer to the same process.

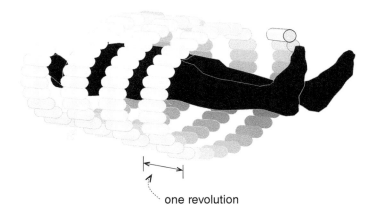

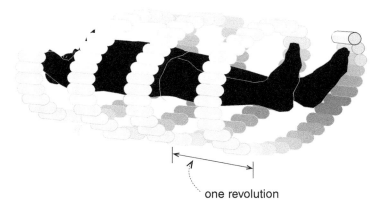

Figure 9.11 Pitch.

There are two advantages to **helical** scanning. The first is the shorter duration of the study due to faster scanning times, and the second is the increased flexibility during data reconstruction. The angle of reconstruction of the axial slices can be chosen by the operator and higher quality coronal and sagittal slices are created from these datasets.

Pitch

The helical motion of the gantry of the scanner can be described by specifying both the rotational speed of the gantry in revolutions per second and the distance the patient bed travels along the long axis of the patient in millimeters for each revolution of the gantry. The latter is called the pitch of the helix, an engineering term for describing the threads of a screw or bolt. The uppermost illustration in Figure 9.11 shows an acquisition with a shorter distance traveled per revolution or a smaller pitch than the lower illustration.

Pitch is mathematically defined as the distance the table travels divided by the summed widths of the detector rows being used for X-ray data collection, which is also the collimated X-ray beam width.

$$\text{Pitch} = \text{table movement per rotation} / \text{beam width}$$

Cone beam CT

Cone beam CT (CBCT), in which the source generates a cone shaped beam of X-rays which travel through the body to a flat panel detector

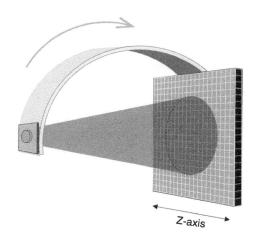

Z-axis

Figure 9.12 Cone beam CT. A large flat panel detector is combined with a cone beam-shaped source of X-rays.

(Figure 9.12) are used in a limited number of applications. In nuclear medicine they are usually used in older SPECT-CT scanners (see Figure 11.3b in Chapter 11, Hybrid Imaging) to obtain nondiagnostic CT scans primarily used for attenuation correction of the SPECT study. They are also used in angiography to obtain three dimensional images of vascular structures.

CBCT is also used for small animal imaging in nuclear medicine and 3-dimensional imaging in dental and oral medicine applications.

The z-dimension or length along the body covered by the cone beam and flat panel is usually big enough to acquire the desired images in a single spin of the detector.

Hounsfield units

CT pixel intensities are given in CT numbers or **Hounsfield unit, (HU)**, and are simply scaled units of attenuation as measured by CT. The Hounsfield unit is named for Sir Godfrey Hounsfield who developed the first practical CT scanner and who, along with Allan Cormack was awarded the 1979 Nobel Prize in Medicine. It is not easily converted to SI units; nevertheless, radiology uses the Hounsfield unit for dose calculation in preference to the attenuation coefficient used by most other disciplines. If μ is the average linear attenuation coefficient for the pixel of interest and μ_w is the value for water, then the CT number of HU is given by

$$HU = 1000 \times (\mu - \mu_w) / \mu_w$$

Tables of Hounsfield units are available. Air, which stops virtually no X-radiation has a value of -1000 HU; water, which moderately attenuates the X-ray beam, has a value of 0 (zero) HU, and bone, which blocks a large fraction of the beam, has a value of 1000 HU and greater. The HU for fat is about -10 while the firmer of the soft body tissues have HU values in the range from about 10 to 60.

A more in-depth discussion of photon attenuation is covered in Chapter 2.

Questions

1. True or false: X-ray production is an efficient process. The majority of electrons striking the tungsten target cause the emission of X-rays.

2. Which of the following statements are true about the X-ray beam produced by X-ray tubes?
   (a) The X-rays are monoenergetic; they all have the same keV.
   (b) The beam is a combination of characteristic and bremsstrahlung radiation.
   (c) The maximum X-ray energy is not affected by the peak voltage applied between the filament and target.
   (d) The number of X-rays produced in the target increases as the current in the filament increases.

3. Which of the following statements are true concerning CT scanning?
   (a) CT images acquired in conjunction with PET images can provide useful correlative anatomic information.
   (b) Helical CT scanning allows for faster acquisition times and greater flexibility in image reconstruction compared to conventional axial CT scanning.
   (c) Current CT scanners consist of a stationary ring of detectors with an inner rotating X-ray source (rotate–stationary) or a rotating arc of detectors that oppose the rotating X-ray source (stationary–stationary).
   (d) All of the above.

4. True or false: A common definition of the term pitch, when used in reference to helical CT scanning, is the ratio of the distance the patient bed advances per gantry revolution divided by the width of the collimated X-ray beam.

5. Select the Hounsfield units (HU) from the values below that most closely correspond to the following:
   (a) Bone.
   (b) Fat.
   (c) Muscle.
   (d) Air.
   (e) Water.

   HU values: $-1000, -10, 0, 30, 1000$.

6. What are the advantages of helical scanning?
   (1) Faster scan times.
   (2) Greater flexibility in angle of reconstruction of axial slices.
   (3) Higher quality coronal and sagittal reconstruction views.
   (4) All of the above.

Answers

1. False, 98% of the kinetic energy of the electrons is lost as heat in the target.
2. (b) and (d) are correct.
3. (d).
4. True.
5. Bone: 1000. Fat −10. Muscle 30. Air −1000. Water 0.
6. (4).

CHAPTER 10

Magnetic Resonance Imaging (MRI)

Magnetic resonance imaging (MRI) is a technique that uses a strong static magnetic field and pulsed radiofrequency electromagnetic waves to elicit a radiofrequency response from the atomic nuclei in the body. This response yields information about the content of the tissue.

Background

A brief review of the spin and magnetic properties of the nucleus (mass and charge were discussed in Chapter 1) and the relationship between electricity and magnetism will provide a basis for understanding how MRI works.

Spin

All protons, neutrons, and electrons have the property of spin. **Spin** is an intrinsic property of these particles and is considered a form of **angular momentum**.

Momentum

Momentum is a property of a moving object and is the tendency of that object to keep moving, mathematically momentum is the product of the object's velocity and mass (momentum = mass × velocity); a large object going slowly can have the same momentum as a small object moving quickly. An object has linear momentum when it is moving in a straight line, it has orbital momentum when it is rotating around another object (like the earth around the sun), and it has angular momentum when it is rotating around its own axis (as the earth does over 24 hours).

However, although spin exhibits the properties of angular momentum, the subatomic particles are not actually spinning (as was originally thought and from whence the name comes). The actual concept of spin is very difficult to grasp as there is no equivalent macroscopic version in the world that we can observe. It can be thought of as an "intrinsic" angular momentum.

For the sake of simplicity, however, spin is usually illustrated as though the subatomic particles are spinning in space. In addition to the circumferential arrow showing the direction of the non-existent rotation of the particle, a vector (arrow) symbolizing the direction of the spin angular momentum is drawn through the center of the sphere representing the particle (Figure 10.1).

Protons, neutrons, and electrons each have spin value of ½.

Magnetism
Electromagnetic fields

Electric fields, designated E, interact with electric charges. Magnetic fields, designated B, interact with magnetic moments as well as with electric charges in motion. Every point in space has a value of E and B, represented by vectors (arrows). The strength of the magnetic field is generally measured in units of Tesla (T).

There is a "close" relationship between electricity and magnetism. Moving electric charge is called an electric current. Current in a wire was originally thought to be due to moving positive charge therefore the direction of current is opposite to the actual movement of electrons in a wire (Figure 10.2). Moving electric charge creates magnetic fields

---

Essentials of Nuclear Medicine Physics, Instrumentation, and Radiation Biology, Fourth Edition.
Rachel A. Powsner, Matthew R. Palmer, and Edward R. Powsner.
© 2022 John Wiley & Sons Ltd. Published 2022 by John Wiley & Sons Ltd.

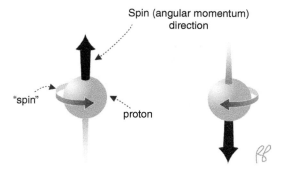

Figure 10.1 Spin (angular momentum) is represented by a vertical arrow through the particle. If you point your thumb in the direction of the arrow and curl your fingers, they will point in the direction of the "rotation" of the particle.

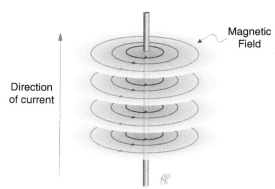

Figure 10.3 Moving electric charge through a straight wire creates a circumferential magnetic field.

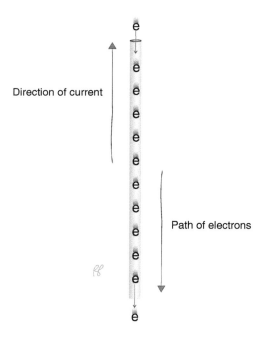

Figure 10.2 Current direction is denoted as moving in the opposite direction to the actual flow of electrons.

(Figure 10.3). An electric current moving through a wire coil creates a magnetic field within the cavity created by the coil (Figure 10.4). Similarly, a moving magnet creates electric current in materials in which electric charges can move (i.e. in materials with a non-zero conductivity); this process is called **Faraday induction**.

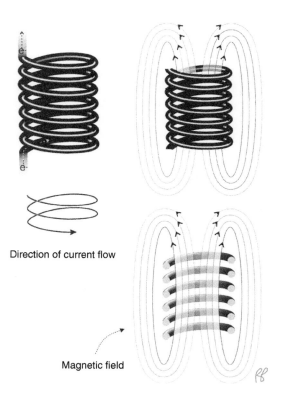

Figure 10.4 Moving electric charge through a wire coil creates a nearly linear magnetic field within the cavity of the coil.

Magnetic moments

Most substances (except for permanent magnets such as bar magnets) only develop measurable magnetism (a **magnetic moment**) when subjected to an external magnetic field; these substances are said

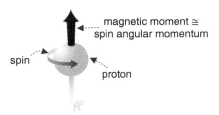

Figure 10.5 The spin angular momentum and the magnetic moment of a subatomic particle are proportional to each other and are both depicted by the same arrow.

to have "inducible" magnetic properties. Subatomic particles (protons, neutrons, and electrons) behave more like permanent magnets. Just like spin, magnetism is an intrinsic property of the particles.

The spin angular momentum and the magnetic moments of the subatomic particles are closely linked. For this reason, it is common for these properties to be referred to interchangeably in magnetic resonance imaging terminology; often the term "spin" is used to represent both spin angular momentum and the magnetic moment (also called the magnetic dipole moment). In addition, it is common to say that it is the spin of the proton (a moving electric charge) that creates the magnetic moment (Figure 10.5).

Introduction to MRI

Magnetic resonance imaging was originally called nuclear magnetic resonance because it depends on

the interactions of the atomic nucleus with a variety of electromagnetic fields created by several magnet coils. From this point on we will focus only on the atomic nucleus and will ignore the interactions of the electrons with these electromagnetic fields.

Magnetic resonance imaging primarily uses information from the interaction with the electromagnetic fields and the nucleus of the ^{1}H hydrogen atom which is composed of a single proton. ^{1}H is used because it is very abundant in the human body and has a net nuclear spin. Imaging of other nuclear species such as P-31 and C-13 is also possible but is not normally performed in clinical MR machines.

Application of the magnetic field

In the absence of an external magnetic field the magnetic moments of the protons (^{1}H) within a sample are randomly oriented in all directions, on average, their magnetic moments "cancel" each other out and the sum magnetization is zero (Figure 10.6a). When a magnetic field is applied to a sample of protons, the magnetic moments of the protons realign either in the direction of the magnetic field (much like a compass needle aligns along the magnetic field of the earth) or in the direction exactly opposite to the direction of the applied magnetic field. Thus, the nuclear magnetic moments have only two possible orientations—with the external field direction or against it. At very low temperatures (close to absolute zero) almost all the moments will align in the direction of the external

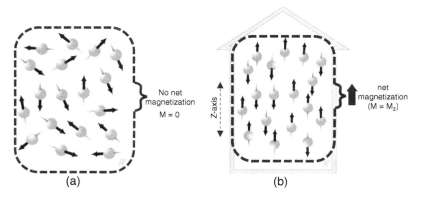

Figure 10.6 (a) Sum magnetization of a sample of protons is zero until (b) an external magnetic field is applied causing parallel or anti-parallel alignment of these magnetic moments. The resulting net magnetization (M) of the sample is equal to M_z since it is aligned with the Z-axis of space.

field giving a very large total magnetic moment in the material. However, at body temperature, only slightly more of the moments are aligned with the external magnetic field (called parallel alignment) than along the direction opposite to the field (called anti-parallel alignment). So at normal temperatures, the sum of the magnetic moments of the group of protons (**M**) is quite a small net moment and is oriented in the same direction as the external magnetic field (which is depicted as being parallel to the Z-axis). This sum is called the **longitudinal magnetization (Mz)** of the sample (Figure 10.6b). This summed magnetization of the protons in the sample is often represented by an arrow labeled **NMV** which stands for the **net magnetization vector**. For simplicity in this text we will instead use M to label this net magnetization vector. As we will see later, M can be tilted away from the direction (Z) of the external magnetic field when excited by a radiofrequency pulse. M_z and $\mathbf{M_{xy}}$ will be used to represent the longitudinal (Z-direction) and transaxial (X-Y plane) components of M.

In equilibrium, M aligns along the direction of the applied external magnetic field. If M gets tipped slightly off the vertical due to variations in the local magnetic field or is tipped even further due to application of a radiofrequency pulse (discussed below) the M precesses or "wobbles" moving at an angle around the direction of the external magnetic field much like a spinning "top" wobbles in the gravitational field when it is slightly tipped away from the vertical direction (Figure 10.7).

The net magnetization vectors (which represent the aggregate of magnetic moments in a small volume) precesses at a frequency (rotational speed or cycles per second) that is both characteristic of the nucleus (in this case a proton) and directly proportional to the applied magnetic field. The frequency of precession is called the **Larmor frequency** (ω_0). The ratio of Larmor frequency and the external magnetic field (B_0) is called the gyromagnetic ratio (γ_0):

$$\omega_0 = \gamma_0\, B_0$$

The unit of magnetic field strength is the Tesla. The strength of the earth's magnetic field at the surface is approximately 1/20,000th of a Tesla.

The gyromagnetic ratio (γ_0) is specific for each type of nucleus, for a proton (the hydrogen ^{1}H

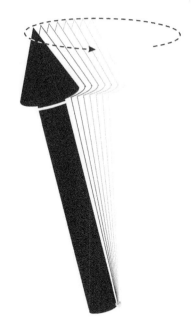

Figure 10.7 The external magnetic field causes M to precess or wobble around the direction of the external magnetic field.

nucleus) it is 42.58 MHz/T. In a 1 Tesla magnetic field the frequency of precession of the proton is 42.58 MHz/T × 1 T which equals 42.58 MHz. In a stronger field, 2 Tesla for example, the frequency of precession is 85.16 MHz.

Application of radiofrequency pulses

After the protons' magnetic moments (spins) reach a state of equilibrium such that M is aligned with the magnetic field, energy in the form of a **radiofrequency (RF)** wave (also called excitation pulse) is applied to the tissue. This energy is applied at the Larmor frequency (actually a narrow band of frequencies centered on the Larmor frequency), in a direction that is perpendicular (90°) to the magnetic field (B_0). Because the energy is applied at the Larmor frequency the magnetic moments can absorb the energy, i.e. they become "excited" and can change their orientation. If the duration of the pulse is chosen carefully, the sum nuclear magnetic vector (M) is tipped perpendicular to the Z-axis, into the X-Y plane (Figure 10.8). A pulse of this type is referred to as a 90-degree pulse. Note that when M is tipped away from the Z-axis it continues to precess around it (Figure 10.9). Similarly, if the excitation pulse is applied for a longer duration, M will

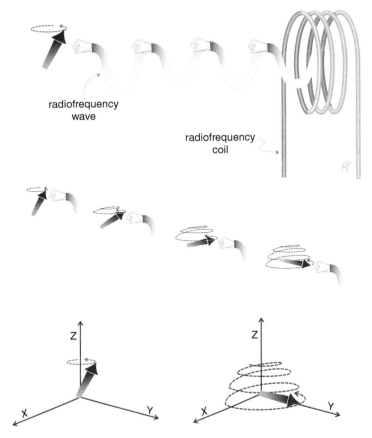

Figure 10.8 Application of a 90-degree radiofrequency pulse perpendicular to the external magnetic field causes M to tip 90°

continue to rotate with respect to the Z-axis and there will be a point where the net magnetization vector is again realigned with the Z-axis but pointing in the opposite direction. This is a 180-degree pulse (Figure 10.10).

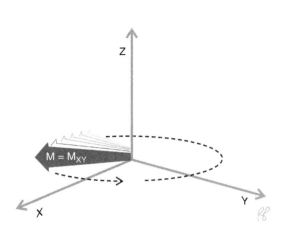

Figure 10.9 Following the RF pulse M precesses in the X-Y plane (therefore it is represented by M_{XY}) perpendicular to the Z direction of the external magnetic field.

Swings and protons

The synchronization between the radiofrequency wave and the frequency of the precessional spin of the protons is often likened to the accurate timing of a parent pushing a child on a swing. If the frequency of the push matches the frequency of the pendulum motion of the swing the push will effectively transfer the energy of the push to the swing increasing the height of the swing.

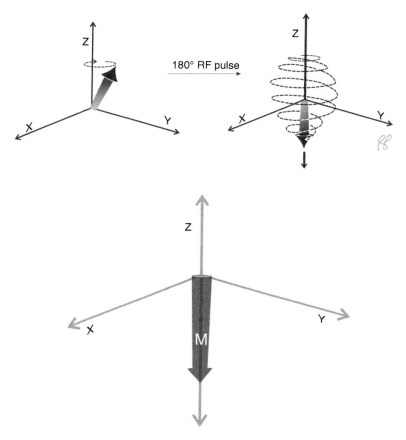

Figure 10.10 180-degree radiofrequency pulse. Top image: A longer RF pulse tips M even further until it is precessing around the Z-axis in the negative projection. M is then aligned opposite to its original direction.

The MR signal

After M is tipped into the X-Y plane by the 90° RF pulse, it continues to precess about the Z-axis. If a conductive metal loop is oriented perpendicular to the X-Y plane (e.g. in the Y-Z plane), the changing magnetic flux through this coil due to the precession of M will induce an electric current in the coil due to Faraday induction, resulting in the MR signal, also called the **echo** (Figure 10.11).

T1 recovery

As the net magnetization vector returns to its original orientation parallel to the Z-axis, the energy that was absorbed from the radiofrequency wave is released into the immediate environment (called the **lattice** as initial experiments were performed in crystalline materials and not body fluids and tissues).

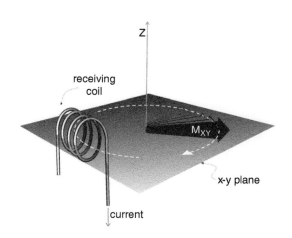

Figure 10.11 The precessing magnetic vector (M_{xy}) generates an electric current in the receiving coil.

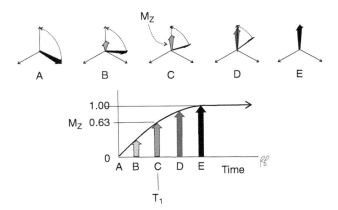

Figure 10.12 T1 recovery after the radiofrequency pulse. T1 is the time it takes for M_z to return to 63% of its value prior to application of the radiofrequency pulse.

The process of the net magnetization vector returning to the Z-axis orientation is called the **longitudinal relaxation** or **spin-lattice relaxation**, and is also known as **T1 recovery**. T1 is the time constant for this recovery and equals the time for M_z to return to 63% of its final value. T1 values in biological tissues range from tenths of seconds to several seconds. The term relaxation refers to the system (in this case, the orientation of the magnetic moments) returning to its prior steady state before the radiofrequency pulse was applied (Figure 10.12).

T2 recovery

When the radiofrequency signal is applied to the tissue not only does **M** tip away from the longitudinal axis, but as it precesses it becomes shorter, representing a loss of the transverse component (M_{XY}) of the net magnetization. This is due to a loss of synchronization of the precessions of the magnetic moments (see top right image of Figure 10.13) due to the influence of microscopic dynamic magnetic field variations including those from neighboring magnetic moments. This loss of synchrony translates to a loss of **phase coherence** in the RF signal. The loss of coherence that results in the shortening of M (and loss of signal) is called **transverse relaxation** or **spin–spin relaxation** (as energy is transferred between the adjacent spins and is not transferred to the immediate environment). Transverse relaxation is also known as **T2 relaxation** as T2 is the time constant for this relaxation and equals the time it takes for loss of 63% of M_{XY}

(see the bottom image in Figure 10.13). Note that this decrease in M_{XY} is irreversible. If it were not for the eventual recovery of the longitudinal component of the magnetization, M_z, there could be no repeated flipping of M and a very limited ability to do any imaging.

Although T1 and T2 relaxation are independent processes they occur simultaneously. T1 and T2 values are different for different types of tissues. In fact, T1 and T2, for many tissues of the body, vary much more than do other bulk physical properties like density, proton density and atomic number. That is what gives MR imaging its capability for **high contrast** imaging. High contrast refers to the ability to distinguish small differences between similar tissues. In particular MRI is particularly good for differentiating normal and abnormal soft-tissues which are generally indistinguishable using CT.

By repeated application of the RF pulse and echo sampling both location of the MR signal and tissue characteristics can be determined.

Signal readout: spin–echo and inversion-recovery

The duration of the echo following a 90-degree RF pulse is extremely brief. Echo intensity diminishes due to T1 and T2 decay but also something called **T2* decay**. T2* decay appears like T2 decay—a loss of coherence in the transverse magnetization, or dephasing—but is faster than T2 and is reversible (by application of the spin–echo method as will be seen). The T2* decay is caused by macroscopic static variations in the magnetic field environment caused by local inhomogeneities. It is because these inhomogeneities do not vary over short times that T2* decay is reversible. These local field strength variations cause spins to have slightly different Larmor frequencies which results in loss of coherence independent of the spin–spin energy transfer.

Since the object of MR imaging is to sample tissue in ways that reflect the T1 and T2 properties of the tissue, pulse sequences have been designed to circumvent this T2* effect that would otherwise dominate the relaxation process. A basic method to accomplish this is with a **spin–echo pulse sequence**. We start by choosing an echo time, TE, at which we would like to sample the decay that has occurred. The sequence begins with a 90-degree excitation pulse after which the spins dephase rapidly due to T2* effects and the echo disappears. After a delay of half the echo time, TE/2, a 180-degree pulse is transmitted. The second pulse has the effect of inverting the net magnetization vector to essentially reverse the T2* effect during the second half of the TE interval and so rephasing occurs and the echo reappears at time TE (Figure 10.14).

To understand this effect, consider a 100 meter sprint. Runners begin the race in synchrony and then, relative to the mean position along the track, they begin to spread out or "dephase", since they are all running at slightly different paces. Now suppose that at exactly 10 seconds from the start,

runners all reverse their direction and continue to run at the same pace. At exactly 10 seconds after reversal or 20 seconds from the start of the race, the runners will all be lined up just like they were at the start of the race.

The spin–echo sequence allows us to sample the T2 decay at time TE. T2 can be estimated directly by sampling at multiple TEs in repeated experiments. In clinical MRI, however, this is not typically done. Instead, a single image is acquired using a spin–echo sequence with a relatively long TE duration. Such a method is said to be T2-weighted as will be discussed later.

In a sequence called **inversion recovery**, the spin–echo sequence described above is preceded with an additional 180-degree pulse and is shown in Figure 10.15. The time between this 180-degree pulse and the subsequent 90-degree pulse is called the **inversion time or TI**. At the end of the 180-degree pulse, the net magnetization is flipped along the negative Z-axis. During the TI interval, M begins to recover from its position along the negative Z-axis towards its equilibrium state along the positive Z-axis. However, before the recovery is complete (M has not reached its maximum value), a 90-degree pulse is applied allowing only part of the full M to be tipped into the X-Y plane for measurement. The portion of the full M that is flipped depends on

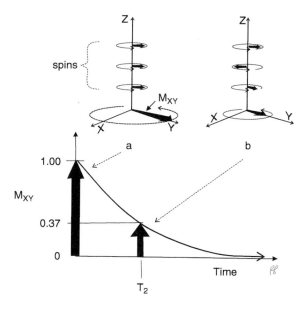

Figure 10.13 T2 recovery. (a) Synchrony between the precessing spins during the radiofrequency pulse (b) decreasing synchrony after the radiofrequency pulse ends. T2 is the time it takes for loss of 63% of M_{XY}.

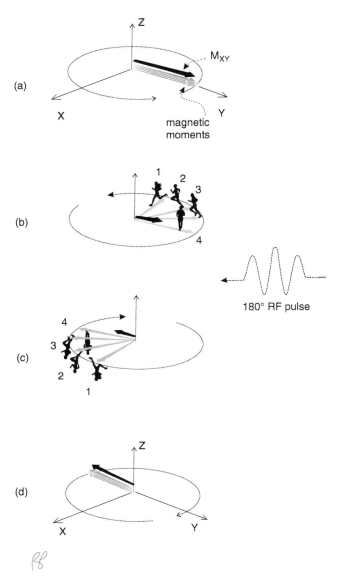

Figure 10.14 A 180-degree radiofrequency pulse is used to reverse T2* decay. (a) Spins are in synchrony. (b) De-phasing of the spin vectors (each runner corresponds to a vector). (c) A 180 degree RF pulse "flips" the vectors 180 degrees (and the relative positions of the runners is now reversed, the slowest runner is first in line). (d) All vectors (and runners) get into phase again.

the recovery time, T1. When the echo is sampled at time TE after the 90-degree pulse, the signal amplitude depends on both T1 and T2. However, if the acquisition is repeated multiple times with the same TE but different TIs, the T1 can be estimated. Again, in clinical MRI it is not typical to measure T1 explicitly as described but rather to use the inversion recovery to obtain T1-weighting.

Signal localization

The process of acquisition and reconstruction of MR data from the body is very different than the techniques we have discussed for SPECT, PET, and CT. Instead of transmitting and collecting X-rays or collecting gamma photons, MRI systems manipulate magnetic fields and transmit and receive radiofrequency (RF) pulses in order to acquire image data.

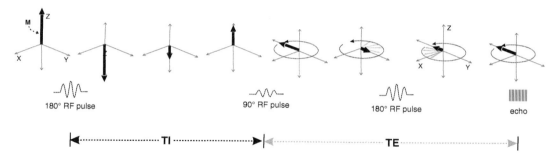

Figure 10.15 Inversion recovery. An initial 180-degree RF pulse inverts M along the Z-axis antiparallel to the direction of B_0 (negative Z-axis), M "recovers" its preferred alignment in the direction of B_0. A 90-degree RF pulse tips M into the X-Y plane, the second 180-degree RF pulse counteracts dephasing caused by T2* and the echo is read. TI is time to inversion and TE is time to echo.

The MR signal waveforms that are collected from the body in response to the RF pulse are stored in a matrix called **k-space**. Once the imaging is complete these waveforms are translated (using "reverse" Fourier transformation [which will be discussed in Chapter 12]) into standard spatial data for display.

Gradient coils

If the field strength (B_0) was the same throughout the body all protons would have the same Larmor frequency and it would not be possible to separate the MR signals coming from different locations within the body. To solve this problem, MR machines are equipped with additional coils called **gradient coils** as well as RF transmitters capable of transmitting RF waves over a range of frequencies.

Gradient coils are designed to add or subtract from the background B_0 magnetic field in a way that varies linearly along the gradient direction (an example of Z-axis gradient coils can be seen in Figure 10.16 middle). While B_0 is in the range of Tesla, gradient coil strengths are in the order of tens of milliTesla per meter. Although the gradient only alters the field strength B_0 slightly at different locations in the body, these changes will be reflected in changes in the Larmor frequencies of the protons in the body and therefore the MR signals arising from tissues at these different locations.

Generation and acquisition of MR signals

The acquisition of MR data involves manipulating gradients, controlling the transmitted band of frequencies, and processing the acquired data in what is called a **sequence** or **pulse sequence**. There are many pulse sequences available on MRI scanners and they have different characteristics, however they all accomplish the basic goal of being able to produce a map in three dimensions of some combination of tissue properties (usually T1, T2 and proton density but a few more are possible). For the purpose of illustration, we will focus on perhaps the simplest pulse sequence called a **2D spin–echo sequence**. The steps in this sequence involve slice selection and then spatial encoding of the tissues within the slice; the latter, spatial encoding, involves two manipulations: frequency encoding and phase encoding.

Slice selection and spin excitation: Gradient coils arranged along the Z-axis of length of the body (any direction can be used but for simplicity we will start with the Z-axis) are turned on in order to slightly vary the B_0 field down the length of the body and therefore change the Larmor frequency of the protons between different Z locations (Figure 10.16).

In order to selectively excite the spins within a particular slab or slice of tissue the MR machine transmits a narrow band of radiofrequency waves containing only frequencies corresponding to Larmor frequencies of the protons within that slice. These excited spins generate MR signals (echoes) that are detected by the radiofrequency receiver.

Slice selection has now reduced the three-dimensional imaging task to a two-dimensional imaging task by selectively exciting spins within a single slice. To build the three-dimensional volume, sequential slices are selected by repeating the entire sequence but increasing or decreasing the mid-point of RF

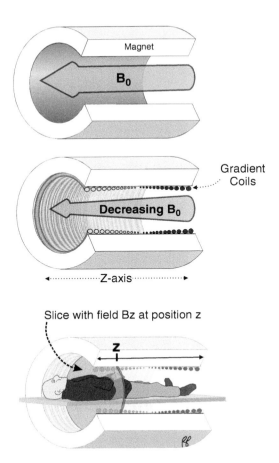

Figure 10.16 Top: MRI without gradient coils—uniform B_0 down the length of the tube. Middle: Gradient coils arranged along the Z-axis alter B_0 at each Z-location such that the spins in a sample body slice at z (bottom) are subjected to a magnetic field labeled Bz. These spins will have a slice specific Larmor frequency which can only be excited by a corresponding RF pulse.

frequency band employed for slice selection. Since the RF pulse repetition rate can be on the order of seconds and the radiofrequency receiver can take readings of the echo (MR signal) every ten to hundred milliseconds, many different slices can sometimes be processed within each repetition interval (TR).

Spatial encoding: Once the slice selection has been accomplished, the Z-axis gradient is turned off and, **spatial encoding** is applied to read-out these excited spins. This is accomplished using the two remaining gradients, one of which is used as a **frequency encoding** gradient (we'll use X-axis

gradient) and the other as a phase encoding gradient (Y-axis) Turning on the frequency encoding gradient alters the frequency of precession, and therefore the frequency of the echo, of the protons along the X-axis (Figure 10.17a). In this way each physical position along the X-axis is represented by a different frequency echo waveform (Figure 10.17b). This representation of a position in space by a wave is a Fourier transformation in one dimension (discussed in Chapter 12). Then, while the X-axis frequency encoding gradient remains on, the **phase encoding** gradient (along the Y-axis) is turned on for a very brief time causing a temporary change in spin frequency along the Y-axis (Figure 10.18a). Once the phase encoding gradient is turned off the spins revert to their Larmor frequencies controlled by the frequency encoding gradient, but have now been altered by a phase step that varies in degree by position along the Y-axis (Figure 10.18b). The information from the MR signals is stored in k-space.

The process above is repeated in entirety for the same slice, however, each time with a different strength phase encoding gradient. After a number of repetitions, usually 128 or 256 (the greater the number the better the resolution but the longer the acquisition), the full two-dimensional transform has been acquired and the final step is to invert that Fourier domain matrix to obtain an image of the slice.

Contrast manipulation in MR imaging

As mentioned previously, in clinical MR imaging, the underlying MR properties of tissues are not really measured but rather an image is formed in which the intensity is derived from some combination of the underlying T1, T2 and proton density. Contrast between different types of tissues can be manipulated by varying the **time to repetition (TR)** of the RF pulses and the TE in a spin echo sequence and TI in inversion recovery with a spin echo readout as described earlier. Some of these variations are explored below.

T1-weighted images

Tissues with longer T1 recovery times (larger T1 values), such as fluid, take longer for their net magnetization, M_z, to return to full strength than tissues with shorter T1 recovery times (smaller T1 values), such as fat. If the radiofrequency pulse

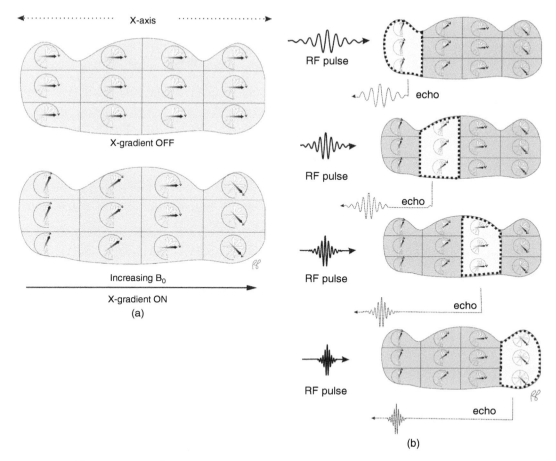

Figure 10.17 (a) Frequency encoding. Gradient coils along the X-axis of the selected slice are turned on and as a result each column (corresponding to each X-position) is subjected to a slightly different B_0 field. Spins at each X-position have identical precessional (Larmor) frequencies. (b) RF pulses that match the precession frequency within each column excite the spins which in turn respond with an echo (MR signal) that is detected by the receiver.

is repeated after a relatively long time (long TR), tissues with long and short T1 recovery times will both have time to recover their full M_z strength so the difference in in the MR signal due to T1 will be minimal. If the time to repetition is short, tissues with longer T1 recovery times will not be able to recover as much of their M_z strength as tissues with short T1 and will therefore appear darker on T1-weighted images; conversely tissues with shorter T1 recovery times generate larger signals and therefore appear brighter on T1 images. In this way tissues with different T1 values can be differentiated using short TR. An illustrated slice from the brain can be seen in Figure 10.19 (T1), the tissue with the shortest T1 recovery time, fat, will appear white, whereas the tissue with the longest recovery time, fluid

(cerebrospinal fluid) will appear black. Tissues with intermediate T1 recovery times will appear in various shades of gray in the images.

Shorter TR times yield a greater impact of the T1 time on the image appearance; therefore, these images are said to have stronger **T1 weighting**.

T2-weighted images

As discussed previously, the echo time can be chosen to sample T2 recovery. If TE is short compared with T2, then the MR signal does not reflect much T2 decay. The shorter the TE the more similar the MR signals from tissues with long and short T2 recovery times. The longer the TE the greater the difference between the signals of tissues with different T2 values. The longer the TE therefore the

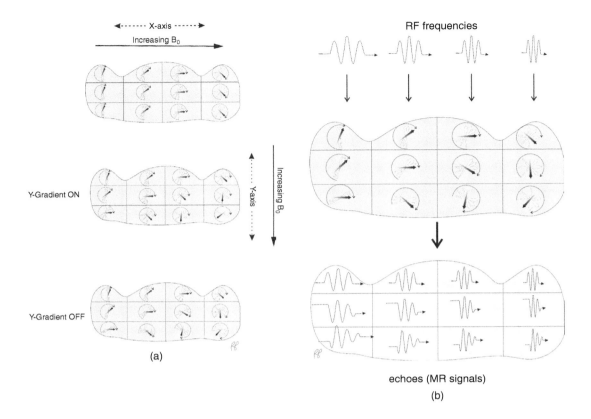

Figure 10.18 (a) The X-gradient remains on and the slice is subjected to a varying B_0 field along the Y-axis created by briefly turning on the Y-gradient (middle image). Each row (y position) of spins is then bathed in a slightly different B_0 magnetic field creating different spin precession frequencies between rows. The Y-gradient is switched off (bottom image) and all of the frequencies return to the baseline X-gradient frequencies, except each row is now out of phase with the other rows. (b) Spins in each X-position will respond to a single matching RF pulse, but the MR signal frequencies will be out of phase with one another and therefore in this very small matrix example each cell will generate a "unique" echo frequency.

stronger the **T2 weighting** in the image. Tissues with smaller T2 times measured at a longer TE will have lost more of their coherence and their signal will appear smaller; they will appear dark on T2-weighted images. Conversely tissues with larger T2 times measured at longer TE times will have retained more of their coherence and their signal will be greater and they will appear bright on T2-weighted images. An illustrated sample of a T2-weighted slice of the brain can be seen in Figure 10.19 (T2).

Combing TR and TE

For images that emphasize T1 weighting, called T1-weighted images, a typical TR/TE combination would have a shorter TR, emphasizing the differences in tissues with different T1 values, and a shorter TE which will de-emphasize the different

signal strengths from tissues with different T2 values. A sample of such a sequence is a TR of 340 ms and TE of 13 ms (labeled TR/TE of 340/13 ms) [1].

Reversing this strategy creates a T2-weighted image, i.e. a longer TR to de-emphasize the signal differences between tissues with different T1 values and a longer TE to emphasize the differences in signals between tissues with different T2 values. A sample sequence for T2-weighted images is TR/TE of 3500/120 ms [1].

Proton density images

A sequence that promotes acquisition of the greatest MR signal response from tissue utilizes a long TR (allowing greatest recovery of the net magnetization vector in the Z axis) and a short TE that "gathers" the MR signal very soon after the excitation pulse before much T2 decay. The magnitude of the MR

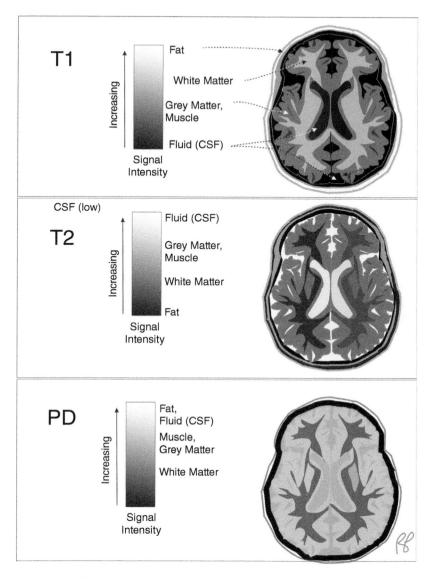

Figure 10.19 Transaxial slice of a brain MRI study: T1-weighted, T2-weighted, and proton density (PD) images.

tissue signal response is therefore dependent on the density of the ^1H protons within the tissues. The tissues with the greatest number of protons will have the greatest signal. A sample of such a sequence is TR/TE of 2000/15 ms [1]. A representative sample of a **proton density weighted** slice of a brain can be seen in Figure 10.19 (PD).

Other sequences

There are a multitude of manipulations of the method of applications of the radiofrequency pulses and variations in the sampling of the tissue responses that are used to reveal other useful tissue characteristics in MR imaging. Further exploration of these techniques is beyond the scope of this text, but is available from many other sources including a reference near the end of this chapter [2].

MRI scanner

A schematic of the relationship of the components of an MRI scanner is shown in Figure 10.20. The majority of MRI magnets which are used to make the homogeneous B_0 field within the scanner are superconducting magnets—coils made of alloys

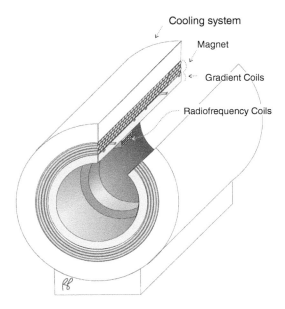

Cooling system

Magnet

Gradient Coils

Radiofrequency Coils

Figure 10.20 Schematic of an MRI scanner.

such as niobium-titanium which are supercooled by liquid nitrogen to nearly absolute zero (4 Kelvin or −269 Celsius or −452 Fahrenheit). The gradient coils, which are not superconducting, are placed along the inner surface of the superconducting magnet. The radiofrequency coil(s) used to generate the RF pulse and receive the MR tissue signal are located along the inner surface of the gradient coils.

References

1. Weishaupt D, Kochli VD, Marincek B. *How Does MRI Work? An Introduction to the Physics and Function of Magnetic Resonance Imaging*, 2nd edn, Section 3.2. Heidelberg: Springer, 2006.
2. Weishaupt D, Kochli VD, Marincek B. *How Does MRI Work? An Introduction to the Physics and Function of Magnetic Resonance Imaging*, 2nd edn, Chapter 7. Heidelberg: Springer, 2006.

Questions

1. True or false: The direction of current in a wire represents the direction of motion of electrons within the wire.

2. Which of the following statements is correct?
   (a) Current within a straight wire creates magnetic fields surrounding the wire.
   (b) A moving magnet can create electric current in metals such as copper.
   (c) A nearly linear magnetic field can be created by an electric current in a wire coil.
   (d) All of the above.
   (e) None of the above.

3. True or false: The spin angular momentum and the magnetic moments of subatomic particles are closely linked and often represented by the same vector which is drawn through the center of the representation of the particle.

4. Which of the following statements are correct?
   (a) An external magnetic field causes all of the protons magnetic dipole moments within the field to either align along the direction of the field or opposite to the direction of the field.
   (b) The net magnetization of the dipole moments of the protons is in the direction of the external magnetic field.
   (c) All of the above.

5. The gyromagnetic ratio (γ_0) for the nucleus of ^{23}Na is 11.26 MHz/T. What is the Larmor frequency (ω_0) for this nucleus in a 2 Tesla magnetic field?

6. Match the following abbreviations with their definitions:
   (a) B_0.
   (b) RF.
   (c) MR signal (echo).
      (i) Radiofrequency wave used to excite protons in the tissue which are precessing under the influence of an external magnetic field.
      (ii) Current generated in a receiving coil as the excited protons realign with the external magnetic field.
      (iii) The external magnetic field applied to a body within an MRI machine.

7. Match the following phrases with one or more of the associated terms:
   (a) T2 recovery.
   (b) T1 recovery.
      (i) Transverse relaxation.
      (ii) Longitudinal relaxation.
      (iii) Spin–spin relaxation.
      (iv) De-phasing.
      (v) Net magnetization vector returning to Z-axis orientation.
      (vi) Spin–lattice relaxation.

8. Which of the following statements are true:
   (a) Using shorter TR times (time to repetition of RF pulses) results in images with greater T2 weighting.
   (b) Using a longer TE (time to echo) yields images with greater T1 weighting.

9. True or false: Gradient coils magnetic strengths are nearly the same strength as the background B_0 magnetic field.

10. Arrange the following steps for localization of an MR signal in the order that they are applied by the MRI scanner when performing 2D spin–echo imaging:
    (a) Phase encoding.
    (b) Slice selection.
    (c) Frequency encoding.

11. True or false: k-space is a matrix containing MR signal wave data that is converted to spatial images using Fourier transformation.

Answers

1. False. The direction of current is the opposite to the path of movement of electrons as it was originally thought that positive charges moved, not electrons.
2. (d).
3. True.
4. (c).
5. $\omega_0 = \gamma_0 \times B_0 = 11.26\,\text{MHz/T} \times 2\,\text{T} = 22.52\,\text{MHz}$.
6. (a) (iii). (b) (i). (c) (ii).
7. (a) (i), (iii), (iv). (b) (ii), (v), (vi).
8. Neither are true: shorter TR times yield T1-weighted images, longer TE times yield T2-weighted images.
9. False, gradient coil strength is about 1/10,000th the strength of B_0.
10. (b), (c), then (a).
11. True.

CHAPTER 11

Hybrid Imaging Systems: PET-CT, SPECT-CT, and PET-MRI

Hybrid imaging systems were created in order to more accurately register the complementary information derived from tomographic nuclear medicine imaging, CT, and MRI.

PET-CT and SPECT-CT imaging

For specific clinical diagnoses positron emission tomography (PET) and single photon computed tomography (SPECT) imaging can detect more sites of disease than conventional anatomical imaging such as X-ray computed tomography (CT) or magnetic resonance imaging (MRI). Interpretation of PET and SPECT can be difficult, however, because these nuclear medicine images have few anatomical landmarks for determining the location of abnormal findings. Combining PET or SPECT with CT images acquired sequentially on their separate devices provided a partial solution to this problem. Unless patient positioning was carefully reproduced between the studies, the nuclear medicine and CT images did not match, and the resulting misregistration led to inaccuracies in determining the anatomic location of the abnormalities seen in the nuclear medicine images. In one approach to correcting for positioning errors, the images from completely separate PET or SPECT camera and a CT scanner were fused manually or by computer software or both.

To further ensure accurate registration of the PET and CT (or SPECT and CT) images the paired imaging scanners are placed adjacent to each other with a shared patient bed that moves through both scanners. This arrangement allows the patient to maintain the same position in both scanners and anatomical registration is much better. These combined devices are called **PET-CT scanners** and **SPECT-CT scanners**. This arrangement of combined units also facilitates the use of the CT data to correct the nuclear medicine images for the attenuation of the gamma radiation as it traverses body tissues en-route to the detectors.

PET-CT

PET-CT scanners are presently configured as sequential gantries, also called in-line cameras, with a shared patient bed, or pallet. An illustration of a combined PET-CT is shown in Figure 11.1. The advantage of this configuration as discussed at the introduction of the chapter is the consistent positioning of the patient between the acquisitions which reduces the risk of misregistration of the images. In addition the CT data can be used for attenuation correction for the PET or SPECT images. Attenuation correction using CT data is discussed in Chapters 8 and 12.

In PET-CT configurations the CT scanner is closer to the patient. The CT scan is acquired in its entirety prior to acquiring the PET scan (Figure 11.2), although the order of acquisition of the studies can be reversed.

SPECT-CT

All PET-CT scanners are currently manufactured with multislice CT units. Hybrid SPECT-CT scanners, however, are offered in a number of different configurations. In addition to the sequential gantry configuration, with the SPECT camera heads on a gantry closer to the patient, there are systems where both the SPECT camera heads and the CT X-ray tube and detectors are supported on a single

Essentials of Nuclear Medicine Physics, Instrumentation, and Radiation Biology, Fourth Edition.
Rachel A. Powsner, Matthew R. Palmer, and Edward R. Powsner.
© 2022 John Wiley & Sons Ltd. Published 2022 by John Wiley & Sons Ltd.

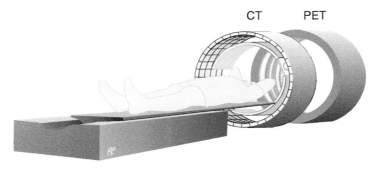

Figure 11.1 PET-CT.

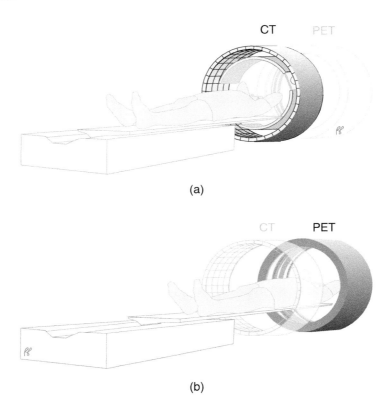

(a)

(b)

Figure 11.2 PET-CT. (a) The entire CT scan is acquired, followed by (b) the PET scan.

rotating gantry (Figure 11.3). The latter solution is more compact (frequently requiring fewer room modifications for installation) and usually less expensive than the dual gantry configurations. In addition, due to lower X-ray tube output, they require less room shielding.

There are some limitations in the single gantry systems. With both the X-ray tube and detectors and SPECT heads mounted on a single rotational system, the speed of rotation is limited and CT acquisition is slower than systems with the CT scanner incorporated as a separate gantry. Consequently, artifacts from patient motion, both voluntary and involuntary, such as peristalsis of the gastrointestinal tract, are more common. As a result of patient motion and the lower X-ray tube output the CT image quality is generally inferior to that of the multislice systems.

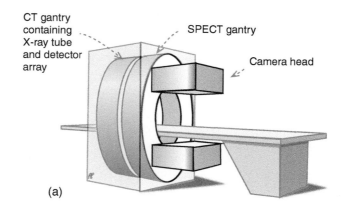

(a)

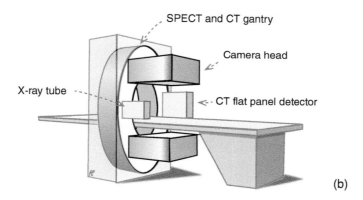

(b)

Figure 11.3 SPECT-CT. (a) Two gantry system with CT contained within one gantry and SPECT heads supported on a second gantry and (b) single gantry system with one gantry supporting both the SPECT camera heads and an X-ray tube and flat plane detector.

Current limitations in SPECT-CT and PET-CT hybrid imaging

Breathing artifacts

Hybrid cameras have mitigated the majority of the PET or SPECT and CT registration problems caused by differences in patient positioning which occur when the patient must be physically moved between independent nuclear medicine systems and CT units. However, due to differences in breathing patterns between CT, where breath-holding is desirable, and PET and SPECT imaging, where breath-holding is not possible, misalignment, particularly near the diaphragm can cause misregistration of images in the lower lungs and upper abdomen. In addition, if the CT data is used for attenuation correction, artifacts may be introduced into the PET and SPECT images in the same areas. To assure better alignment of the diaphragm some institutions instruct patients to breathe normally, or shallowly, during both CT and PET or SPECT acquisitions.

Contrast agent artifacts

The use of intravenous and oral contrast during CT imaging can improve anatomic localization; however, contrast is relatively dense and can alter the attenuation maps that are constructed from

CT data. In particular the X-ray attenuation will be greatly increased at sites of greater concentration of contrast, such as pooling of the oral contrast in the colon, or vascular filling with an intravenous bolus. Although the gamma photon emissions in both PET and SPECT imaging are also attenuated by contrast, the distribution of the contrast can change between the time of acquisition of the CT and PET or SPECT studies. As a result, the CT attenuation map may not correctly approximate the gamma photon attenuation in these specific areas.

In addition, the HU, or amount of X-ray attenuation, will also be somewhat increased in the soft tissues into which the contrast diffuses. As a result, the attenuation coefficient scaling factors (see Chapter 12, section on attenuation correction) for soft tissue which are based on noncontrast CT X-ray attenuation are not as accurate. For the above reasons use of attenuation correction data from contrast enhanced CT studies to correct attenuation in PET and SPECT studies may result in artifacts in the final images.

In cases where a contrast CT is needed it is not uncommon to first acquire a low-dose CT study for attenuation correction of the gamma photon images, and then, after the PET or SPECT study is acquired, to inject contrast media and acquire a better quality diagnostic CT study.

PET-MR imaging

Introduction

MR scanners produce images with greater soft tissue contrast and resolution than CT scanners. This added information combined with metabolic information from PET scanning has shown promise for better localization and characterization of tissue in certain diseases. Since MR image data takes a lot longer to acquire than CT, artifacts due to organ motion (such as in the lungs and bowel) reduce image quality. MRI has greater utility in organs that do not move, such as the brain, the extremities, and the prostate. Imaging the heart is possible, however, because data acquisition is timed to the cardiac cycle by using an electrocardiogram attached to the patient (just like gated

image acquisition in nuclear medicine illustrated in Figure 6.26).

PET-MR scanner design

Some PET-MR scanners are similar to PET-CT scanners with independent sequential units sharing an imaging table. Due to the problems discussed below the scanners are shielded from each other (Figure 11.4a). This system design results in very long imaging times as both MR and PET acquisition are time-consuming.

Newer PET-MR scanners have incorporated the PET scanner within the MR scanner to allow simultaneous acquisition of images. The design of these merged units is technically challenging; the strong magnetic fields created within the MRI tube disrupt the flow of the electrons in the conventional vacuum photomultiplier tubes (PMTs—see Chapter 4) of PET detectors. In addition, certain materials used in standard PET camera design can disrupt the homogeneous MR magnetic field causing distortion of the MR images. These problems have been resolved by replacing PMTs with semiconductor-based photomultipliers, for example silicon photomultipliers (SiPM), which are not affected by, nor do they cause disruption in, the MRI magnetic field (Figure 11.4b). Silicon photomultipliers (SiPM) are described in Chapter 4.

Attenuation correction

One of the more difficult problems to overcome in PET-MR design has been creating accurate attenuation maps from the MRI data to use for attenuation correction of the PET images. Attenuation correction using CT data is more straightforward as both the X-rays used to generate the CT data and the gamma photons imaged with gamma and PET cameras are attenuated by electrons in the tissue being imaged. Air, water, soft tissue, and bone can be differentiated on CT images and the attenuation coefficients derived from this data can be applied to correct the SPECT and PET data (see Chapter 12).

However, the signal intensity of MRI imaging is related to the density, and the magnetic field-induced behavior, of protons in tissue and not to the electron density of the tissue. MRI signals, therefore, cannot be easily used to estimate attenuation of gamma photons.

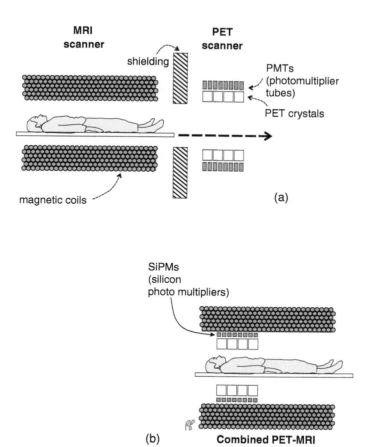

Figure 11.4 PET-MRI. (a) Older scanner design with shielding between the MRI scanner and PET scanner to protect the PET vacuum photomultiplier tubes from the MRI magnet, and to protect the magnetic field in the MRI from disruptions caused by the components of a standard PET scanner. (b) Newer design with silicon photomultipliers permits placement of the PET scanner components within the MRI magnetic field.

For example, on CT, bone, which is dense and causes the highest attenuation of gamma photons and X-rays, has a much higher attenuation coefficient than air, which has a low density and low attenuation coefficient. In contrast, on standard MRI imaging bone and air are indistinguishable as both contain few freely mobile protons (the majority of freely mobile protons in tissue are the hydrogen nuclei contained in water molecules).

Previously, transmission scans using a germanium-68/gallium-68 source to estimate tissue attenuation or imported axial CT scans segmented into bone, soft tissue, and air regions were used for attenuation correction of the PET images from an MRI-PET scanner.

Newer techniques utilize MRI data for attenuation correction. One such solution utilizes T2-weighted imaging with an ultrashort echo time (UTE), which can detect the signal emitted during the very short T2 relaxation times of cortical bone (less than 10 milliseconds compared to, for example, 1000 milliseconds for muscle). Using this technique MRI axial images can be segmented, like CT images, into air, soft tissue, and bone regions and these regions can be assigned predetermined attenuation coefficients for the three different tissues for correction of the PET images.

Questions

1. Artifacts in SPECT-CT hybrid imaging can occur as the result of which of the following?
   (a) Breath-hold following deep inspiration during CT acquisition followed by normal breathing during PET or SPECT acquisition.
   (b) Attenuation correction of PET or SPECT images with contrast CT images.
   (c) (a) and (b).

2. True or false: Semiconductor photomultipliers are used instead of vacuum photomultiplier tubes in PET/MR scanners because the magnetic field disrupts the current flow in vacuum photomultiplier tubes.

3. What are some of the advantages of using a hybrid imaging system?
   (a) Misregistration as a result of patient motion is reduced as the patient remains on the same imaging pallet (bed) during acquisition of both the CT or MRI and PET or SPECT images.
   (b) The CT or MRI images can be used both for attenuation correction and for localization of the PET findings and CT images can be used for both attenuation correction and localization in SPECT imaging.
   (c) (a) and (b).

Answers

1. (c).
2. True.

3. (c).

CHAPTER 12

Image Reconstruction, Processing, and Display

In the modern nuclear medicine clinic, computers are highly integrated into the clinical workflow. Software algorithms are responsible for the critical tasks of image reconstruction from projections and the display of digital data on computer monitors. In addition, specialized software may be employed in the processing of data for such tasks as reformatting, filtering to enhance or de-emphasize certain features in the images, and for rendering surfaces or calculating specialized projections.

Reconstruction

Reconstruction is the process of creating transaxial slices from projection views. There are two basic approaches to creating the transaxial slices: **filtered backprojection** and **iterative reconstruction**. Filtered backprojection, which in the past was the dominant method for nuclear medicine tomographic reconstruction and is still widely used for CT reconstruction, will be covered in depth in this chapter. Iterative reconstruction, now ubiquitous in SPECT and PET reconstruction algorithms and appearing widely in the CT domain, is more computationally intensive. Iterative reconstruction will presented at the end of this section.

Filtered backprojection

The process of backprojection will be introduced, followed by a discussion of filtering.

Backprojection

In backprojection, the data acquired by the camera are used to create multiple **transaxial slices**. Figure 12.1 is a representation of this process; the 10 projection views are cut into seven bands and shown pulled apart. The bands forming each view are then shown smeared along a radius, like the spokes of a wheel. It is this smearing back toward the center that gives us the term backprojection. The smears of the middle bands (shown in dark gray) are seen in translucent gray.

A simplification of the processes of projection and backprojection is illustrated in Figures 12.2 and 12.3. Figure 12.2 is a representation of data obtained in the acquisition of the projection views of a thin radioactive disk. In this figure, an imaginary grid is placed over the disk (Figure 12.2a), the disk is imaged (Figure 12.2b), and the counts for each pixel are recorded (Figure 12.2c). The counts in each of the cells of a column are summed and stored in an array shown above the matrix (Figure 12.2d). In a similar manner, all of the rows are summed and stored in an array of sums to the right of the matrix (Figure 12.2e).

During backprojection, the two arrays of projection data are used to recreate an image of the original disk. In the upper panel of Figure 12.3, the upper array is spread or backprojected across the columns of a blank matrix so that each of the values in any single column are identical. The array to the right of the matrix is backprojected across the rows, and these values are added cell by cell to the values of the preceding set (middle panel). If the counts in each

Essentials of Nuclear Medicine Physics, Instrumentation, and Radiation Biology, Fourth Edition.
Rachel A. Powsner, Matthew R. Palmer, and Edward R. Powsner.
© 2022 John Wiley & Sons Ltd. Published 2022 by John Wiley & Sons Ltd.

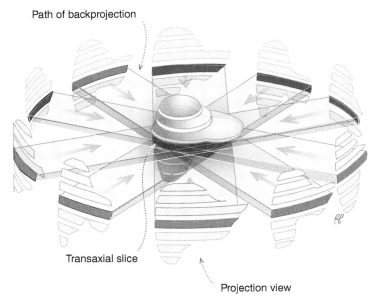

Figure 12.1 Projection views of a liver are backprojected to create transaxial slices.

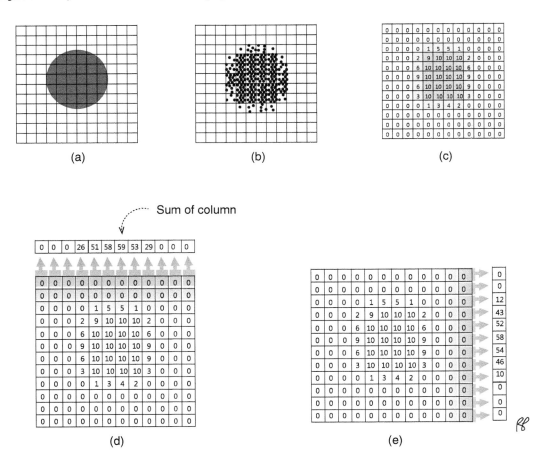

Figure 12.2 Acquisition of projection views (as numerical arrays) of a disk.

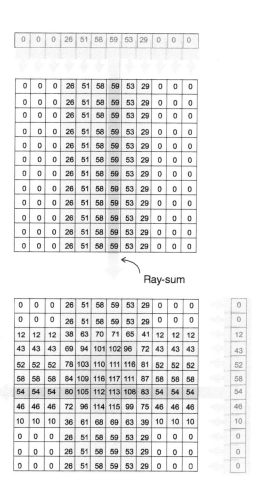

Ray-sum

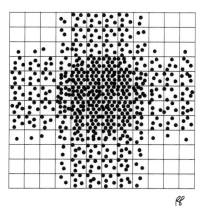

Figure 12.3 Projection views of the disk are backprojected.

pixel are represented by dots (for the ease of illustration each dot represents five counts) one begins to see a relatively dense central area that corresponds generally to the size and the location of the original disk (lower panel). The wide bands of dots extending in four directions from this central density and forming a cross shape are an artifact of the backprojection process; they are residual counts from the backprojection of the arrays.

Backprojection artifact

As the number of projection views used to create the image is increased the residual counts from the backprojections discussed above give the appearance of a star surrounding the object, the so-called **star artifact** illustrated in Figure 12.4a. Increasing the number of projection views removes the star appearance and improves definition of the object (Figure 12.4b, c), however an overall "blur" remains surrounding the object (Figure 12.4d). This blur, which will be referred to from this point on as the **backprojection artifact**, is a demonstration of how backprojection does not really re-create the original object and is not the inverse of the process of projection (see Figure 7.3 and associated text in Chapter 7).

Filtering

Filtering is a mathematical technique applied during reconstruction to improve the appearance of the image. In particular, for our purposes, filters are used to reduce the effects of the backprojection ("blur") artifact and to remove image noise (see box).

When image data is represented in familiar terms, such as in counts per pixel, this data is said to exist in the **spatial domain**. Filtering can be performed on this data as it is. Alternatively, the data can be represented as a series of sine waves and the filtering performed on these. In the latter case, the data is said to be transformed into the **frequency domain**. Before we discuss this transformation of data from the spatial domain to the frequency domain, we will apply some simple filters to data represented in the spatial domain in order to reduce the backprojection artifact and noise in images.

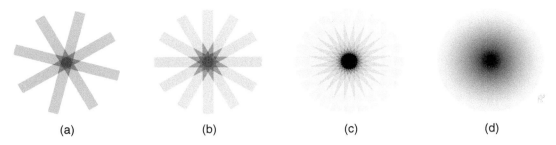

Figure 12.4 Star and backprojection "blur" artifact.

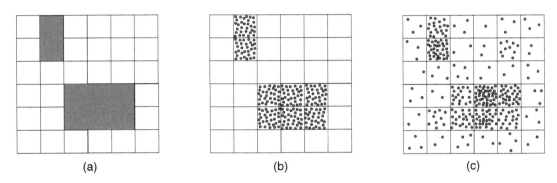

Figure 12.5 Statistical variation in counts.

Signal vs. Noise

The **signal** is that part of the information that produces the actual image; **noise** is extraneous data and may have no direct relation to the actual image. Noise reduces the quality of the image. Statistical variation in counts and random electronic fluctuations are among the sources of noise, which can be reduced by improved collimation, longer acquisition times, and better design of the circuitry.

Filtering in the spatial domain

Spatial filtering to reduce noise: nine-point smoothing: Figure 12.5 demonstrates the effects of noise on the images of two rectangles. In Figure 12.5a, a grid is placed over the two rectangles being imaged. Figure 12.5b is a representation of an ideal image with uniformly distributed counts. Figure 12.5c is a more realistic representation of an acquired mage of the rectangles. The counts are greater over the rectangles than the background, but noise contributes to inhomogeneity in uptake in the rectangles and background.

Smoothing partially redistributes the counts from the pixels with the highest counts to its immediate neighbors, in this way the more extreme irregularities in pixel counts are "blunted." The nine-point smoothing technique is demonstrated in Figure 12.6. The counts from the central pixel and eight immediately adjacent pixels are averaged (Figure 12.6a). The count in the central pixel is replaced by this average. This process is repeated pixel by pixel (Figure 12.6b, c).

In one variation of this technique, the central pixel is given a different weight than its eight immediate neighbors. This smoothing filter is applied to pixel (2,2) in Figure 12.7a. The nine pixel elements centered on pixel (2,2) are multiplied pixel by pixel by the corresponding elements in the so-called **filter kernel** (central weight of 10) as shown in Figure 12.7b. The sum of all nine values in the resulting matrix (in this case 339) is divided by the sum of the nine elements of the filter kernel, 18. The resulting value, 19, is the filtered value for pixel (2,2) (Figure 12.7c). In this way, the original value

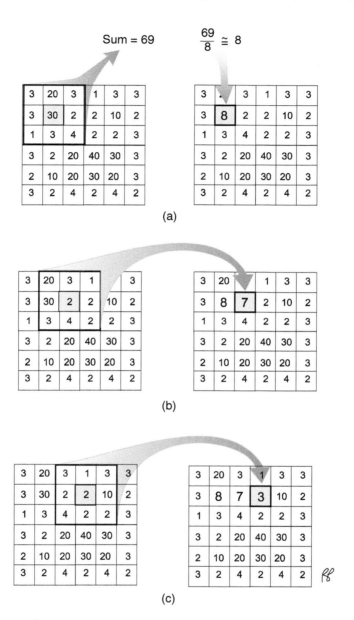

Figure 12.6 Nine-point smoothing.

of pixel (2,2), 30, is modified by the influence of its nearest neighbor pixels. This process is applied to each pixel of matrix.

The result of applying this process to each pixel in the matrix can be seen in Figure 12.8 (upper panel). If a kernel with a less heavily weighted central value of 2 is applied to the matrix, the final image is "more smoothed," that is, the edges of the rectangle are less distinct (lower panel).

Spatial filtering to reduce the backprojection artifact: A somewhat different effect can be achieved by a technique similar to that just described, except that the kernel is given negative values for the peripheral pixels and a positive value in the center. This filter tends to enhance the edges and reduce the intensity of the backprojection artifact. A simple version of this filter can be applied to the previous example depicted in Figure 12.3. This kernel consists of a

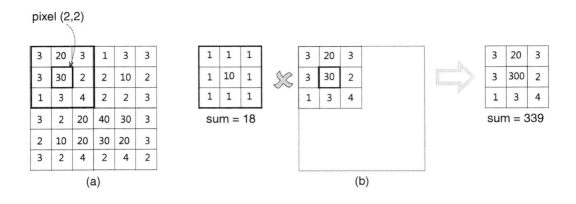

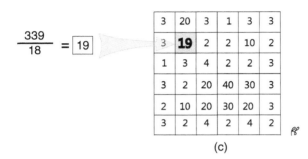

Figure 12.7 Weighted nine-point smoothing.

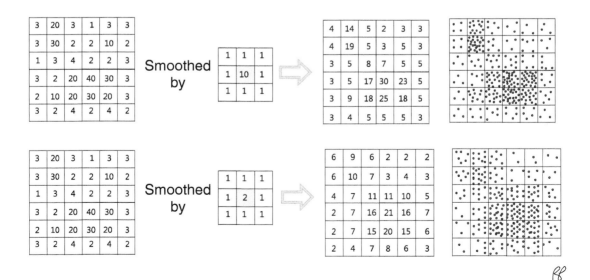

Figure 12.8 Nine-point smoothing using kernels with central weights of 10 and 2.

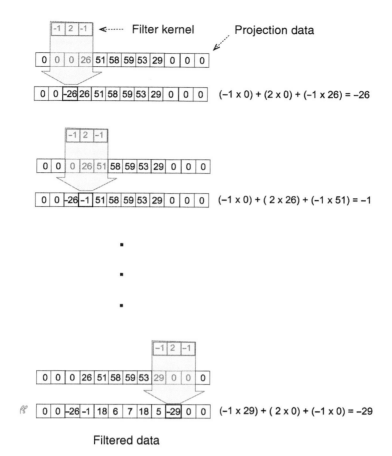

Figure 12.9 Edge-enhancing filter in numerical form.

central value, +2, surrounded by values of −1 (Figure 12.9). This kernel is sequentially applied to each pixel of the array. In the resulting array, the outer values are zero or negative. In a similar fashion, the kernel is applied to the second array of the example in Figure 12.3. When these filtered arrays are backprojected, their peripheral negative values cancel counts in a manner that removes the portion of the rays adjacent to the image of the disk (Figure 12.10). The relative depression of counts surrounding the backprojected disk helps to separate it from the background.

Figure 12.11 is a graphic representation of this process. The top panels demonstrate the process of backprojecting rectangles to create a disk. Each swipe of the paint roller represents a ray. In the upper right image, the combined rays create a disk with indistinct edges. The bottom images demon-

strate the effects of a simple edge enhancement filter in which negative values are used to border each rectangle prior to backprojection (represented by the small white squares on either side of each rectangle). These negative values cancel contributions from adjacent ray-sums and the circle's edge is seen more clearly (bottom right). The filter kernel used here is similar to the kernel in the prior example.

Filtering in the frequency domain
Filtering in the spatial domain proves to be computationally burdensome. In general it is easier to perform filtering in the frequency domain, once the data has been transformed. The following is meant to clarify this process.

Until this point we have discussed data only in the most familiar terms, usually as counts per unit time or counts per pixel—in other words, in

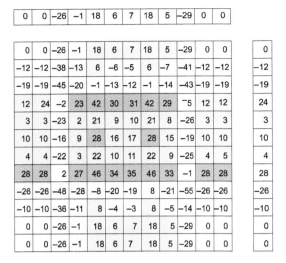

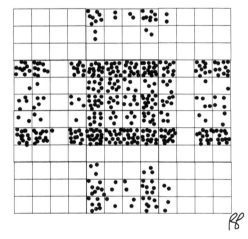

Figure 12.10 Backprojection following application of an edge-enhancing filter.

the **time domain** or in the **spatial domain**. We may look at the data principally in terms of time, for example, the 24-hour uptake in the thyroid gland, or we may view an image of the spatial distribution of the activity in the thyroid. Although they serve different purposes, these two domains are not entirely independent. In fact, they only represent different views of the underlying data.

Now we propose to extend this concept of domains beyond the familiar ones of time and space to another—the **frequency domain**. In this rather unfamiliar domain, the distribution of counts across the image is expressed by a spectrum of spatial frequencies. The frequencies themselves are given in **cycles per centimeter** or **cycles per pixel**. This transformation of data facilitates the computations necessary for filtering.

The first step is the representation of an object as a sum of sinusoidal waves rather than the arrangement of small dots that we usually refer to as an image in the spatial domain. Just as any sound pattern in air can be represented by a combination of sine and cosine waves given in cycles per second, any image pattern can be represented by a combination of sine and cosine waves in cycles per pixel. This use of sinusoidal waves to represent a simple object is illustrated in Figure 12.12. The original rectangles (seen in the top row of column C) can be plotted as a square wave (column A). The three-dimensional view of this square wave is drawn in column B. Column C can be thought of as a bird's-eye view from the top of the three-dimensional square wave. The subsequent rows depict the process of the sequential addition of sine waves to approximate the square waves. The first sine wave (seen in column A of the second row) is a very rough approximation of the square wave, and when viewed from above poorly represents the original rectangles. A second sine wave (of higher frequency) is added to the first sine wave (shown in the third row). Each subsequent addition of a higher frequency sine wave serves to sharpen the image of the rectangles in column C.

In contrast to the original dot image, which can be described by the number of dots at each location, the amplitude of the wave at each frequency now describes the new image (Figure 12.13). This would be the object (in our example, the two rectangles) described in the frequency domain, and a plot of amplitudes of the wave at each frequency is called its **frequency spectrum** (Figure 12.14). Amplitude, the height of the wave, is expressed in counts; frequency is measured in cycles per pixel.

The information obtained by the camera is not changed by this transformation of the collected data from the spatial to the frequency domain; all that is changed is the method of describing the data. More generally, we can say that data can be transformed from one domain into another with neither gain nor loss of the contained information.

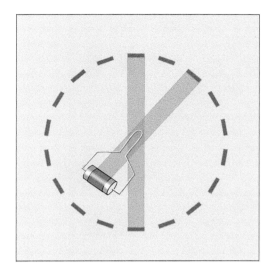
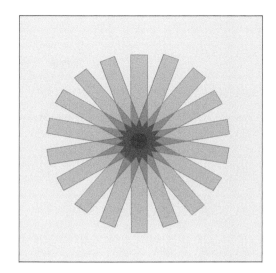
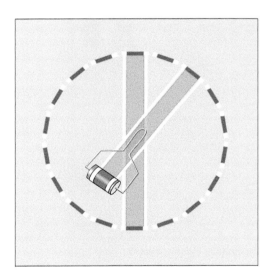
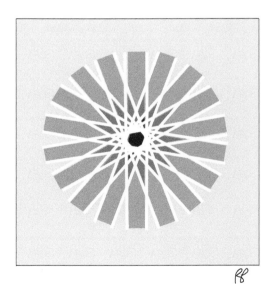

Figure 12.11 Graphic representation of an edge-enhancing filter.

While we are interested here in mathematical methods of transforming data, it is worth mentioning that common physical devices, optical lenses for example, can also be used to transform data. The most pertinent data transformation from the spatial to the frequency domain is based on a method developed about 200 years ago by the French mathematician and physicist Joseph Fourier and is now referred to as the **Fourier transformation**. Its importance lies in the fact that very efficient algorithms are available for computing the Fourier transform and so it saves time when filtering image data.

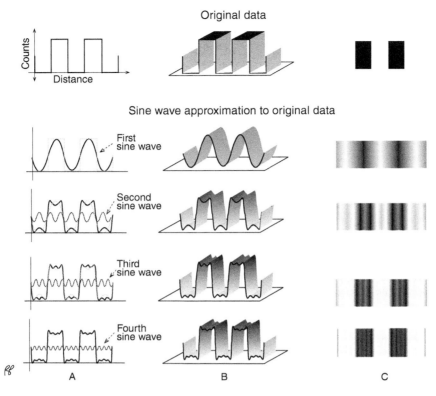

Figure 12.12 The use of sine waves to represent an image: a key step in the transformation of data from the spatial to the frequency domain.

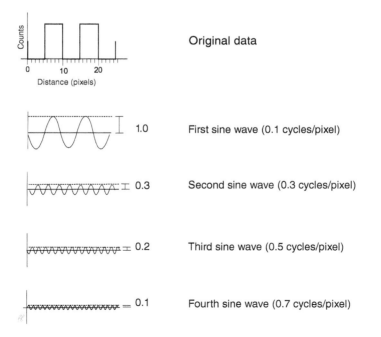

Figure 12.13 Sine waves used to approximate the image of rectangles seen in Figure 12.12.

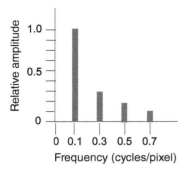

Figure 12.14 Frequency spectrum.

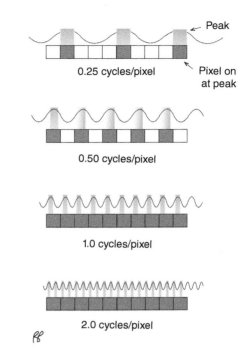

0.25 cycles/pixel

0.50 cycles/pixel

1.0 cycles/pixel

2.0 cycles/pixel

Figure 12.15 The Nyquist frequency of 0.5 cycles/pixel is the smallest discernible frequency for a matrix.

Nyquist frequency: The highest fundamental frequency useful for showing that two adjacent points are separate objects is 0.5 cycles/pixel, which can be demonstrated by showing the effect of higher frequencies. In the top panel of Figure 12.15, a frequency of 0.25 cycles/pixel will cause every fourth pixel to turn on. For demonstration purposes, we have assumed here that only the most positive portion of any sine wave can turn on a pixel. For the frequency of 0.5 cycles/pixel, every other pixel will be on. At still higher frequencies (1.0 cycles/pixel, 2.0 cycles/pixel, and so on), every pixel will be on; in this situation one sine wave peak cannot be separated from the next. The frequency of 0.5 cycles/pixel is referred to as the **Nyquist frequency**; it is the highest fundamental frequency useful for imaging.

Although the Nyquist frequency is always 0.5 cycles/pixel, when expressed as cycles/cm the numeric value is a function of the pixel size. The smaller the pixel size the greater the Nyquist frequency in cycles/cm. As shown in Figure 12.16, for a pixel size of 0.5 cm, 0.5 cycles/pixel is 1.0 cycle/cm; for a pixel size of 0.25 cm, it is 2 cycles/cm; and so on.

Signal, noise, and the backprojection artifact in the frequency domain: To understand the design of filters it is necessary to look at the frequency distribution of the important components of an image. Figure 12.17a is a distribution of frequencies derived from a hypothetical image; the image itself is not shown. The darker gray bars derive from the signal data that are composed principally of frequencies in the low to middle

range; white bars represent noise, which is nearly uniform across the spectrum. Following backprojection (Figure 12.17b) the spectra of both the signal and noise are altered by the effect of backprojection. In essence, backprojection acts as a kind of smoothing filter that diminishes higher frequencies and enhances the lower frequency components of the signal and noise. An ideal filter would remove the backprojection artifact to restore the original signal spectrum and at the same time, remove all of the noise. Unfortunately, the frequency ranges of the signal and noise overlap. Practical filters used in filtered backprojection operations are designed to trade-off between restoring the image detail and suppressing noise.

Frequency filtering to reduce the backprojection artifact: The **ramp** filter is named for its shape in the frequency domain. This filter was designed to reduce the artifact resulting from backprojection. Figure 12.17c demonstrates that the ramp filter effectively removes this artifact while retaining both signal and noise data.

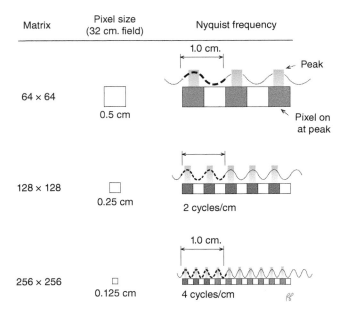

Figure 12.16 The Nyquist frequency expressed in cycles/cm.

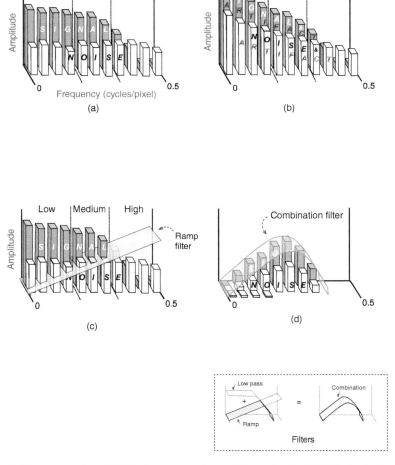

Figure 12.17 Effect of the ramp and combination low-pass and ramp filter on signal data, statistical noise, and the backprojection artifact.

Frequency filtering to reduce noise: Filters can be described by the portion of the frequency spectrum that they transmit. The most common examples are the low- and high-pass filters. **Low-pass** filters retain (or "pass") low-frequency data and reject high frequency data; **high-pass** filters retain high-frequency data and discard low-frequency data. The ramp filter just described is an example of a high-pass filter.

In general, the use of a low-pass filter results in an image with indistinct edges and loss of detail (Figure 12.18, top right panel). High-pass filters accentuate edges and retain finer details, but can be difficult to interpret due to their "grainy" appearance caused by high-frequency noise (Figure 12.18, bottom right panel).

Low-pass filters: Although the ramp filter is an excellent means of removing the backprojection artifact the image still contains noise that can interfere with interpretation of the images. Noise due to statistical variation in counts is more of a problem in low-count images, such as SPECT projection images, than it is in a standard high-count planar view. A low-pass filter is used to reduce noise in the higher frequency ranges while retaining signal which is predominantly composed of low and middle range frequency data.

• *Types of low-pass filter:* There are many low-pass filters available to process nuclear medicine data, and all are named after their inventors, for example, Hann (or vonHann), Hamming, Butterworth, Weiner, and Parzen. Each filter has a different shape (albeit some are quite similar), and when applied will modify the image differently.

Some typical low-pass filters used to reduce high-frequency noise are plotted in Figure 12.19. The Parzen filter is an example of a low-pass filter that greatly smooths data; generally it is not used for SPECT. The Hann and Hamming filters are low-pass filters with some smoothing but a relatively greater acceptance of mid- and high-frequency data than the Parzen filter. The commonly used Butterworth filter allows the user to adjust the relative degree of high-frequency wave acceptance (see below). The Butterworth and Hann filters are also "flexible" filters in that their shape can be altered by specifying certain parameters. The very light gray broad band in Figure 12.19 roughly delineates the possible range of shapes of the Hann filter; the darker gray band delineates possible shapes of the Butterworth window.

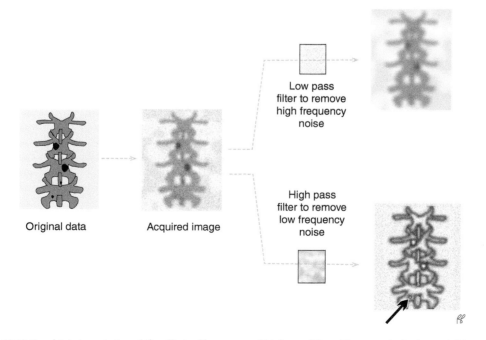

Original data   Acquired image

Low pass filter to remove high frequency noise

High pass filter to remove low frequency noise

Figure 12.18 Graphic interpretation of the effects of low-pass and high-pass filters. The arrow in the lower right panel points to an image detail preserved by the use of a theoretical high-pass filter.

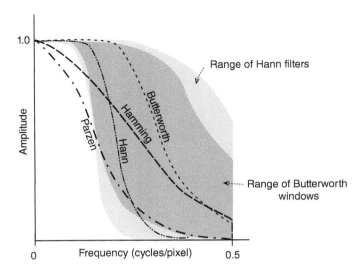

Figure 12.19 Characteristics of commonly used low-pass filters.

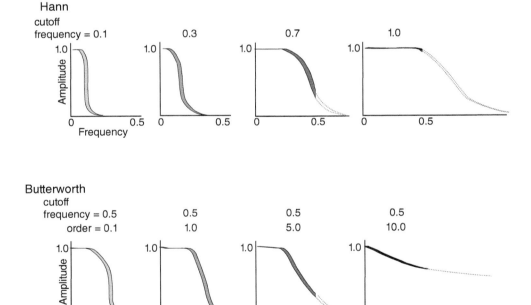

Figure 12.20 The Butterworth and Hann windows (or prefilters) can be modified to match the characteristics of the data set. The curves representing the filters are extended as dotted lines beyond the maximal accepted Nyquist frequency of 0.5 cycles/pixel.

• *Cutoff frequency and order:* The cutoff frequency, often referred to as the power of the filter, is the maximum frequency the filter will pass. If the cutoff frequency is greater than the Nyquist frequency, the filter is abruptly terminated at the Nyquist frequency of 0.5 cycles/pixel. A Hann filter is depicted with different cutoff frequencies in the upper panel of Figure 12.20. An additional parameter, the **order**, can be specified for Butterworth filters. The order controls the slope of the curve (lower panel of

Figure 12.20). Reconstructed images of a bone scan using a Butterworth filter with varying cutoff frequencies can be seen in Figure 12.21.

Sequence for applying filters: Filters can be applied to the data prior to backprojection (**prefiltering**), during backprojection, or to the transaxial slices following backprojection. Often the low-pass filters (Butterworth, Hann, Hamming, Parzen, and others) are applied as prefilters to remove high-frequency noise. The ramp filter is then applied during backprojection to remove the backprojection artifact. The prefilter and ramp filter can be applied in a single step (see Figure 12.17d). This **combination filter** is either referred to by the filter's name, for example "Parzen," or by a description such as "ramp–Parzen filter."

Filter selection: The selection of the optimal filter depends on both the characteristics of the data and on the user's personal preference. In general, a high-pass filter is better suited for higher count data, whereas a low-pass or smoothing filter is better for data containing a small number of counts.

Butterworth filter, order 6

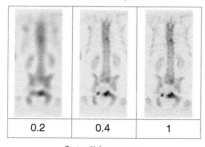

| 0.2 | 0.4 | 1 |

Cut-off frequency

Figure 12.21 Sample images of reconstructed bone scan using Butterworth filters with varying cutoff frequencies.

With respect to preference, some users like smoother, less-detailed images; others are willing to tolerate the "grainy" appearance following the use of a high-pass filter in order to retain the finer details of the signal data.

Attenuation correction

Attenuation: Photons originating from inside the body are more likely to be absorbed or scattered by the surrounding tissue than photons originating near the surface. The attenuation coefficient for ^{99m}Tc in tissue (see discussion of attenuation in Chapter 2) is 0.15/cm. This means that every centimeter of tissue between the source and camera will absorb or scatter approximately 15% of entering photons. Attenuation of photons will reduce counts from the middle of the body. In Figure 12.22 the photons from the deeper portions of the myocardium are less likely to exit the surface of the body than photons from the more superficial portions.

Correction: Attenuation correction in the past was routinely performed by calculation techniques which assumed uniform tissue density across the body and therefore uniform attenuation. Transmission imaging for measuring attenuation, which is rarely uniform across the body, has nearly completely replaced calculation techniques, especially in the chest where soft-tissue, lung, and bone densities coexist in the same transaxial slices. However, calculated attenuation correction is still useful for brain imaging where the consistency of the tissue is fairly uniform.

Calculated attenuation correction: Attenuation correction can be performed by applying a correction factor that takes into account source

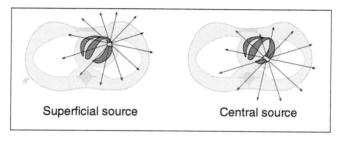

Superficial source   Central source

Figure 12.22 Attenuation of photons.

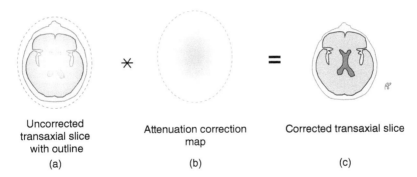

Uncorrected transaxial slice with outline

(a)

Attenuation correction map

(b)

Corrected transaxial slice

(c)

Figure 12.23 Attenuation correction using a calculated attenuation map.

depth and the tissue attenuation coefficient. The tissue attenuation coefficient is assumed to be a constant value throughout the cross-section of the body.

There are several algorithms available for calculated attenuation correction. A simplified application of one such mathematical technique, the Chang algorithm, is the most commonly used method. Figure 12.23 highlights the major points of the method. An approximation to the outline of the head is drawn by computer or manually (Figure 12.23a). Within the outline, a correction matrix is constructed; this is shown symbolically by the shading (Figure 12.23b) in which the darker area indicates greater correction. As seen in Figure 12.23c, the greater correction increases the number of counts in the deeper portions of the brain.

Transmission correction: In this technique, attenuation correction factors are obtained directly from **transmission** measurements. Transmission measurements are tomographic projections obtained from a radionuclide source positioned outside the patient on the side directly opposite the camera (Figure 12.24). Attenuation of photons through the body from this external source is dependent on tissue thickness and attenuation coefficient along the transmission rays. As the camera head and source are rotated around the patient, the attenuation of photons through the body varies between the source and the camera head. The transmission projections are then reconstructed to obtain an images of attenuation coefficients much like what is done in a CT scan. Unlike CT scans however, the quantity of transmission photons recorded by the detector is

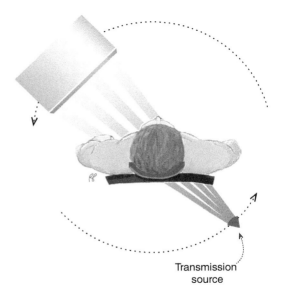

Figure 12.24 Transmission image using a rotating gamma emitting source.

severely limited and the images are very noisy. For that reason, transmission images are usually segmented and voxels are classified as constituting one of a number of allowed tissue types—usually just bone, air, and water—and the known attenuation coefficient for that tissue is substituted for the noisy estimate.

Attenuation corrections for SPECT-CT and PET-CT scanners are derived from the CT axial images. CT inherently measures attenuation—the HU is a scaled and biased estimate of the linear attenuation coefficient for X-ray photons. In order to use CT images for attenuation correction of SPECT or PET data, the coefficients need to be adjusted, or transformed, to reflect the difference in attenuation of the

X-rays energies (used to produce the CT scan) and the gamma photon. X-ray photon energies are generally less than 140-keV and most SPECT gamma photon energies and all PET photon energies are greater than 140-ke V. If attenuation was due to density alone, a simple scaling factor could be applied to the CT data in order to transform it to the appropriate gamma energy. However, attenuation is highly dependent on the atomic number of the absorber. At CT X-ray energies, higher Z materials are strongly attenuating but at higher energies, Z is less important. For this reason, the gamma photon attenuation is estimated using the assumption that values with CT numbers less than water (HU = 0) represent a mix of air and soft-tissue, values greater than water are a mix of bone and soft-tissue, and values greater than some threshold represent pure bone. A graph of the attenuation coefficient scaling factors for 511-keV annihilation photons is shown in Figure 12.25. Of note, if contrast material is used for the CT scan, these scaling factors are adjusted to incorporate the effects of contrast.

The transformation is applied to the pixels in the CT data to create attenuation maps. For PET data the attenuation for each pixel along each line of detectors is identical (see Figure 8.15). These attenuation factors are applied to the PET emission data prior to reconstruction. For SPECT data it is somewhat more complex. The attenuation along any line (ray) is different for each pixel along the ray. As a result, the attenuation factor for each pixel of SPECT data is not a constant but depends on the angle—i.e. different for each ray that projects back to the detector. For that reason, an attenuation coefficient image or map is an approximation usually represented as the average of attenuation factors from the CT attenuation map for each ray.

Iterative reconstruction

A relatively elegant technique called iterative reconstruction has steadily replaced filtered backprojection. Images reconstructed with this technique exhibit significantly less backprojection artifact (see Figure 12.4) than those created using filtered backprojection.

In iterative reconstruction, the computer starts with an initial "guess"-estimate of the data to produce a set of transaxial slices. These slices are then used to create a second set of projection views which are compared to the original projection views as acquired from the patient. The transaxial slices from the computer's estimate are then modified using the difference between, or ratio of, the two sets of projection views. A new set of transaxial slices reconstructed from this modified, or second, estimate are then used to create a set of projection views which are compared to the original projection views. Again these projection views are compared

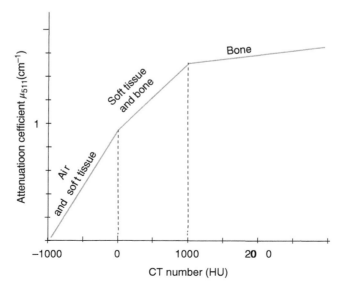

Figure 12.25 Attenuation coefficient scaling factors for ^{18}F PET based on CT numbers.

to the original projection views. If the process proceeds efficiently, each iteration generates a new set of projection views that more closely approximate the original projection views. The process is complete when the difference between the projection views of the estimated data and the original data is below a predetermined threshold.

Figures 12.26 through 12.28 are simplified illustrations of this process using a single transaxial slice shaped like a squared-off horseshoe to represent a transaxial slice of a heart, and a simple square object to represent the computer's initial estimate of this transaxial slice. Figure 12.26 illustrates the creation of the original and estimated data projection views. Figure 12.27 illustrates the comparison of the projection views for the first estimate with those of the original data (Figure 12.27a), and the subsequent creation of the correction projection views from their ratio (Figure 12.27b). A transverse correction slice is then constructed by "backprojecting" these projection views (Figure 12.27c) (the correction slice and projection views are mathematical entities and as such are shaded-in with an ambiguous pattern). The estimate of the first slice is then multiplied by this correction slice to create the second estimate slice (Figure 12.27d) from which a new set of projection

views are created (Figure 12.27e). Subsequent iterations proceed in the same manner using each new set of projection views in conjunction with the original data set to create a new set of estimated projections. Figure 12.28 summarizes the results for five iterations of this idealized model; at the fifth iteration the estimated transaxial slice equals the original data and the process is complete.

In practice most iterative reconstructions are terminated at a predetermined number of iterations i.e., when the physician reading the studies is satisfied with the overall image quality, instead of allowing them to progress until the difference between the estimated and projection views reaches a set value. In general, the image resolution improves with increasing number of iterations, as demonstrated in Figure 12.29 using a single coronal slice of a lumbar spine from a SPECT bone scan. However, beyond a certain reasonable number of iterations, further improvements in resolution can only be accomplished at the cost of increased image noise.

The use of iterative reconstruction techniques was limited in the past because of lengthy computation times; faster computers and "short-cut" mathematical techniques such as OSEM have mitigated this problem.

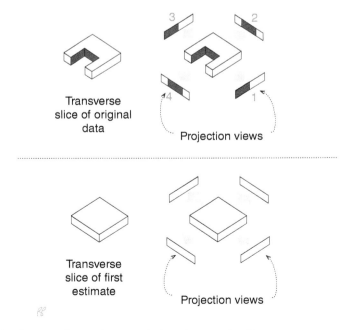

Figure 12.26 Original and estimated projection views for iterative reconstruction.

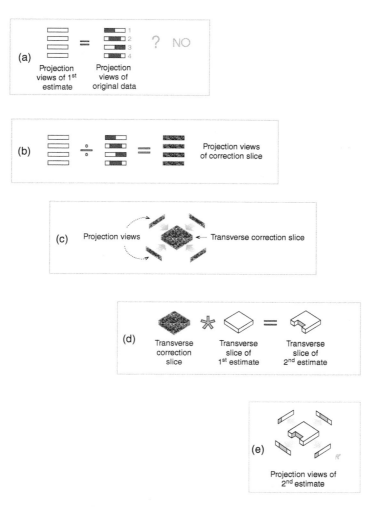

Figure 12.27 (a) Projection views from the first estimate are compared to the projections views from the original data. Note that projection views are oriented as seen by an outside observer looking toward the transaxial slice of the original data shown in Figure 12.24. (b) Correction projection views. (c) Transverse correction slice. (d) Second estimate transverse slice. (e) Second estimate projection views.

OSEM

One widely used iterative reconstruction technique is **the maximum likelihood expectation maximization (MLEM)** algorithm. The computation time is very lengthy when all of the projection views are used in each iteration to create the correction slices. To shorten the processing time a smaller group, or **subset**, of matched projection views from the estimated and original datasets are used for each iteration to create the correction slices. For each iteration, a different group or subset is used. Each subset consists of projection views sampled evenly over the entire arc of the acquisition, 180 or

360 degrees. For example, the first subset might contain every 12th projection view beginning with the first projection view. The second subset might contain every 12th projection view beginning with the sixth projection view, and so on. The process of using subsets for expectation maximization is called **ordered subsets expectation maximization (OSEM)**.

Another advantage of iterative reconstruction compared to filtered backprojection is that corrections for factors that degrade images such as attenuation, scatter, and even collimator and detector spatial resolution can be incorporated directly.

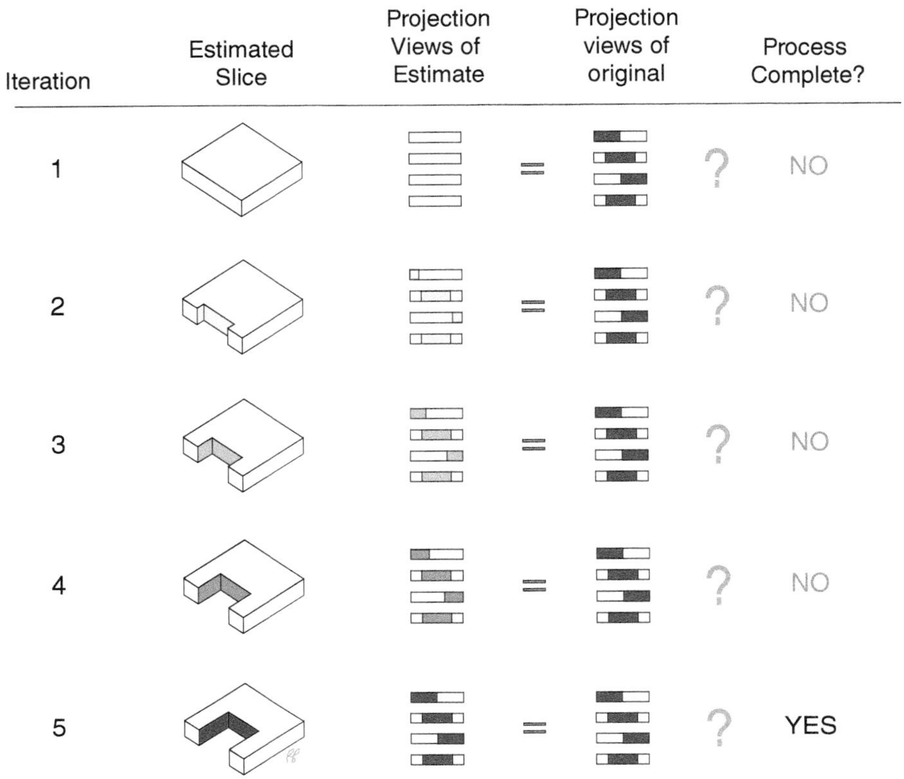

Iteration	Estimated Slice	Projection Views of Estimate		Projection views of original		Process Complete?
1			=		?	NO
2			=		?	NO
3			=		?	NO
4			=		?	NO
5			=		?	YES

Figure 12.28 Progression of five iterations.

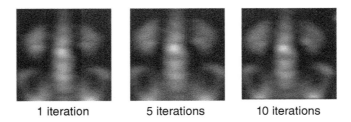

| 1 iteration | 5 iterations | 10 iterations |

Figure 12.29 Resolution improves with increasing iterations.

Iterative reconstruction internalizing correction of image degradation factors

Early implementations of iterative reconstruction algorithms were designed to replace filtered-backprojection algorithms and fit into the image reconstruction process in exactly the same way. As such, if corrections were to be made, for example for attenuation correction or for scatter, they would be performed on the projected data prior to reconstruction.

Designing algorithms to correct acquisition projection data for effects such as attenuation and scatter can be challenging and corrections for degradations such as the depth-dependent blurring due to collimator response, for example, might be impossible. With advances in iterative reconstruction, however, it is possible to achieve these corrections by simulating the degradation inside the iteration loop.

This iteration update essentially applies the correction by supplying an image estimate that when projected and degraded produces similar projections to the acquisition projections. Instead of corrected acquisition projection data being involved in the step that produces an update, the uncorrected acquisition projections are used in conjunction with the degraded projections of the image estimates to produce the update. This is illustrated in Figure 12.30.

Attenuation, scatter, variable spatial resolution (resolution degrades in the center of the field of view due to increasing distance from the collimator in SPECT imaging and degrades towards the edge of the field in PET imaging due to parallax error (see Chapter 8, PET)), random coincidences (in PET), even detector normalization (used for correction of variable crystal sensitivity in PET) can all be modeled fairly accurately and so applying this strategy in PET and SPECT generally results in improved image quality and quantitative estimates. The penalty is of course computational complexity. Correcting for photon attenuation is fairly simple computationally, however, scatter correction is complex and to model it accurately can be computationally burdensome. Also, scatter is a three-dimensional problem and fields of view are typically restricted to only a portion of the data set to be reconstructed so scatter due to activity outside the field won't be modeled properly.

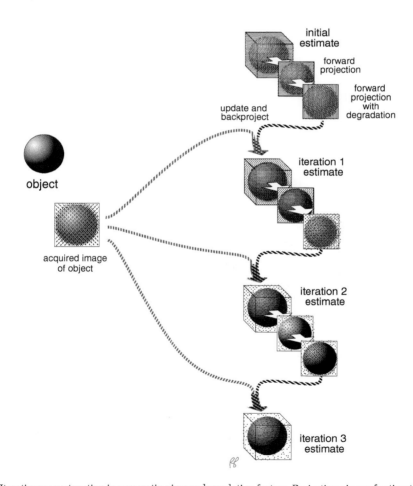

Figure 12.30 Iterative reconstruction incorporating image degradation factors. Projection views of estimates of the data are first altered by degradation factors, then combined with acquisition projection views for an updated projection view which is then backprojected into a new estimate of the object. The process is repeated for a predetermined number of steps, in this illustration for three iterations.

Resolution recovery

The term **resolution recovery** (also called **point-spread-function modeling or processing)** refers to a set of additional algorithms used during reconstruction that attempt to correct for "blurring" in the image data—essentially improving the spatial resolution. In a system that uses a traditional reconstruction approach, it is possible to employ a high-pass filter (for example the ramp filter in Figure 12.17 and the high-pass filter in Figure 12.18) which produces an image with better preservation of detail but greater noise. In modern iterative reconstruction, resolution recovery can be achieved by applying the blurring (resolution loss) to the projection estimates created during iterative reconstruction (as illustrated for other degradation factors in Figure 12.30). An additional advantage of this is that the model can be quite comprehensive—in other words, instead of a global, approximate burring model, blurring can change its character spatially which more accurately approximates what happens in a real imaging environment.

Postreconstruction image processing

Multiplanar reformatting

Stacks of transverse images can be resliced or resampled in a process called multiplanar reformatting.

From these reconstructed transverse images, **sagittal**, **coronal**, and oblique views can be generated. By convention, the transaxial slices are oriented perpendicular to the long axis of the body. Sagittal and coronal slices are oriented parallel to the long axis of the body and at right angles to each other (Figure 12.31). In a similar way, the axes of the heart are defined relative to the heart's long axis, understood to be the line running from base to apex. The **horizontal long axis view** and **vertical long axis view** are oriented parallel to the long axis of the heart. The **short axis view** is oriented perpendicular to the long axis of the heart (Figure 12.32). Multiplanar reformatted sliced images can be computed and saved in the computer or they can be produced live, at the time of display.

Advanced display techniques

Contrast enhancement

X-ray CT and some nuclear medicine images possess information over such a range of intensities that they cannot be displayed for a human observer to be able to see the intensity variations in the brightest and darkest portions of the image. This property of the image is referred to as **dynamic range**—formally defined as the ratio between the largest and smallest possible intensity changes.

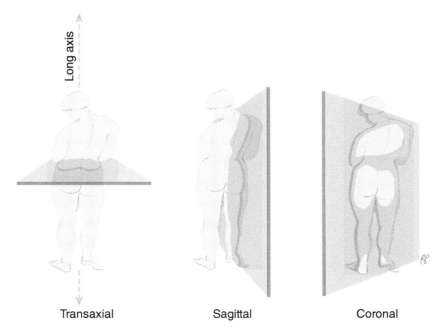

Figure 12.31 Transaxial, sagittal, and coronal images.

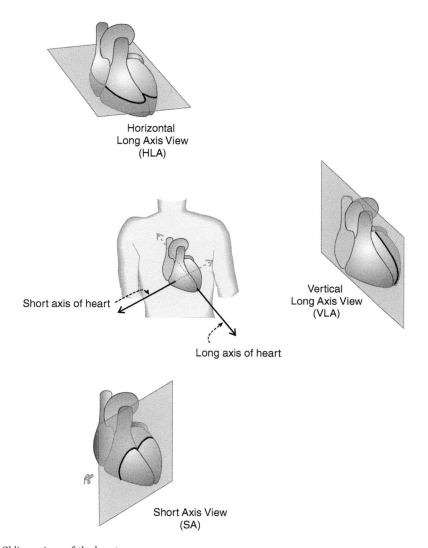

Figure 12.32 Oblique views of the heart.

Display monitors are usually setup to display 256 intensities (gray levels) and the mathematical operation of how to map the image values (perhaps thousands of intensities) onto the 256-level scale is known as contrast manipulation or **contrast enhancement** (not to be confused with the other common use of this phrase in reference to use of injected or ingested contrast materials for enhancing characteristics of anatomy during CT imaging). Contrast enhancement schemes can be quite sophisticated such as a mapping that exaggerates the differences between the darkest objects in an image and diminishes the differences between the brightest objects in the image.

Why reformatting works

Cross-sectional nuclear medicine image data acquired with SPECT or PET scanners typically have what is referred to as cubic or near-cubic voxels (voxels are the three dimensional equivalent of two dimensional pixels. A cubic voxel means that each side of the voxel is identical in length. As a result the spatial resolution in all three planes (axial, sagittal, and coronal) is identical. Therefore the stored image data can be sliced in any of the planes and retain consistent distances between points.

Another approach to contrast enhancement involves compressing the broad ranges of intensities within the entire image to fit into 256-levels. One can also expand the scale to cut off low and high intensities, such that anything below a certain value appears black and anything above another value appears white. This latter scheme is referred to in radiology as **windowing** (not to be confused with windowing in the filtering sense) where the mapping of contrast is defined by a window level—the data intensity value that will be assigned to 128 (half-intensity)—and the window width—the range of data intensities that fill the displayed brightness scale.

As discussed in Chapter 9 each pixel of a CT image can be assigned a Hounsfield unit which ranges from −1000 HU (air) to greater than 1000 (dense cortical bone). Portions of the dynamic range from −1000 to 1000 are mapped onto the 0 to 256 range of the display monitor. This greatly improves the image contrast for the type of tissue of interest. For example, selecting "lung windows" on the workstation might set the window level to −500 and width to 1500 and "bone windows" might set the level to 500 and width to 2000.These selections center the displayed intensity in the mid-range for the expected or typical CT number in that anatomical feature, i.e. −500 for lung features and 500 for bone features, and then a window width that preserves a broad range of intensities. Alternatively, the interpreter might select "liver windows" with a level of 95 and a width of only 100, thereby amplifying small intensity changes above and below the expected intensity in the liver. The three most commonly used windows, soft tissue, lung, and bone are depicted in Figure 12.33.

Windowing is so important in the analysis of CT images that the viewer can usually select a number of predefined window settings on the workstation.

Maximum intensity projections
Both SPECT and X-ray CT image data are so-called three-dimensional data because they represent underlying anatomy or physiology over three spatial dimensions. Conventional workstation display technology is really only capable of displaying two dimensional data. The conventional method of rendering three-dimensional data is to scroll through a set of consecutive slices.

These slices can be displayed as they are or they can be combined mathematically in a number of ways to form new images. Images formed from a number of underlying slices are called projections. If the formula used to form the computed slice takes the average of the projected slices then this is the **average projection**. If computation involves taking the maximum value through the slices that form the projection then this is called the **maximum intensity projection or MIP**.

MIP images formed for nuclear medicine image display and for CT imaging appear to be different but are really just slight variations of the same underlying scheme. The MIP image is most useful when the brightest features are the features of interest. Low-intensity features tend to get lost in the formation of the MIP. In nuclear medicine SPECT and PET, the MIP images are usually computed at a number of equally-spaced angles perpendicular to the long axis of the body (Figure 12.34) and then played back as a movie or a dynamic sequence called a cine-loop. In playing back the views, the observer has the impression that anatomical features are suspended in a somewhat transparent three-dimensional space that is rotating. The rotational motion is processed by the observer to give a sense of depth.

In CT imaging when very thin slices are acquired, maximum intensity projections are usually formed by processing groups of consecutive slices. Again, this is most useful in applications where the most intense features in images are of most interest, for example when intravenous contrast is used for imaging, or in cases where small details seen on only one slice would be lost by averaging information over several slices. The MIP collapses the most intense features of individual slices (indicated by arrows on slices A and B in Figure 12.35) onto two-dimensional depictions that contain these features (arrows in transverse MIP slice C in Figure 12.35) while still retaining some anatomical detail. Figure 12.36 demonstrates how a small pulmonary nodule is accentuated in a CT MIP image compared to an average intensity projection image.

Surface and volume rendering
Other types of three-dimensional displays of SPECT or CT data can be used to enhance presentation and can aid in interpretation. Two standard methods of

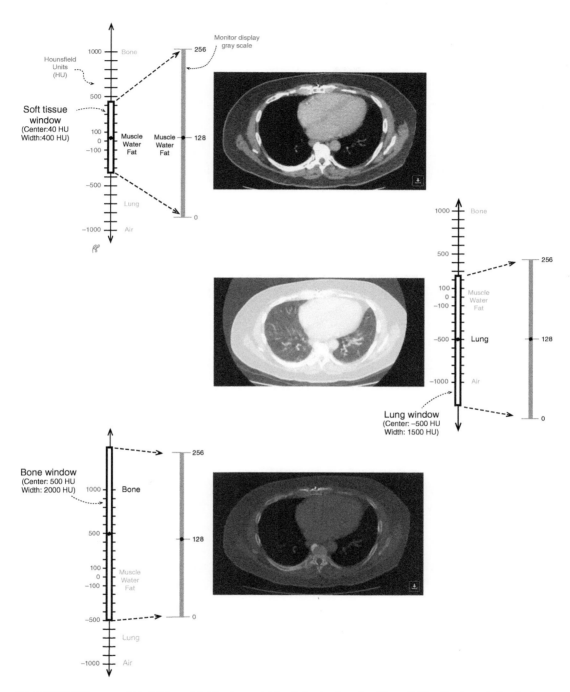

Figure 12.33 CT image contrast enhancement using variable windowing based on Hounsfield unit values. A standard range of Hounsfield units used to display soft tissue with a sample transaxial slice are shown at the top, ranges and images for lung and bone are shown in the middle and bottom respectively.

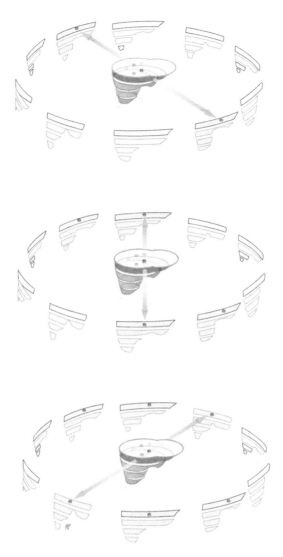

Figure 12.34 Nuclear medicine maximum intensity projection (MIP) image. The most intense feature (depicted by a dark gray sphere) along any ray is projected onto MIP images.

display surface rendering (visualization of the surface of the data), and volume rendering (a more transparent view of the data set) are available on many workstations.

Both surface and volume rendering depend on, as the first step, the ability to segment the image data into multiple separate regions. This process is performed automatically and works best when image features are easily classified by intensity. Such is the case for example in bony structures and airways in CT or for specific lesions or tracer-avid anatomy in SPECT images. When three-dimensional data are segregated into distinct regions representing tissue types they can then be

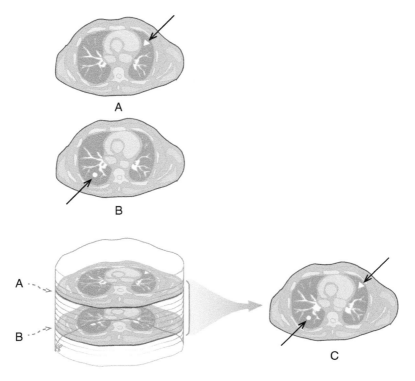

Figure 12.35 Maximum intensity projection (MIP) CT image collapses most intense features from several sequential slices into a single image.

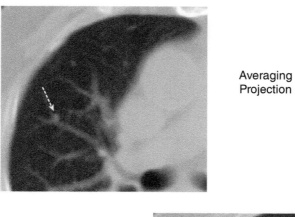

Averaging
Projection

Maximum Intensity
Projection

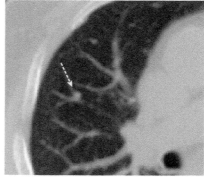

Figure 12.36 Maximum intensity projection image for lung CT image accentuates image detail.

processed by computer-graphics algorithms and depicted as virtual scenes. In this step, the tissues are treated as though they have real-world optical qualities such as color and texture. The graphics rendering assumes a position of the illumination source and computationally recreates what the observer would see by tracing light rays, transmitted from the source, get reflected off the surface model or get transmitted through and attenuated by portions of the volume model. An example of surface rendering of a portion of the skeleton from a CT scan is seen in Figure 12.37.

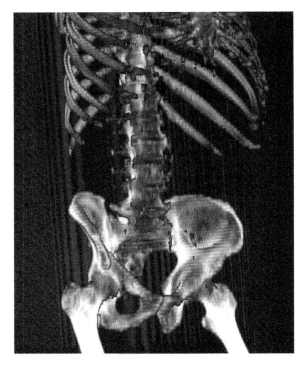

Figure 12.37 Skeletal tissue from a CT scan displayed using surface rendering. The tubular structures in the mid abdomen and in the pelvis are calcifications in the walls of the aorta and common iliac vessels.

Questions

1. Which of the following statements about filtering used in reconstruction is correct:
   (a) Filtering is used to reduce noise and preserve signal data in the image.
   (b) Filtering can only be applied to the data prior to back projection.
   (c) Filtering is used to reduce artifact created during backprojection.

2. True or false: The frequency domain can represent a spatial image as a sum of sine waves.

3. Match the following statements with either "low-pass filter" or "high-pass filter":
   (a) Used to remove high-frequency noise such as noise from statistical variation in counts.
   (b) Used to remove the "blur" from the backprojection artifact.
   (c) Can create "grainy" images, but preserve detail.
   (d) Creates "smoother" images, but image detail may be lost.

4. Which of the following statements about filters is correct?
   (a) The Nyquist frequency is 5.0 cycles/pixel.
   (b) The cutoff frequency of a filter is the minimum frequency the filter will pass.
   (c) Nyquist filters have an additional parameter called the order of the filter which controls the slope of the curve.
   (d) All of the above.
   (e) None of the above.

5. Which of the following statements are true about iterative reconstruction:
   (a) Due to long computational times "short-cut" techniques such as ordered subsets expectation maximization are often used in iterative reconstruction.
   (b) Successive iterations are performed until the projection views of the estimate closely approximate the original data or until a predefined number of iterations have been completed.

   (c) Newer iterative reconstruction algorithms incorporate image degradation factors (such as scatter, attenuation, etc).
   (d) All of the above.
   (e) None of the above.

6. Which of the following statements are true about resolution recovery:
   (a) Resolution recovery is applied during reconstruction to improve image resolution by reducing image "blurring".
   (b) Low-pass filters can be used during traditional filtered backprojection to improve resolution and preserve image detail.
   (c) Resolution recovery algorithms in iterative reconstruction improve image resolution by directly incorporating the blurring factor into projection estimates.

7. To correct for attenuation effects in SPECT imaging with ^{99m}Tc, the correction matrix might be based upon:
   (a) The transmission data from a single photon emission radionuclide source.
   (b) The known attenuation coefficient for 140 keV photons in tissue.
   (c) The transmission data from a CT X-ray beam.
   (d) None of the above.
   (e) All of the above.

8. True or false: MIP (maximum intensity projection) images for SPECT and PET are used to accentuate the brightest details in a study.

9. Windowing is important in CT imaging because:
   (a) The range of pixel values in a CT image is much greater than the 256 gray scale range available on a computer monitor.
   (b) The range of X-ray energies used to create the images must be reduced in order to see detail.
   (c) Only a small section of a CT image can be viewed at one time.

Answers

1. (a) and (c). Filtering can be applied before, during, and after backprojection, so (b) is incorrect.
2. True.
3. (a) Low-pass filter. (b) High-pass filter. (c) High-pass filter. (d) Low-pass filter.
4. (e) The Nyquist frequency is 0.5 cycles/pixel, the cutoff frequency refers to the maximum frequency the filter will pass, and only the Hann and Butterworth filters have the additional parameter called the order of the filter.
5. (d).
6. (a) and (c). (b) has nothing to do with resolution recovery and is not correct because low-pass filters produce smoothed images with less detail. High-pass filters produce "noisier", higher resolution images with greater image detail.
7. (e).
8. True.
9. (a).

CHAPTER 13
Information Technology

Just as we encounter every day in our world resources that are increasingly interconnected by an electronic infrastructure, so has the radiology and nuclear medicine environment evolved. Imaging devices are no longer stand-alone pieces of equipment but now operate as intelligent nodes in a networked environment. A sample networked radiology environment is shown in Figure 13.1.

Network

Imaging devices, work stations and computers are connected within the hospital or department over a **local area network** (LAN) using a set of standards built upon Ethernet communications. The basis of Ethernet communications is that communicating devices share a common medium for communication and that data is broken up into packets that are sent out over the network and then reassembled at the destination. When a device wishes to send an information packet to another device then it essentially attaches an address to the data and sends it out on the network. The network takes care of routing it to the destination whether it's across the room or across the world.

For a number of reasons to do with security and efficiency, rather than the entire world (or **wide-area network**, WAN) communicating on the same medium, the Ethernet is organized as a set of inter-connected local-area networks (LANs). Data flows unimpeded between nodes of the same LAN but must go through a gate-way when it needs to be delivered to another LAN or to the WAN. In addition, the gateway might perform some security operations to, for example, make certain destinations inaccessible or to block certain types of communications from

entering the LAN. This is particularly important in a hospital environment where images and patient-related data must be protected from being accessible to people beyond those directly involved in patient care. In fact, when information flows on the WAN, there is no way to control what other machines do with it. Therefore, if images or data were to be sent out over the network, even if the destination was a trusted computer for example in a referring doctor's office, there is no way to ensure that a copy wasn't made by one of the machines that was involved in routing the packets.

As the utility of a broadly connected network architecture has grown over the years, the issues associated with security and protecting data have become more pressing. It is not uncommon in hospital environments to have to connect imaging equipment at a remote location into the clinic's LAN structure. One example of this situation might be a SPECT camera located at a remote clinic. Another example might be the diagnostic worksta-tions used on holidays and off-hours for performing emergency image interpretation. In both situations you have two LANs that must be connected over the public WAN while maintaining a secure environ-ment. The technology for this structure is referred to as a **virtual private network** (VPN). Software operating on both LANs intercepts all the traffic and encrypts it for communication before it is released onto the public internet. This way, even if an unau-thorized computer were to make a copy of the data during transit, the data would be nonsensical with-out access to the encryption details.

Just like the internet itself, hospital networks have evolved to become part of the critical infrastructure

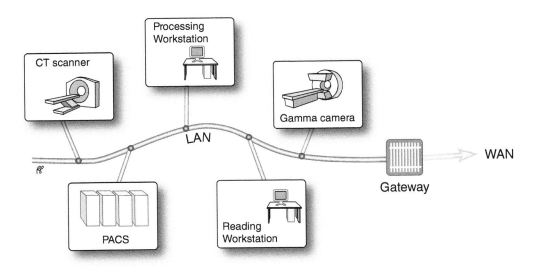

Figure 13.1 Simplified network diagram for a radiology department.

that binds increasingly distributed, flexible, and often mobile resources. The term **cloud computing** is used when the physical location of the devices that enable the image workflow becomes unimportant—they are virtually present merely by connecting to the network. PACS storage is increasingly cloud-based and some computing resources like 3D rendering computers for example are implemented as cloud services, i.e. the software runs on a virtual computer whose location is unknown and can change. There are several advantages of this type of architecture.

DICOM

Most modern diagnostic imaging devices are now built to communicate using a standard referred to as DICOM (digital imaging and communications in medicine). The DICOM standard is a set of rules that establishes the manner in which image data is transmitted from one machine to another and also imposes a structure on the radiological data. A **DICOM information object** consists of image data and associated information such as, for example, patient name, date of birth and time of acquisition. The nonimage portion of the DICOM data is often referred to as the "header," the pieces of information are "fields" and these fields have names that are referred to as "tags." The tag names are generally descriptive. For example, the patient's date of

birth is stored as an eight-character sequence representing year, month and day in a DICOM field with the tag-name "PatientBirthDate." A diagram representing a DICOM information object is shown in Figure 13.2.

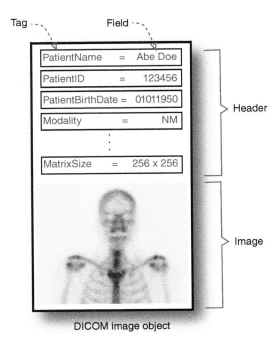

Figure 13.2 DICOM information object containing image and header.

The DICOM image and header data are packaged for communication or storage in a manner that they cannot be easily separated. A single DICOM object contains a large and variable number of header tags but contains only one image—say one radiographic view or one slice from a multislice CT scan, but this image can have multiple frames. In nuclear medicine studies packaged as DICOM objects, it is common to use the multi-frame format to encode the sequence of projections from a SPECT study as well as the sequence of frames recorded in a dynamic study.

Many of the DICOM header tags are common to all examination types. Some examples of such fields are the patient name (PatientName), date of birth, (PatientBirthDate) and the name of the institution where the examination was performed (InstitutionName). Other tags are modality-specific such as the kVp (KVP) and mA (XrayTubeCurrent) of a CT scan. The modality itself is coded as a two-letter sequence in the modality tag. Modality codes for CT, PET, MRI and nuclear medicine are CT, PT, MR and NM respectively. All DICOM-compliant devices can generally understand the structure and store or send DICOM information objects regardless of modality but they do not need to be capable of interpreting and displaying each object. For example, a particular display workstation might be able to receive and display planar X-rays and slices from a CT examination and receive PET images, but might not be able to display PET images correctly.

DICOM is, strictly speaking, a communications protocol that has evolved to also function as a universal storage format. Its adoption by all the major vendors of medical imaging devices has helped to impose a uniform structure on how a radiological exam is structured. In DICOM terminology medical images are grouped into one or more **series** which are then grouped together as a **study**. Studies and series have **unique identifiers** (UIDs) which consist of a long sequence of numerals. Study, series and image UIDs are generated by the scanner at the time of creation in such a way as to be globally unique. They are never reused and they can never be duplicated by any other scanner in the world. Studies and series usually have names (StudyDescription, SeriesDescription) which are either chosen at the discretion of the technologist, or selected from a standard set used in an institution. An example of this type of hierarchical organization

is shown in Figure 13.3. In this exam the study is a SPECT/CT parathyroid scan which consists of four series with the series descriptions, "Ant Pinhole", "Transverse NM", "Transaxial CT", and "Fused Transverse". Each series contains one or more dicom image objects. By convention, as discussed above, the transverse slices from the SPECT scan are stored as a single multiframe dicom image object whereas each transaxial CT slice and each transverse fused slice are stored as individual dicom image objects.

Images acquired by a hybrid machine such as SPECT/CT or PET/CT, will have an additional DICOM tag, the "**FrameOf ReferenceUID**", with a unique value common to both series. This lets a reading workstation know that the two series share a common reference frame or axes coordinates and so the workstation software can perform the image fusion at the time of display.

Since image fusion is a relatively sophisticated and special-purpose function, many reading workstations don't have fusion capability. It's therefore common in PET/CT and SPECT/CT workflows to perform the fusion once and then save the fused series. Such a synthetic image is referred to as a **secondary capture** and is tagged with the modality code '**SC**' or alternatively "**SS**" (save screen). SC images series are picture objects that typically lose their quantitative information (CT data is no longer readable in HUs for example it just becomes a grayscale image that looks like the CT data with a fixed window width and level setting). The series labeled "Fused Transverse" in Figure 13.3 is a set of secondary capture DICOM objects. They are a particular view (window width and level settings and color map choice) of a fused version of the NM transverse and CT transverse series that have been recaptured as a sequence of pictures.

In addition to image objects, DICOM defines a number of other information objects, an example of which is a **structured report** (SR). There are many kinds of DICOM SR objects but one example is the radiation dose structured report (RDSR) that is associated with CT exams. The RDSR is a series object within an exam and is communicated and stored just like an image. It cannot be rendered on a reading workstation unless the workstation software is able to decode the structure and interpret and present the contents. RDSR objects are used to store technique factors and additional data about the exam that enables calculation of radiation dose.

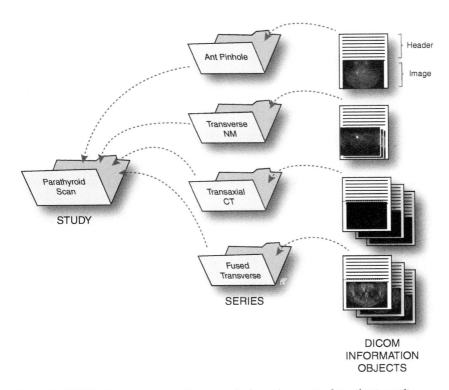

Figure 13.3 DICOM objects are grouped in series which are then grouped together in studies.

PACS

At the heart of the modern electronic radiology or nuclear medicine clinic is a **picture archiving and communications system** (PACS). The PACS in a large radiology department can consist of a large number of computers with various specialized roles or it could be just a single computer attached to the network that communicates information between a few imaging devices and workstations. One of the central roles for the PACS is the storage of image data and in this respect, it is the functional equivalent of what used to be the film archive. Image information is stored in the PACS archive, usually on hard disk drives but also on various types of media such as DVDs. As discussed earlier in this chapter PACS storage is becoming increasingly cloud-based.

In general, the DICOM format is used for PACS storage and communication. This enhances the compatibility of the various systems since modality computers, workstation and various other imaging components generally have DICOM capabilities. This may not be the case throughout the system however as vendor-specific formats and protocols might be used to gain a speed advantage or to compress data for storage.

The set of networked computers and associated software that comprises the PACS might also have various other capabilities. It is common in modern hospital environments for the PACS to be capable of transferring image data to CDs or DVDs that can then be sent to referring doctors or given to patients. In addition, there is sometimes a need to print hard-copy (paper, photographic paper, or maybe film) of images that reside in the PACS archive. The computers used by radiologists for diagnostic read-out and by technologists for management and quality control purposes are also often considered to be part of the PACS infrastructure. And finally, many PACS networks have the ability to modify their images in such a way that they can be viewed with a standard web-browser or with a simple piece of software referred to as a thin-client.

Information systems

The modern electronic clinic needs to communicate not just image information but also information to assist the clinical workflow. Information such as radiology reports and scheduling and billing procedures are examples of electronic information that isn't part of the image object and for which there are no DICOM capabilities. The management and communication of this type of information is the job of the **radiology information system** (RIS). The RIS computers are also connected via the network and use a language called **HL7** (health level seven, an international standard for communication) to code the information.

Other departments in the hospital such as pathology or various clinics are also typically highly integrated and dependent on digital information and computer communication. The collection of computers that manage information at the hospital level and communicate with the RIS and department-level information systems are referred to as the **hospital information system** (HIS).

Information systems for hospital environments are developed in a highly dynamic milieu. The exact information responsibilities of the HIS, RIS or PACS are not well defined or "nailed-down" by standards and so they vary by vendor and product. An international collaboration referred to as **Integrating the Healthcare Environment** (IHE) is an effort to promote standardization for information sharing within the hospital environment. IHE has representation from governments, industry and professional organizations and in particular from the radiology and nuclear medicine community. Standardization of information sharing will facilitate communication between components of the information systems within hospitals while reducing the need for extensive local customization.

Figure 13.4 shows a sample topology for a radiology department working within a HIS/RIS environment.

Additional DICOM capabilities

There are two DICOM functions that are not really integral to the coding and communication of image data but are important for facilitating the flow of information between modalities, the PACS and the HIS/RIS. These are the **DICOM modality worklist** (DMWL) and the **modality performed procedure step** (MPPS). The associated structure and protocols are defined as part of the DICOM standard.

A **worklist server** is a computer on the network that obtains scheduling and demographic information from the radiology information system (RIS) and sends this information out in the form of DMWL messages to modality workstations in response to "worklist queries". From this message the modality computer obtains an accurate set of patient and study-related data that can be used to populate the subsequent DICOM information fields. In this manner the DMWL message ensures information precision and reduces the problems caused by errors during manual entries. For example, in preparing the scanner for a patient study, the technologist might simply query the worklist server and select the next patient by name or medical record number. The DMWL message would then transmit other information such as date of birth, exact patient name, various control numbers, the exact name of the procedure and so on.

The MPPS on the other hand, provides a way for the modality-related computers to pass information back to the RIS or the PACS containing information about progress within a study. Essentially there are two types of messages, one to inform the system that a procedure has been started (N-CREATE) and another to convey that a procedure has been completed (N-SET). The MPPS completion message also contains a list of all the images created during the procedure which makes it possible for the PACS or RIS to determine whether it received a complete study.

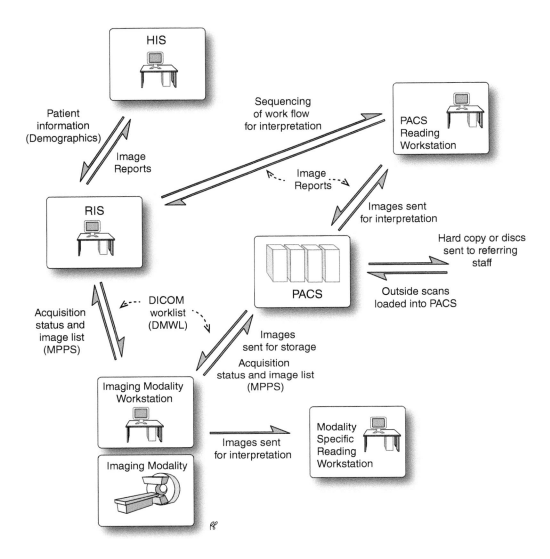

Figure 13.4 Schematic of the information exchange between components of the radiology and hospital computer systems.

Questions

1. A physician in California wants to send SPECT images across the country to her colleague in Massachusetts for a second opinion on a case. To insure privacy, she could do which of the following:

   (a) Send a CD containing the images using a trusted courier service.

   (b) Attach snapshots of the images to an e-mail.

   (c) Upload the snapshots of images to a web-based picture-sharing service and simply not tell anyone else except the physician colleague how to access the images.

   (d) Send the DICOM images using the VPN that was set up by IT departments in the two institutions.

2. If the DICOM worklist server computer is temporarily not functioning correctly, which of the following scenarios might ensue and have an impact on the clinic?

   (a) Packets get lost or routed incorrectly and drop-out artifacts may appear in the images.

   (b) Patient scheduling information will not be available and so the front-office staff cannot book future appointments.

   (c) Technologists will have to enter patient information manually in the modality worksta-

   tion computers and may make typographical errors that will need to be fixed at a later time.

   (d) The record of which studies were performed will be lost and so billing information will have to be entered manually.

3. When the physician is accessing a SPECT/CT study on the PACS system, he encounters some missing CT slices. Which of the following is the likely cause and potential solution?

   (a) The CT scanner likely stopped collecting data for a brief period during the study. Put the patient back into the scanner and reacquire the study.

   (b) The PACS workstation that the physician is using is probably faulty. The physician should log in to another workstation and re-access the study.

   (c) Due to a network error, some CT slices were lost when the study was transmitted from the modality workstation to the PACS system. Retransmit the study.

   (d) There may be simply a delay somewhere in the system. Wait for 5 minutes and try to access the study again on the PACS.

Answers

1. (a) and (d). E-mail is not generally secure and could be intercepted by a third party. Web-based photo or picture sharing-sites are not generally secure even if it seems unlikely that a third party would view the images.
2. (c) The worklist server communicates patient demographics from the RIS or HIS and avoids errors associated with manual entry.
3. (c) is the most likely. (d) is possible—in a congested network environment and complicated transfers of large amounts of data between multiple computers, it is possible to accumulate significant delays.

CHAPTER 14

Quality Control

To ensure dependable performance of equipment, each nuclear medicine department is required to perform a routine series of tests on each device. These tests comprise the quality control program for the department.

Nonimaging devices

Dose calibrator

The testing performed on dose calibrators is quite rigorous to ensure that correct radiopharmaceutical doses are administered to patients. Dose calibrators are checked for accuracy, constancy, linearity, and geometry.

Accuracy

Accuracy is a measure of the readings of the dose calibrator in comparison to well-accepted standards. Two long-lived nuclide sources, such as ^{137}Cs (half-life = 30 years) and ^{57}Co (half-life = 270 days), are measured repeatedly in the calibrator and the average readings are compared to values issued by the **National Institute of Standards and Technology (NIST)** for that particular source. If a reading differs from the standard by more than 10%, the dose calibrator should not be used. Accuracy should be checked at *installation*, *annually*, and *after repairs* or *when the instrument is moved* to a new location within the clinic.

Constancy

To ensure that the calibrator readings are constant from day to day, a long-lived nuclide such as ^{137}Cs is measured in the dose calibrator. The reading should not vary by more than 10% from the value recorded at the initial accuracy test corrected for the decay of

the standard. In addition, a test called a "channel check" is usually performed in conjunction with the constancy measurement. With the source in place, the dose calibrator is measured on a number of predefined settings (or "channels")—e.g. ^{99m}Tc, ^{131}I, ^{67}Ga, etc. This test is a hold-over from the days when the dose calibrator relied on stable gains to be maintained for the separate analog circuits (the channels) used to scale the ionization current measurement. Each of those channels needed to be calibrated independently. In a modern dose calibrator, scaling of the ionization current is done digitally and there so there is only one common gain and a single constancy measurement should suffice. However, many calibrators do have the ability to alter the calibration constants associated with individual radionuclides through a setup procedure. The channel check, which has become a nuclear medicine hot lab morning ritual, does serve the purpose of checking that the instrument hasn't been reprogrammed inadvertently.

The channel-check results are recorded and compared to previous readings. **Constancy** (including the channel checks) is performed *daily*.

Linearity

Linearity tests the calibrator over the range of doses used, from the an activity higher that what would ever be administered to a patient (in the 10 s of mCi to hundreds of mCi depending on the clinic) down to a value lower than would ever need to be measured clinically (usually 10 μCi). One method of checking linearity is to measure the maximum activity such as 7.4 GBq (200 mCi) of ^{99m}Tc, and to repeat the measurement at regular intervals such as 6, 24, 30, and 48, and 96 hours. A more rapid technique is to

Essentials of Nuclear Medicine Physics, Instrumentation, and Radiation Biology, Fourth Edition.
Rachel A. Powsner, Matthew R. Palmer, and Edward R. Powsner.
© 2022 John Wiley & Sons Ltd. Published 2022 by John Wiley & Sons Ltd.

measure the dose unshielded, then repeat the measurement of the same dose shielded within **lead sleeves** of varying thickness. The thickness of the sleeves is such that when used both individually and in combination they effectively reproduce the decline in activity of the ^{99m}Tc seen over 96 hours (Figure 14.1). The sleeves should be carefully examined prior to use; they will not yield accurate readings if there are any cracks or dents. The initial

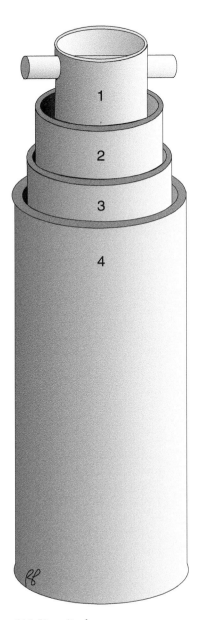

Figure 14.1 Linearity sleeves.

linearity check should be performed with the slower method of measuring a sample as it decays. Linearity should be checked at *installation* of the device, *quarterly*, and *after repairs* or *when the instrument is moved* to a new location within the clinic.

Geometry

The apparent activity of a dose might vary with the volume and shape of the container and the position of the dose within the chamber. The effect of sample **geometry** can be tested by placing a small amount of activity at the bottom of a container and progressively adding a diluent such as water. This procedure should be repeated for each type of container used within the laboratory—vials, syringes, bottles, and so on. The left side of Figure 14.2 illustrates photon absorption in a relatively large volume of diluent; the right side illustrates photon loss through the calibrator opening when the sample is placed in a taller container. If measurements vary by more than 10% for certain geometries then the measurement can be used to derive a correction factor to apply to subsequent samples with that specific geometry. Geometry should be checked at *installation* and *after repairs*.

Survey meters

Constancy

Daily battery checks and constancy tests should be performed. For the constancy test a long-lived radioactive source should be checked *daily* to ensure that the meter reading of the source is constant (within 10% of its original value). If the reading differs by more than 10% of the original value, the survey meter should be recalibrated. Typically, a tiny amount of radioactivity, a "check-source" is attached directly to the side of the survey meter to make it quick and easy to perform the constancy check.

Calibration

All survey meters, including Geiger counters, must be checked for accuracy. To do so, readings are taken from two long-lived sources (^{57}Co and ^{137}Cs) at incremental distances (such as every tenth of a meter up to one meter) from the sources. The sources should be radioactive enough to generate readings at approximately one-third and two-thirds of full scale. The readings must be within 20% of their expected measurement. This test should be

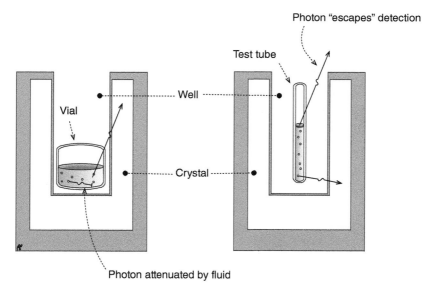

Figure 14.2 Variation in sample geometry.

performed at *installation*, *after repairs*, and *annually*. A typical nuclear medicine clinic usually doesn't possess the sources required to perform the calibration and so the survey meters are usually sent out to an accredited calibration laboratory.

Crystal scintillation detectors: well counters and thyroid probes

Calibration

On a *daily* basis or prior to each patient measurement the photopeak is checked using a long-lived nuclide reference source (usually ^{137}Cs) which is placed in the well counter or in front of the probe. The voltage or gain settings are adjusted manually or, more commonly automatically for the maximum peak (count rate); the settings and the peak count rate should be recorded. The count rate should not differ from the previous average values or a similarly established value by more than 10%. The full-width half-maximum (FWHM) of the photopeak should be <10% of the energy of the photopeak. In addition to daily checks, calibration should be routinely performed as well *annually* and *following repairs*.

Efficiency

This *annual* test of the sensitivity of the detector is performed using reference standard sources with similar energy emissions to the nuclides measured routinely in the well counter or in front of the thyroid probe. For

example for the thyroid probe barium-133 (principal gamma emission 356 keV) can be used as a reference for iodine-131 (364 keV) and cobalt-57 (122 keV) can be used for iodine-123 (157 keV).

A tiny amount of radioactivity (a few hundred nCi to a few µCi) is placed in the well counter or on the face of or inside the collimator of the thyroid probe. The activity must be low enough so that the deadtime losses are minimal and large enough to get a few thousand counts within the count interval.

The **efficiency** of the thyroid probe or well counter can be calculated using the following equation:

$$\frac{\text{Efficiency in cpm}}{\text{dpm}} = \frac{\left[\binom{\text{counts per minute}}{\text{of standard}} - \binom{\text{counts per minute}}{\text{of background}} \right]}{\binom{\text{activity of standard in}}{\text{Bq} \times 60\, \text{s / min}}}$$

This result is often multiplied by 100 and expressed as a percent value. Remember that one becquerel equals one decay per second.

Chi-square test

The chi-square test is a simple statistical method for checking the reliability of the thyroid probe or well counter. Since nuclear decay is a random phenomenon the precision of measurement is limited by relatively low counts and is therefore referred to as

count-limited. Repeated measurements of a sample of radioactivity yield estimates that form a statistical distribution. The name of the distribution is the Poisson distribution and when the expected number of counts per sample exceeds about 10 (almost always the case), the shape of a Poisson distribution is well approximated by a Gaussian (normal or bell-shaped) distribution. In a chi-square test, a sequence of samples is tested to determine if the variability in the measurement is well characterized by a Gaussian shape. The chi-square test is performed with a long-lived source, usually ^{137}Cs. The recommended frequency of this test varies by manufacturer. It's performed at least annually for well-counters and thyroid probes and sometimes more frequently.

See box for an example of a chi-square calculation.

Sample chi-square test

A ^{137}Cs source is counted 10 times by the thyroid probe and the sum of the counts, the mean of the counts, the difference between the counts and the mean, and the square of each count minus the mean is calculated (last column). The latter values are summed and divided by the mean.

Sample	Counts (N)	Mean ($\bar{N}$)	Counts-$\bar{N}$	(Counts-$\bar{N}$)²
1	32392	3257	−178	31684
2	32523	3257	−47	2209
3	32597	3257	27	729
4	32795	3257	225	50625
5	32666	3257	96	9216
6	32619	3257	49	2401
7	32593	3257	23	529
8	32887	3257	317	100489
9	32240	3257	−330	108900
10	32387	3257	−183	33489

Sum of the counts (Σ) = 325700			Sum of (Counts $-\bar{N}$)² =	340271
The mean $\bar{N}$			χ^2 = Sum of (Counts	
= Σ/10 =	**32570**		$-\bar{N}$)² / $\bar{N}$ =	10.4

The formula representing this calculation is

$$\chi^2 = \frac{\sum_1^N \left(N - \bar{N}\right)^2}{\bar{N}}$$

For the equipment to pass the chi-square test the χ^2 value (called the chi-square statistic) the probablility that this statistic describes a group of samples that comply with a normal distribution typically must be between 10% and 90% (which are sample acceptable threshold values for this test). Probabilities for chi-square values are found in a table of chi-square critical values. To use the table one must first calculate the degrees of freedom (DF) for the data. In this case DF = (number of samples) − 1 = 10−1 = 9. Chi square statistics corresponding to probability values from the table for a DF of 9 are:

Probability	99%	95%	**90%**	**10%**	5%	1%
χ^2	2.088	3.325	**4.168**	**14.684**	16.919	21.666

The chi-square statistic from our example is 10.4 which is between the chi-square values for 10% and 90% probability and therefore the equipment passes the test.

Imaging

Planar gamma camera

Photopeak

Prior to imaging, the pulse-height analyzer may require adjustment to properly center the window of photon energies accepted. The procedure of adjustment differs from camera to camera.

One simple procedure for checking the location of the energy window is to place a vial or syringe containing a small quantity of isotope against the collimator. The computer screen displays a plot of counts vs. energy and the current location of the window (see Figure 5.6). The user can then adjust the location and width of the window. For example, a standard setting for technetium-99m is a photopeak of 140 keV and a window of 20%. The window is set between 126 keV and 154 keV. A narrower window rejects more scattered photons but also reduces the number of acquired counts. Newer cameras automate this process by identifying the photopeak of ^{57}Co (122 keV) from the flood source.

Drift of the energy windows away from the peak will lead to significant artifacts in images. Off-center windows will yield relatively "hot" or "cold" photomultiplier defects on the daily uniformity floods. Figure 14.3 presents images of a uniform source acquired with varying energy windows. In the upper images the energy window is centered above the photopeak, in the lower images the window is centered below the photopeak.

Uniformity floods

Ideally, a scintillation camera should produce a uniform image of a uniform source. Unfortunately, this ideal is not met due to imperfections in the collimators, variations in crystal response, differences among photomultiplier tubes' response, and minor fluctuations in the electrical circuitry.

The uniformity of the camera's response can be checked by imaging a uniform distribution called a "flood source". There are two ways to create a flood source: **extrinsically** (i.e. with the collimators in place) using a planar source of radioactivity large enough to cover the entire field of view and, **intrinsically** (collimators removed) using a point source of radioactivity located centrally but far

enough from the detector so that it appears to be uniform (typically five times the largest detector dimension). In a variant of the intrinsic flood geometry, a point source located closer to the detector can be imaged and then an image processing step called a "curvature-correction" can be applied to convert what looks like a large bright spot at the center of the image to a uniformly illuminated field. The advantage of this is that the point can be located inside the gantry and both detectors flooded at the same time. The disadvantage is that while the expected counts can be restored mathematically using the curvature correction algorithm, the statistical variations in those peripheral pixels is greater since that signal has been amplified. This means that curvature correct floods usually need more counts to achieve uniformity check with required precision.

Sheet-sources are most commonly constructed as large plastic plates with 5 to 20 mCi of ^{57}Co uniformly distributed throughout their extent. Fillable sheet sources have been used in the past but these are now obsolete. The typical routine for daily floods is to acquire a 5- to 30-million-count image. The minimum acquisition will be recommended by the manufacturer.

Daily assessment of uniformity

Images of the flood source should be collected and examined *daily*. The human eye can discern some degree of variation in counts. A uniform flood image is shown in Figure 14.4. If the image is not uniform, corrective action is required. An example of nonuniformity is shown in Figure 14.5, where a large, rounded defect suggests malfunction of a photomultiplier tube. This corresponds to a similar defect in an image of the thyroid. Less common, but more serious, is the sharply demarcated defect caused by a crack in the crystal (Figure 14.6). These defects are detectable with or without the collimator in place. A subtler example of nonuniformity, from slow drift in the energy window circuitry over a period of three weeks, is shown in Figure 14.7. A damaged collimator can cause linear photopenic defects.

In addition to the visual inspection of the flood image, software is usually available on the camera or workstation to perform mathematical uniformity analysis. The steps involved in this analysis are defined by NEMA [1] and are as follows:

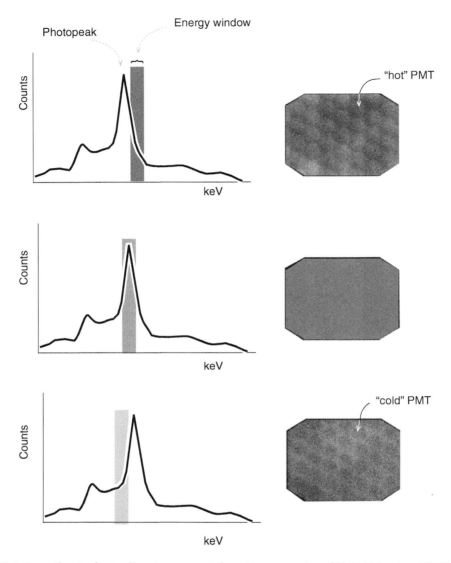

Figure 14.3 Nonuniformity due to off-center energy windows. (Images courtesy of Philip Livingston, CNMT.)

1. The image is re-sampled or "re-binned" onto a 64 × 64 grid.
2. The 64 × 64 pixel image is slightly smoothed by a simple filter.
3. The **field of view** (FOV) is categorized in two regions—the **useable field of view** (UFOV) which is the entire image FOV minus perhaps one or two pixels along the edges, and the **central field of view** (CFOV) which is defined as the central area with sides of 75% of the dimensions of UFOV. Note that the UFOV and CFOV relate to the uniformly-flooded portion of the image which may not have completely filled the image matrix.

4. Two types of **uniformity indexes** (UIs) are defined: The **integral uniformity** refers to the uniformity index over all pixels in the respective FOV and the **differential uniformity** which is calculated on sliding "bands" of five rows or columns at a time. For each FOV, a single integral uniformity is calculated and a large number of horizontal and vertical differential uniformities are calculated with the worst case (highest index) being reported as differential uniformity.

In each case, the formula employed is Index = $100\% \times (\text{max} - \text{min}) / (\text{max} + \text{min})$.

Figure 14.4 Uniform flood field.

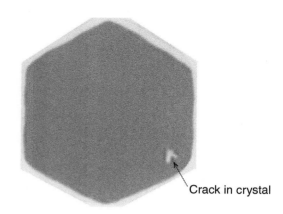

Crack in crystal

Figure 14.6 Cracked crystal.

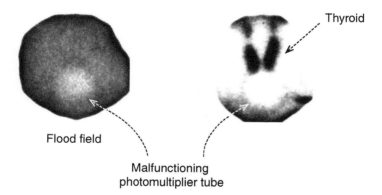

Thyroid

Flood field

Malfunctioning
photomultiplier tube

Figure 14.5 Defective photomultiplier tube.

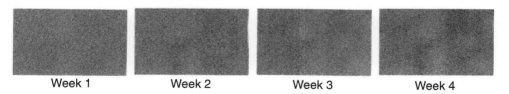

Week 1   Week 2   Week 3   Week 4

Figure 14.7 Nonuniformity due to a drift in circuitry.

An example of this uniformity analysis is seen in Figure 14.8.

Correction of nonuniformity

Even when perfectly tuned, a gamma camera detector does not intrinsically acquire a uniform image when it is flooded uniformly. Achieving that requires multiplication of acquired data by a **uniformity correction matrix**. This correction matrix is determined when the camera is setup and periodically during operation—either at fixed intervals like every six months for example or following maintenance, or when the uniformity begins to degrade. To establish the correction matrix, a source is located exactly as it would be for a uniformity testing and a large number of counts acquired—typically 50 to 100 million for a large area detector. The system then retains a scaled, possibly smoothed and inverted version of this high-count image as the correction map, or set of

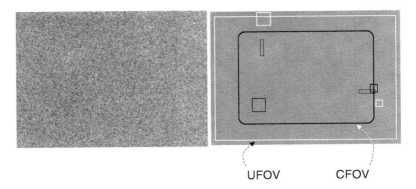

UFOV   CFOV

Figure 14.8 Uniformity analysis image. The acquired image of the flood source is seen on the left and a smoothed version on the right. UFOV and CFOV are labeled. The maximum global counts for each FOV can be found in the center of the larger squares and the minimum global counts in the center of the smaller squares (coded by outline shade to match the UFOV and CFOV outlines). These values are used to calculate the integral uniformity. The narrow rectangles outlined in dashed lines identify the columnar and row regions of greatest variability in counts and are used to calculate the differential uniformity.

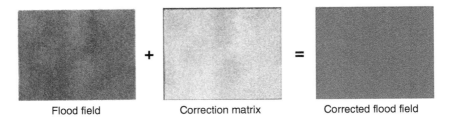

Flood field   Correction matrix   Corrected flood field

Figure 14.9 Uniformity correction matrix.

correction factors applied to subsequent acquired images.

Figure 14.9 is a simplistic representation of the application of a uniformity correction matrix.

Spatial resolution

Bar phantom: The resolution of the imaging system can be evaluated visually by imaging a **bar phantom**. One type of bar phantom is made of lead bars encased in lucite. The phantom is divided into four quadrants, and the bars within each quadrant are spaced in regular intervals; the bar spacing is different in each quadrant. The intervals illustrated in Figure 14.10 are an example of one such phantom, however, the spacing of the bars varies between manufacturers.

The flood source is imaged with the bar phantom placed between it and the collimator. The quadrant with the closest bar spacing that can be distinguished

is a measurement of the resolution of the system. The spatial resolution is checked *weekly* (or at intervals recommended by the manufacturer) for degradation of resolution.

With the bar phantom depicted in Figure 14.10, placed directly on the collimator and illuminated from above by the sheet source, you will typically be able to see bars spaced at 3.5 mm and maybe even 3.18 mm. The example in Figure 14.10 was performed with the collimator removed, the resolution is better than that which will be seen with the collimator in place, in this case bar spacing at 3.18 mm is clearly seen and 2.5 mm spacing is faintly visualized.

Linearity
Linearity of the gamma camera image is tested by examining the image of the bar phantom obtained with a high-resolution collimator in place. The lines in the image should be straight and unbroken. Note

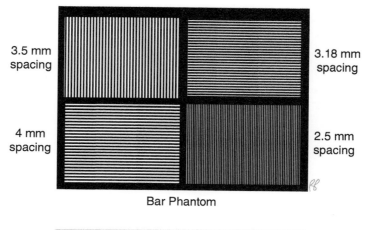

3.5 mm
spacing

3.18 mm
spacing

4 mm
spacing

2.5 mm
spacing

Bar Phantom

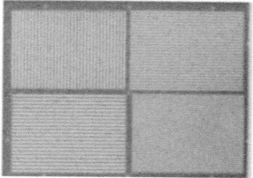

Image with Bar Phantom placed
between flood source and crystal

Figure 14.10 Bar phantom.

that linearity here refers to the appearance of the bars as lines, whereas the same word in reference to the dose calibrator refers to the relationship between dose and meter reading.

Spatial resolution and distance from source

The bar phantom can be used to demonstrate that spatial resolution decreases as the distance between the source and the camera increases, as shown in Figure 14.11. In the images on the left, the bar phantom is placed directly on the collimator; the minimum resolvable bar spacing is 3.2 mm. On the right, the phantom is positioned 12 cm away from the collimator, and the minimum resolvable bar spacing is 4.8 mm.

SPECT

The following additional quality control procedures are necessary for SPECT cameras. The frequency of performance of these tests will vary according to the manufacturer recommendations.

Uniformity

SPECT images are degraded by small degrees of nonuniformity in the flood field that do not adversely affect planar images. It is important to acquire the **flood uniformity correction** for approximately 100 million counts (depending on manufacturer's recommendations) to reduce nonuniformity caused by statistical variations in count rate. During backprojection, relatively minor defects will become quite prominent and sometimes appear as ring artifacts in the reconstructed transaxial slices. The camera head effectively "drags" the

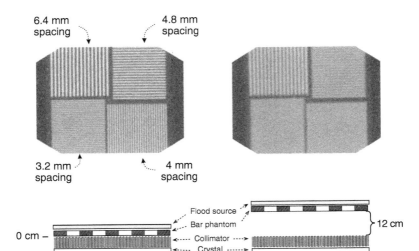

6.4 mm spacing 4.8 mm spacing

3.2 mm spacing 4 mm spacing

Flood source
Bar phantom
Collimator
Crystal

0 cm –

12 cm

Figure 14.11 Degradation of resolution with distance.

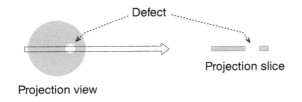

Defect

Projection slice

Projection view

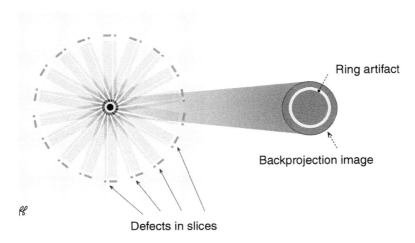

Ring artifact

Backprojection image

Defects in slices

Figure 14.12 Ring artifact created during backprojection of an area of nonuniformity.

defect with it as it circles the patient. Figure 14.12 illustrates this effect.

Center of rotation

It is assumed that the camera heads will rotate in a near perfect circle and that heads will remain almost precisely aligned in their opposing positions. It is also assumed that the predicted or "electronic" center of the path of rotation will match the "mechanical" or actual center of the camera head rotation. Deviation from either expectation will degrade image resolution and can be seen as a displacement of the **center of rotation** (COR). Probably the most common cause of apparent displacement of COR is a result of inadvertent errors (not leveling the camera head, bumping the table, and so on) during data collection.

The most common cause of true shift of the COR is electronic malfunction. Mechanical problems, such as the use of a collimator that is too heavy for the gantry, are less common. Figure 14.13a illustrates a near perfect circular rotation path for a camera. The predicted COR (cross) is aligned with the actual (mechanical) COR (circle); Figure 14.13b illustrates an "unintended" elliptical orbit caused by a heavy camera head that at the bottom of its orbit drifts downward under the influence of gravity. The center of this elliptical orbit (circle) is offset from the center of the predicted circular orbit (cross).

Measurement of COR: The test for center of rotation varies by manufacturer but in general a simple scheme consists of placing on center or off center (per manufacturer) a point source on the patient bed. Projection views are obtained over a 360° arc (upper panel of Figure 14.14). COR tests for dual headed cameras should be performed for each of the head configurations used for imaging, such as the 90° configuration used for cardiac imaging and the 180° configuration used for whole body SPECT.

There are several ways to analyze the difference between the actual and predicted COR. One common approach is to plot the position of the point source as a function of camera head position along the circle of rotation and compare this to the predicted values. The location of the point source is plotted in the x (perpendicular to the long axis of the bed) and y (parallel to the long axis of the bed) directions. The position of the source plotted in the

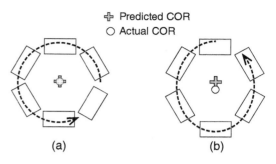

Figure 14.13 Deviation of the mechanical COR.

x direction should closely approximate a sine wave (lower panel of Figure 14.14). The plot of the image of the source in the y direction (not depicted) should be a straight line.

The plot of the source on a camera with a normal COR is illustrated in the upper portion of Figure 14.15. The bottom graph plots the same source in the camera with the elliptical orbit depicted in Figure 14.13. This plot deviates by several pixels from the expected sine wave (dashed lines). Along a portion of the rotation, the measured position differs by several pixels from the expected position of the source. This COR test is abnormal. Deviations of greater than one half pixel from the expected position of the source are considered abnormal and should be checked with a second collection. A persistent abnormality will require repair prior to collection of further SPECT studies. The results of the COR calculation are stored in the computer and used to correct subsequent SPECT scans.

Assessing spatial resolution and contrast in SPECT

Phantoms are fillable objects that are used to assess camera resolution. A phantom can be as simple as a plastic bag or as complex as a model of a slice of the brain. SPECT phantoms are cylindrical lucite containers in which are interspersed different sized rods, cylinders, and/or cones of lucite. The container is then filled with water containing a small amount of radioactivity. Tomographic images of the phantom are collected and the reconstructed slices are inspected for visibility of the lucite objects. The images should be compared to prior acquisitions for evidence of degradation in resolution. Figure 14.16 shows an image of a phantom.

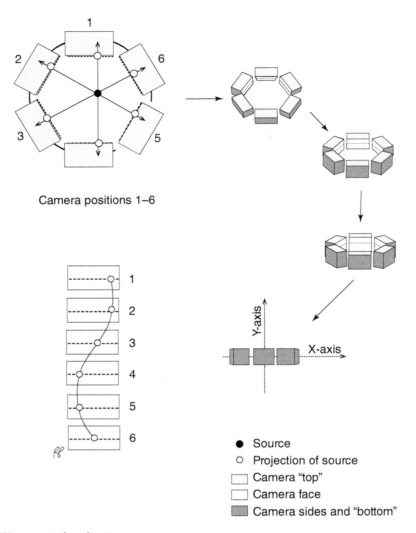

Camera positions 1–6

- ● Source
- ○ Projection of source
- ▢ Camera "top"
- ▢ Camera face
- ▨ Camera sides and "bottom"

Figure 14.14 COR curves in the *x* direction.

PET

The quality-control protocols for PET cameras can be quite simple or quite extensive depending on the manufacturer and the quality control protocols of the clinic. Some examples of routine procedures are summarized briefly in this section as an introduction to this topic for the reader.

Daily QC

A common *daily* quality control procedure is the acquisition and evaluation of a scan using an internal source or a separate low activity source without the patient in the scanner (sometimes called **a blank scan**). The blank scan is evaluated automatically by the computer as well as by direct inspection for evidence of defective detectors. A sample display of quality control results can be seen in Figure 14.17a. Other representations of the blank scan include the data displayed in a cine view (Figure 14.17b) and as a sinogram (Figure 14.17c).

Timing resolution test

For PET-CT scanners which utilize time-of-flight circuitry to approximate the location of annihilation events the time delay between event detection in paired opposing detectors is measured and compared to expected values.

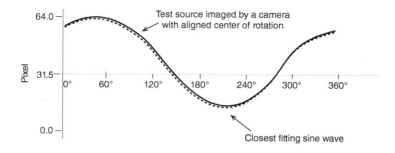

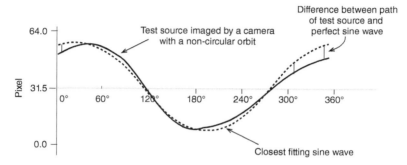

Figure 14.15 Normal and abnormal COR tests.

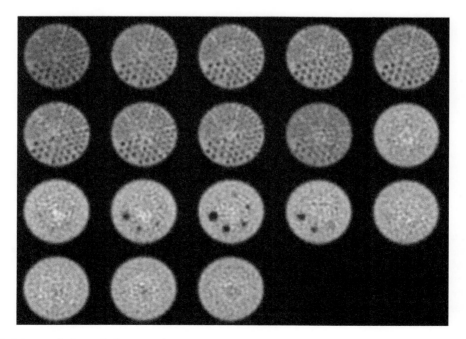

Figure 14.16 Image of a Jaszczak phantom. The top two rows contain cross-sectional images of lucite rods of varying size used to measure resolution, the lower two rows contain lucite spheres of varying sizes to evaluate image contrast.

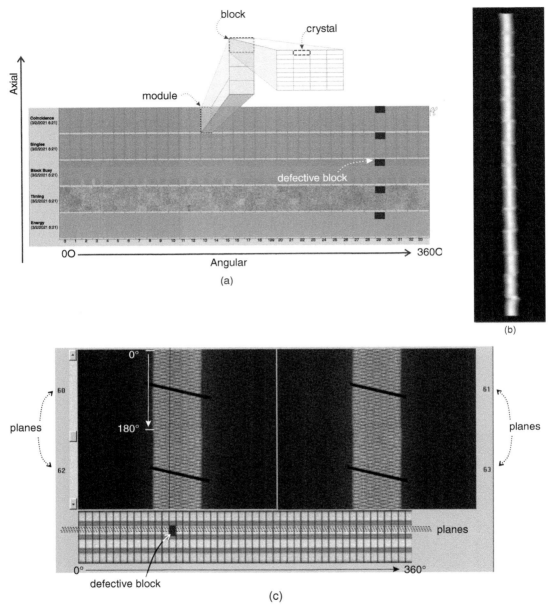

Figure 14.17 PET Daily QC image. (a) Multiple tests (one per labeled row) are run on the PET detectors by imaging a source placed in the center of the gantry. In this scanner 36 crystals comprise a block and four blocks comprise a module. Malfunctioning detectors can be easily identified and then located by their position in the image. The axial direction is the z-axis perpendicular to the ring of detectors; the angular axis "wraps" around the circular ring of detectors from 0 to 360 degrees. (Abnormal result created by overlying graphics on a normal blank scan from a 4-ring GE Discovery MI PET/CT. Original image courtesy of Arda Konic, PhD.) (b) A cine view of a partitioned rod source (higher activity "centroids" with lower activity spaces between the centroids) is examined for nonlinearity and defects which, if present, would indicate a need for service. (Image from a Philips Gemini TF PET/CT.) (c) Altered QC image from a Siemens Biograph mCT. A defective block is represented as a rectangle on the lower portion of the image (as in (a) this portion is an "unwrapped" representation of the circular ring of detectors). The upper portion of the image is a series of four sinograms obtained at four different planes through the ring of crystals. The defective block appears in the sinograms as a diagonal thick line. Because of coincidence detection the sinogram from 180–360 degrees contains the same information as the sinogram from 0–180 degrees so only the latter is displayed.

During the transmission and emission testing described above a number of tests might be conducted automatically by the system. Detector gains can be adjusted, energy windows checked and adjusted and timing can be tuned up.

Cross-calibration and SUV validation

Periodically the PET scanner is subjected to a test and possible adjustment of calibration factors that enable the quantitative ability of PET. To accomplish this, a small amount of carefully-measured positron emitter is diluted in a standard water-filled phantom of known volume. The measured activity and time of calibration as well as the phantom volume expressed as a weight are entered at the console. If the PET scanner is properly calibrated, the mean SUVs measured in relatively large regions of interest placed throughout the uniform cylinder will be equal to 1.0 ml/g. Deviations from 1.0 can be used to derive a correction factor which can be applied to subsequent SUV measurements. This new correction is usually handled internally by the scanner software and not applied explicitly by the user.

The procedure consisting of placing known activity (i.e. "known" in the sense of it having been assayed by the same dose calibrator that will be used for assaying patient doses) inside the PET scanner and determining the calibration factor that converts PET measurements (counts per second per ml) to Bq/ml is often referred to as a well-counter calibration (discussed in more detail in Chapter 7). This is by analogy to the efficiency determination that's done for a well-counter—i.e. to derive the scaling factor for a particular nuclide to convert counts per second (CPS) to Ci or Bq.

Image quality

Most quality control programs involve scanning periodically (typically quarterly and at least annually) a phantom containing hot and cold features. This enables a periodic assessment of scanner performance and protocol settings in terms of image quality (noise, spatial resolution and contrast) and quantitative capability (SUV accuracy). An image of a phantom is shown in Figure 14.18. This is a standard quality control phantom used by all sites that are accredited by the American College of Radiology and is based upon the design typically used to evaluate SPECT scanners (Jaszczak

phantom, also used for the ACR's SPECT accreditation). It consists of sectors of rods arranged in patterns and of decreasing diameter and a series of cylindrical features that are filled with activity of 2.5 times the background (8 mm, 12 mm, 16 mm and 25 mm diameter) and with cold cylindrical features of various materials (air, water and Teflon that simulates bone).

CT

Like PET, CT quality control procedures vary among manufacturers. Although a comprehensive discussion of CT quality control is beyond the scope of this text a brief introduction to some of the more common procedures is included below.

Tube conditioning

Daily quality control begins with a period of tube conditioning, during which the x-ray tube is gradually warmed-up by applying stepwise increments in power (combinations of kV and mA). This gradual acclimation prolongs the life of the tube by reducing the risk of cracking and electrical arcing.

Air calibration

Daily scanning without a phantom in place is called air calibration and this is performed with varying combinations of kVp and mAs to adjust the gain on the detectors so that the output or response to the X-ray flux is uniform among detectors. These images are inspected for artifacts as are the phantom images discussed next.

CT phantoms

Although individual phantoms could be used to perform each of the following quality control procedures most CT phantoms are composed of multiple smaller phantoms, and different portions are used for different tests.

CT number QC

CT number for water, calculation of noise, and visual inspection: A water filled phantom or a phantom composed of a plastic with a density similar to that of water is scanned and a large central region of interest is drawn on an image slice. The mean CT number (Hounsfield unit) for the region should be at, or near, the expected CT number of the material,

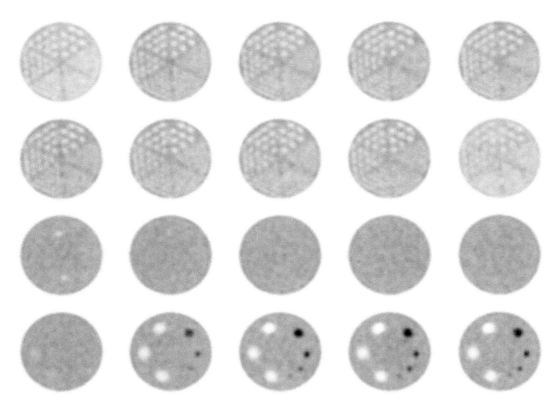

Figure 14.18 Image of PET phantom. The top three rows contain cross-sectional images of lucite rods of varying size used to measure resolution. The bottom row shows cross-sectional images of cylinders of different diameters containing either a solution of radioactivity (appearing as black) as well as a cylinder each of nonradioactive water, air, and Teflon (all appearing as white). These features are used to assess contrast.

for water the value is 0, for plastics the value will be specified by the manufacturer. The standard deviation of the CT number for the region is a measure of the signal **noise** in the image and should be compared to the manufacturer's specifications. An example of a region of interest used for calculating the CT number and standard deviation is depicted with a dashed white circle in Figure 14.19. The image of the phantom is visually inspected for artifacts.

CT number uniformity: Uniformity of the CT number across the slice is measured by comparing central and peripheral CT numbers within the phantom, these should be within close range of each other per manufacturer's specifications. Sample central and peripheral regions of interest are delineated with dashed black circles in Figure 14.19.

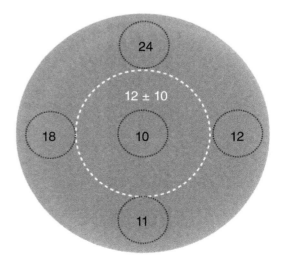

Figure 14.19 Regions of interest used to calculate CT number uniformity and noise. The phantom used for this example is made of plastic.

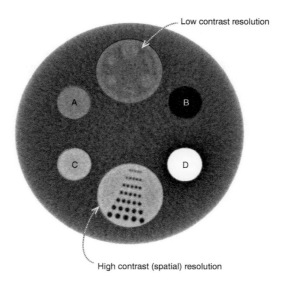

Figure 14.20 Slice of a phantom used to determine CT number accuracy over a wide range of materials (depicted by regions A–D). The low contrast resolution phantom is seen at the top of the image and the high contrast spatial resolution phantom on the bottom.

CT number linearity: A separate phantom, or portion of a larger phantom, containing materials of different densities, such as Teflon, nylon, and water is scanned to ascertain accuracy of CT numbers over a wider range of numbers similar to those encountered in scanning the human body. The image of four regions composed of materials of different densities are labeled A–D in Figure 14.20.

Low-contrast resolution
A phantom containing objects of steadily decreasing size made of a materials with similar CT numbers to the background (such as polystyrene cylinders in water, or water filled holes in a polystyrene background) is used to evaluate the resolution when there is little contrast between an object and the background. This phantom simulates the small differences in contrast between different types of soft tissue found in the human body. An example of an image of a low-contrast resolution phantom is seen at the top of Figure 14.20.

Spatial (high-contrast) resolution
Spatial resolution can be tested using a phantom somewhat similar to the bar phantom used in SPECT imaging. These phantoms are composed of patterns of alternating equally sized pieces of materials.

The pattern is repeated with elements of steadily decreasing size. Unlike the low-contrast phantom, the materials have significantly different densities, such as holes or lines (containing air) cut into an aluminum or acrylic glass disc. The phantom is scanned and the image is examined for the smallest resolvable pattern. One example of this type of phantom is seen in the bottom of Figure 14.20.

Hybrid system testing
Intermittently SPECT-CT and PET-CT scanners are checked for accuracy of PET and CT or SPECT and CT image registration. One method uses a frame or phantom containing paired radionuclide and radiopaque sources arranged within the field of view. The phantom is scanned in emission and transmission modes just as a patient would be and then the reconstructed images are analyzed for registration of the sources. Alignment could be confirmed visually but is more often analyzed automatically by the computer. The calculated offset between the SPECT or PET and the CT images can be expressed as shift and rotation parameters and are typically stored in the machine calibration database. Subsequent clinical data are corrected by applying the inverse of these shift and rotation parameters prior to reconstruction.

Reference

1. NEMA NU-01 2007 standards. Performance measurements of gamma cameras. National Electrical Manufacturers Association, Rosslyn, Virginia, Section 2.4.4.2 (A newer version of this document is available as NEMA NU-01 2018).

Questions

1. Match each of the following quality control procedures with recommended frequency of performance:
   (a) Dose calibrator linearity.
   (b) Dose calibrator constancy.
   (c) Survey meter constancy.
   (d) Dose calibrator geometry.
   (e) Well counter efficiency.
     (i) Daily.
     (ii) Quarterly.
     (iii) Annually.
     (iv) At installation and after repairs.

2. True or false: A 5-million count daily uniformity flood can be used to create the uniformity correction matrix for SPECT imaging.

3. Which of the listed QC procedures might detect the following camera problems (more than one answer per question is possible).
   Camera problem:
   (a) Drift of the energy window.
   (b) Malfunction of a photomultiplier tube.
   (c) Collimator damage.
   (d) Decrease in spatial resolution.
   Quality control procedure:
   (1) Extrinsic flood.
   (2) Intrinsic flood.
   (3) Extrinsic flood source with bar phantom.
   (4) Checking the photopeak.

4. True or false: In assessing the results of the center of rotation test, a deviation of the measured position of the source less than two pixels from the expected position does not need further investigation.

5. Match the following quality control procedure with the imaging system:
   Quality control procedure:
   (a) SUV validation.
   (b) Tube conditioning.
   (c) Air calibration.
   (d) Center of rotation.

Imaging system:
(i) PET.
(ii) CT.
(iii) SPECT.

6. True or false: Tube conditioning is performed at the start of CT quality control to warm up the X-ray tube and thereby prevent tube cracking or electrical arcing.

7. Which of the following two procedures are used to test dose calibrator linearity?
   (a) A long-lived radioactive source such ^{137}Cs is placed in the dose calibrator and is measured at each energy setting to make sure the response is linear from day to day.
   (b) A vial containing 200 mCi of ^{99m}Tc pertechnetate is placed in the dose calibrator and measured at regular intervals for several days to make sure the readings match predicted decay values for the sample.
   (c) A vial containing 200 mCi of ^{99m}Tc pertechnetate is placed within lead sleeves of different thickness which are then combined such that the overall thickness of the lead reproduces the decline in activity of the source over time.

8. Match the name of the CT QC test with the composition of the phantom:
   (a) Low contrast resolution.
   (b) Spatial (high contrast) resolution.
     (i) Objects of decreasing size made of a material with a similar density to the background material used to simulate the small differences in densities of soft tissues.
     (ii) Patterns of two alternating materials of steadily decreasing size. The two materials are of markedly different densities.

9. Calculate the efficiency of a well counter for Cobalt-57 given the following information:
   The reading for a 500 Bq source is 25,000 cpm and the background reading is 200 cpm.

Answers

1. (a) (ii). (b) (i). (c) (i). (d) (iv). (e) (iii).

2. False: a high count flood, approximately 100 million counts, is necessary for SPECT uniformity correction.

3. (a) (1), (2), and (4). (b) (1), (2), and (3). (c) (1) and (3). (d) (3).

4. False: Deviations greater than one half pixel are abnormal and should be checked with a second collection. A persistent abnormality will require repair prior to further SPECT studies.

5. (a) (i), (iii) (on some systems). (b) (ii). (c) (ii). (d) (iii).

6. True.

7. (b) and (c). Choice (a) is a description of the dose calibrator constancy test.

8. (a) (i). (b) (ii).

9. $(25,000 - 200)$ counts/min/$(500$ decays/s $\times$ 60 s/min$) = 24,800/30,000$ cpm/dpm $= 0.83$ cpm/dpm or 83%.

CHAPTER 15

Radiation Biology

The biologic effect of radiation can be understood in terms of the transfer of energy from radiation (photons and particles) to tissue. When the energy of radiation is deposited in the body, it can disrupt the chemical bonds and alter tissue. It is important to understand some of the details of this transfer. The interaction of radiation and tissue is governed by the energy and mass of the incident radiation (alpha and beta particles, gamma ray, or X-ray) and the properties of the tissue.

Radiation Units

Radiation absorbed dose (rad)

The radiation absorbed dose, or **rad**, is a measure of energy transferred to any material from ionizing radiation. The corresponding Système International (SI) unit is the **gray** (Gy), named after the English physicist Louis Harold Gray. Remember that ionizing radiation is a term that applies to any radiation that is sufficiently energetic to create ion pairs; it includes X-rays, gamma rays, alpha and beta particles, and neutrons and protons.

One gray is equal to 1 joule of energy absorbed per kilogram of tissue; one gray is equal to 100 rads. For example, a bladder wall receives approximately 0.04 Gy (4rad) from its contained urine following the excretion of a 740 MBq (20 mCi) intravenous dose of ^{99m}Tc-pertechnetate.

Roentgen-equivalent man (rem)

The roentgen-equivalent man, or **rem**, is the unit of absorbed energy that takes into account the estimated biologic effect of the type of radiation that imparts the energy to the tissue. Particles with higher linear energy transfer, such as alpha particles, protons and neutrons, produce greater tissue damage per rad than beta particles, gamma rays, or X-rays. The relative damage for each type of radiation is referred to as its **radiation weighting factor** (W_R), the values for which are given in Table 15.1.

The **dose equivalent** (or **absorbed energy**) is represented by the letter H (or H_T) and is the product of the dose times the radiation weighting factor, or

$$H = \text{dose equivalent (in rem)} = \text{absorbed dose (in rad)} \times W_R$$

And, in SI units,

$$H = \text{dose equivalent (in sieverts)} = \text{absorbed dose (in Gy)} \times W_R$$

The quantities and units used to measure radiation in nuclear medicine are given in Table 15.2.

The effects of radiation on living organisms

The effects of radiation on living organisms can be described at the level of the cell, a tissue, an entire organism, or a whole population.

Essentials of Nuclear Medicine Physics, Instrumentation, and Radiation Biology, Fourth Edition.
Rachel A. Powsner, Matthew R. Palmer, and Edward R. Powsner.
© 2022 John Wiley & Sons Ltd. Published 2022 by John Wiley & Sons Ltd.

Cellular effects

Individual cells

Cellular structure: Cells are the building blocks for living matter and are composed of a nucleus and cytoplasm. The nucleus contains the genetically important chromosomes that are composed of **deoxyribonucleic acid** (DNA), which is a large molecule consisting of thousands of small subunits (nucleotides) coiled into a double helix. Each nucleotide is composed of a sugar, phosphate, and a base. The genetic code for the cell and the entire organism is held in the sequence of pairs of bases along the two strands of the double helix. During the process of cell division, called **mitosis**, the DNA reproduces itself so that a complete set of chromosomes is deposited within each cell. In this way the genetic code is propagated. Since DNA plays such a pivotal role in cellular multiplication and function, radiation damage to DNA has a profound impact on living tissue. Chromosomes are particularly radiosensitive (vulnerable to radiation damage) during mitosis.

DNA contains two chains of alternating sugar molecules and phosphate groups. The sugars of the chains are linked by pairs of **bases**—thymine, cytosine, adenine, or guanine. The term base refers to the basic, as opposed to acidic, nature of the isolated compounds. These four bases are commonly referred to by their initial letters—T, C, A, and G. The chains and bases are arranged in two long, coiled, and intertwined strands, which are tightly packed to form a **chromatid** (Figure 15.1). Two identical chromatids are "attached" to a centromere and form a **chromosome**. As shown at the bottom of Figure 15.1, the bases form pairs across the strands as follows: adenine pairs with thymine and guanine with cytosine. The genetic code for the cell and, indeed, for the entire organism is held in the sequence of the nucleotides with their base pairs.

The human cell contains 23 pairs of chromosomes, one of each matched pair is inherited from each of an individual's parents. One of the pairs of chromosomes determines the individuals sex; male children inherit an X chromosome from their mother and a Y chromosome from their father and female children inherit an X chromosome from each of their parents. The long strand of DNA within each chromosome contains thousands of genes, each of which contains the information from which the cells can manufacture specific proteins.

Table 15.1 Radiation weighting factors (W_R) for ionizing radiation

Ionizing radiation	W_R
Alpha	20
Neutrons	Varies with neutron energy
Protons	2
Beta (electrons and positrons)	1
Gamma and X-rays	1

Source: ICRP, 2003. Relative Biological Effectiveness (RBE), Quality Factor (Q), and Radiation Weighting Factor (w_R). ICRP Publication 92. Ann. ICRP 33 (4) p. 11. (Adapted from Table 1.2 Radiation weighting factors.)

Table 15.2 Quantities and units used in nuclear medicine

Quantity	Système International (SI) Unit	Conventional unit	Equivalence	Meaning
Activity (A)	becquerel (Bq)	curie (Ci)	$1\ Bq = 2.7 \times 10^{-11}\ Ci$	Number of disintegrations of radioactive material per second
Absorbed dose (D)	gray (Gy)	rad	$1\ Gy = 100\ rad$	Energy absorbed from ionizing radiation per unit mass of absorber
Exposure	coulombs per kilogram (C/kg)	roentgen (R)	$1 C/kg = 3.9 \times 10^3\ R$	Amount of charge liberated by ionizing radiation per unit mass of air
Dose equivalent (H)	sievert (Sv)	rem	$1 Sv = 100\ rem$	Absorbed dose times the radiation weighting factor (Dose $\times\ W_R$)

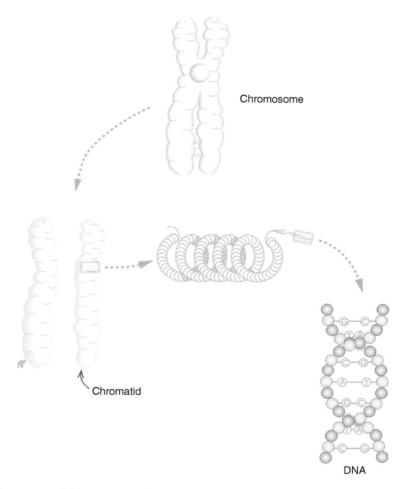

Figure 15.1 The structure of chromosomes and DNA.

Mechanisms of radiation damage to DNA: Ionizing radiation can cause deletions or substitutions of bases and/or actual breaks in the DNA chain. Ionizing particles (neutrons, alpha and beta particles) are responsible for biologic damage. Photons (X-rays and gamma rays) transfer energy to "fast" electrons (via Compton scattering and the photoelectric effect), which in turn cause biologic damage through ionization.

Base deletions or substitutions can have variable effects on the cell line. DNA strand breaks, if not repaired, cause abnormalities in chromosomes that may result in cell death. **Single breaks**, caused by low-LET (linear energy transfer; see Chapter 3) radiation given at a low-dose rate, are relatively easily repaired by using the other strand of DNA as a template. Radiation of relatively high-LET, or a

high-dose rate of low-LET, may produce single breaks in close proximity to each other in both strands (called **double or multiple strand breaks**), which are more difficult to repair (Figure 15.2).

Direct and indirect action of radiation: DNA damage can occur as a result of a **direct action** in which the particulate radiation (such as alpha particles) or fast electrons produced by photons in Compton and photoelectron interactions strike the DNA molecules (Figure 15.3). Alternatively, damage may be caused by **indirect action** in which the radiation interacts with the water molecules in the cell to form free radicals (see box), which in turn damage the DNA strands (see Figures 15.3 and 15.4). Most DNA damage caused by low-LET radiation is a result of indirect action. Most DNA damage by high-LET radiation is via direct action.

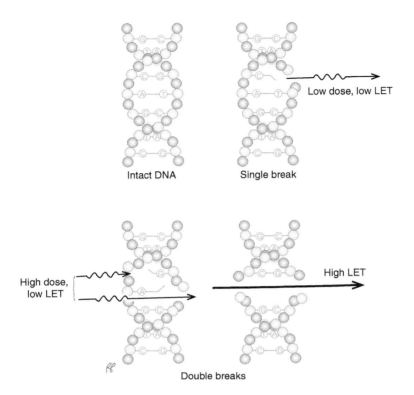

Figure 15.2 Single strand and double strand breaks.

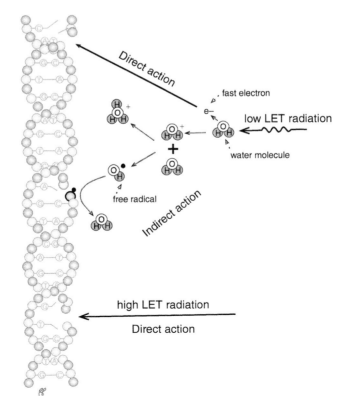

Figure 15.3 Direct and indirect action.

Radiosensitivity and cell cycle: The normal mitotic cycle of the cell is illustrated in Figure 15.5. The **cell cycle** can be divided into four segments, the length of which varies as a function of cell type. During **mitosis** the cell divides into two individual cells. This is followed by **interphase G1** during which only one copy of the cellular DNA is contained in a chromatid. The **synthetic** (S) **phase** is a period of DNA replication. In **interphase G2** the chromatid has duplicated and the DNA is doubled and is located in chromosomes.

Experiments have shown that the cell is relatively resistant to radiation damage during the latter part of the S phase, the period of DNA synthesis. It is hypothesized that during this portion of the cell cycle, the relative abundance of repair enzymes (DNA polymerase and ligase) facilitates DNA repair. Other experiments have shown that the greatest amount of damage occurs during the period of mitosis; the dose needed to halt mitotic activity in a dividing cell is much less than that needed to destroy the function of a differentiated cell. The latter portion of the G_2 phase is nearly as sensitive as the mitotic phase.

Cell survival curves

Thus far we have outlined the effects of radiation on individual cells. Since it is likely that cells will be randomly damaged, it is more useful to consider the overall effects of radiation on groups of cells.

The effects of radiation on cell populations is often expressed as a semi-logarithmic plot of the fraction of surviving cells vs. radiation dose. The surviving cell fraction is plotted along the y-axis using a logarithmic scale and the radiation dose as a linear scale along the x-axis (see Figure 15.6). The actual biophysical mechanisms underlying the observed cell survival curves are felt to be complex and are not fully understood. The following explanations for the curve shape, although simplistic, are useful.

Cell survival as a function of radiation dose is exponential (appearing as a line on the semi-logarithmic plot) for high-LET radiation (bottom plot in Figure 15.6). A likely explanation for this appearance is that most DNA damage with high-LET radiation is via multiple breaks that are generally not repaired. In contrast, cells exposed to lower doses of low-LET radiation can often repair the single strand breaks caused by this type of radiation. For the lower doses of this radiation, therefore, the fraction of the cells surviving is greater than for a similar dose of high-LET radiation. The initial, relatively more horizontal slope in

the low-LET curve likely reflects the cells' ability to repair the single breaks caused during low doses of low-LET radiation (top plot in Figure 15.5). At increasingly higher doses of low-LET radiation multiple DNA breaks are more likely and the slope of the curve becomes steeper, more closely approximating that of the high-LET radiation.

Free radicals

Indirect DNA damage is mediated by free radicals. When particulate or photon radiation interacts with water (H_2O) an ion pair is formed (H_2O^+, e^-). The electron will combine with H_2O to form H_2O^-. The H_2O^+ and H_2O^- are called ion radicals (not to be confused with free radicals). Ion radicals are very unstable and rapidly dissociate: H_2O^+ becomes H^+ and $OH^•$, and H_2O^- becomes $H^•$ and OH^-. $OH^•$ and $H^•$ are free radicals.

A free radical is an atom or molecule that has no electrical charge, but is highly reactive because it has an odd number of electrons with an unpaired electron in its outer shell. Free radicals tend to quickly recombine to form stable electron configurations. However, in high enough concentrations in the cell, they can create organic free radicals ($R^•$) and $H_2O_2^•$ (hydrogen peroxide), a toxic molecule. $OH^• + RH$ become $R^• + H_2O$ and two $OH^•$ become H_2O_2. Organic free radicals in DNA lead to breakage of the strands and cross-linking. $OH^•$, since it oxidizes (removes electrons), is more damaging than $H^•$, which is a reducing agent (gives up its electrons).

Factors affecting cell survival

Dose rate:

Low-LET radiation: The degree of damage incurred by administering a dose of low-LET radiation is dependent on the rate at which this dose is delivered. With delivery of a given dose over a longer period of time (lower dose rate), most DNA damage is via single strand breaks and the cell has time to repair the damage. At high-dose rates there are more multiple strand breaks and less time to repair single strand breaks. As a result, the initial more horizontal portion of the curve becomes smaller (Figure 15.7).

High-LET radiation:

High-LET radiation causes such a high incidence of multiple strand breaks that repair is negligible at any rate.

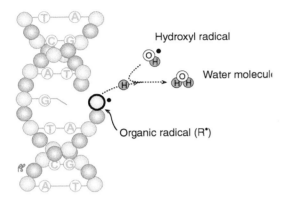

Figure 15.4 During indirect action the hydroxyl free radical interacts with the DNA strand creating an organic free radical and in the process acquires a hydrogen atom to form a water molecule (see top Figure 15.7).

Chemical interventions: The introduction of certain chemicals in the medium in which the cells exist can alter the cell population's response to administered radiation doses. These chemicals alter the indirect effects (via free radicals) of radiation on DNA.

Radiosensitizers: These substances increase the amount of radiation damage to cells at a given radiation dose and are used in radiation therapy to increase death of tumor cells. Radiosensitizers include oxygen, halogenated pyrimidines, and nitroimidazoles.

- *Oxygen*: Oxygen enhances the indirect action of low-LET radiation by binding to the free radical $R^{\bullet}$. The resulting $RO_2^{\bullet}$ is a more stable free radical, and the damaged ends are less likely to be repaired (Figure 15.8). Oxygen has less effect on the radiotoxicity of high-LET radiation, which is more likely to damage DNA by direct action. The effects of oxygen as a radiosensitizer is most pronounced in anaerobic tissues such as the center of tumor masses.

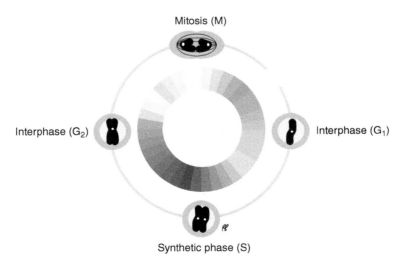

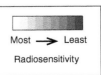

Figure 15.5 The cell cycle and relative radiosensitivity.

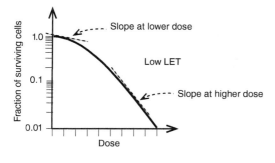

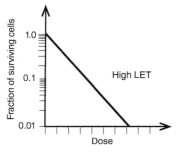

Figure 15.6   Cell survival curves for low and high-LET radiation.

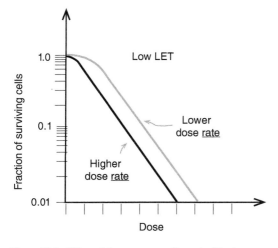

Figure 15.7   Effect of dose rate on cell survival for low-LET radiation.

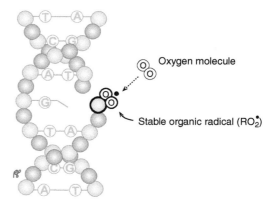

Figure 15.8   Oxygen binds to damaged DNA.

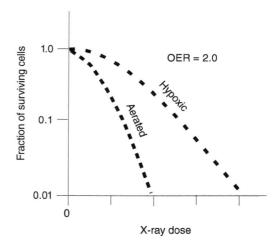

Figure 15.9   Effects of oxygenation on cell survival during low-LET radiation.

The **oxygen enhancement ratio** (OER) is the ratio of the dose in hypoxic tissue to the dose in aerated tissue required to cause a given tissue effect. For photon or X-ray irradiation, this ratio is approximately 2.5 to 3.5 at high doses [1]. For high-LET radiation (alpha particles), the ratio approaches 1.0, since most of the damage is via direct action. Figure 15.9 illustrates an OER of 2.0 from a hypothetical X-ray dose. Half of the X-ray dose is needed during oxygenation to kill the same proportion of the cell population radiated in anaerobic conditions.

• *Halogenated pyrimidines:* The halogenated pyrimidines, 5-iododeoxyuridine and 5-bromodeoxyuridine, are very similar to thymine and are easily incorporated in its place into DNA. However, the substitution "weakens" the DNA making it more susceptible to radiation damage.

• *Nitroimidazoles:* The nitroimidazoles, including misonidazole, and etanidazole, mimic the action of oxygen by binding to the free radical R· on the damaged ends of a DNA break. They are effective in

Table 15.3 Radiosensitivity of cell types

Relative radiosensitivity	Examples
Highly sensitive	Spermatogonia, erythroblasts, lymphocytes
Relatively sensitive	Epidermal basal cells, intestinal crypt cells, myelocytes
Intermediate sensitivity	Osteoblasts, spermatocytes, chondroblasts
Relatively resistant	Liver cells, spermatozoa, granulocytes, erythrocytes, osteocytes
Highly resistant	Neural cells, muscle cells

hypoxic tumors as they can penetrate more deeply; unlike oxygen they are not metabolized by surrounding tissue.

• Radioprotectors: Radioprotectors such as cysteine and amifostine (also known as WR-2721) "scavenge" or combine with free radicals, thereby reducing the likelihood of low-LET DNA damage.

Tissue effects

The radiosensitivity of different types of tissues is largely dependent on the mitotic rate of the cells. In general, cells with a higher mitotic rate and those that are less differentiated are more radiosensitive. Mature lymphocytes are an exception to the general rule and are very radiosensitive as apoptosis (programmed cell death) during interphase is increased in lymphocytes following exposure [2]. Table 15.3 lists cell types and their relative radiosensitivity.

Organ toxicity

Table 15.4 outlines the effects of acute exposure on selected organs with threshold doses.

Embryo and fetus: Prior to and during early implantation of the embryo, when the cells are pluripotential, it is generally accepted that the embryo will either succumb to radiation or will survive without significant abnormalities. After the time of implantation and during the time of rapid organ development (organogenesis), organ malformation may occur. Most observed organ damage from radiation during human embryonic and fetal development involves the brain. Table 15.5 outlines the effects of radiation during formation of the embryo and fetus.

Acute whole-body radiation toxicity: Radiosensitivity varies between species. It is expressed as the lethal dose which will kill half of the individuals within a specific time period. Human lethal doses are expressed over 30 or 60 day intervals. The $LD_{50/60}$ (50% deaths in 60 days) for humans is between 3 and 5 Gy [3]. Acute radiation sickness following whole body radiation is discussed in Chapter 19.

Heritable and cancer effects

The adverse effects of radiation exposure include death and tissue damage, the development of cancer and inherited genetic effects. The risk of developing an adverse effect is classified as either stochastic or nonstochastic.

Stochastic and nonstochastic risks

Cancer and genetic effects of radiation are examples of **stochastic risks**. A stochastic risk is the probability that exposure to radiation will result in damage to an exposed organism. The likelihood than an individual will develop cancer or suffer from her parent's gonadal exposure to radiation is dose dependent; the greater the dose the more likely the adverse effect. However, these are only statistical probabilities; within a population exposed to radiation it is not known which particular individuals will develop cancer or a genetic defect (unless of course the dose is high enough to create a 100% risk). On the other hand, dose-related risks, also known as **nonstochastic** or **deterministic** risks do not result from exposure alone, but from **dose-related** exposures. In the latter case, there are thresholds below which the radiation damage will not occur in exposed individuals, for example the threshold for future cataract development from radiation exposure to the eyes is 0.5 Gy [4], the previous estimated threshold was 2 Gy. Increasing doses are associated with decreasing latency periods (time between exposure and cataract formation); for patients receiving 2.5 to 6.5 Gy to the eye, the latency period is approximately 8 years and this decreases to an average of 4 years for doses of 6.51 to 11.5 Gy [5]

Heritable effects

Estimates for heritable effects of low-LET, low-dose radiation in humans have of necessity been derived in part using mutation rate data from irradiated

Table 15.4 Organ toxicity from acute exposure

Organ	Type of damage	Threshold Gy (rad)
Ocular lens	Cataract formation	0.5 (50)[a]
Bone marrow	Depression of hematopoesis	0.5 (50)[a]
Reproductive organs	Permanent male sterility	3.5–6 (350–600)[b]
	Permanent female sterility	2.5–6 (250–600)[b]

Sources: [a] ICRP, 2012. ICRP Statement on Tissue Reactions/Early and Late Effects of Radiation in Normal Tissues and Organs—Threshold Doses for Tissue Reactions in a Radiation Protection Context. ICRP Publication 118. Ann. ICRP 41(1–2).
[b] ICRP, 2007. The 2007 Recommendations of the International Commission on Radiological Protection. ICRP Publication 103. Ann. ICRP 37 (2–4).

mice as there is a lack of conclusive data from retrospective studies of human irradiation. The estimated spontaneous or baseline genetic mutation rate in the human population is approximately 3×10^{-6} mutations per gene per generation. The **doubling dose** is the dose of low-LET, low-dose radiation that will induce, or cause, an equivalent number of genetic mutations as the spontaneous rate. Using the human spontaneous mutation rate combined with the average rate of radiation induced mutations in mice (approximately 3.6×10^{-6} per gene per generation) the doubling dose (DD) for humans has been estimated as approximately 1 Gy [6].

For such diseases as retinoblastoma or Huntington's chorea, a single mutation in a gene inherited from one parent will cause disease, even in the presence of normal DNA in the comparable gene of the other parent. Inheritance through the

Table 15.5 Radiosensitivity of the human embryo and fetus up to week 25

Stage	Characteristics	Time period	Effect	Level of exposure to low-LET radiation below which the effect is unlikely[a]
Pre-implantation and implantation	Implantation begins on Day 6	Days 0–14	"All or nothing": termination or survival without apparent defects[a,b]	100 mGy
Embryogenesis (organogensis)	Most major organ systems are formed	Weeks 3–8	Potentially severe organ abnormalities including growth retardation[a,b]	100 mGy
Fetal stage	Rapid nervous system development with increased mitotic activity, neuronal cell proliferation	Weeks 8–15	Highest risk for severe mental retardation[c]	300 mGy
			IQ decreases 21 points/Gy[d]	100 mGy
	neuronal cell differentiation and formational of synapses	Weeks 16-25	Continued risk for severe mental retardation[c]	
			IQ decreases 13 points/Gy[d]	

[a] ICRP, 2007. The 2007 Recommendations of the International Commission on Radiological Protection. ICRP Publication 103. Ann. ICRP 37(2–4), pp. 130, 169.
[b] Data based on research in rodents.
[c] ICRP, 2003. Biological Effects after Prenatal Irradiation (Embryo and Fetus). ICRP Publication 90. Ann. ICRP 33(1–2), p. 106.
[d] ICRP, 2003. Biological Effects after Prenatal Irradiation (Embryo and Fetus). ICRP Publication 90. Ann. ICRP 33(1–2), p. 108.

single gene constitutes **autosomal dominance**. Similarly, a male child can inherit a genetic mutation on the X chromosome acquired from his mother where there is no matching gene on the Y chromosome inherited from his father. These are called **X-linked** diseases.

The combined baseline incidence for autosomal dominant and X-linked diseases is approximately 16,500 per million births. An additional 750–1500 cases are estimated to be born to parents who have been exposed to radiation for each gray of exposure [7]. Therefore the increased incidence per gray of radiation for these inherited diseases is approximately 6%.

There are, however, many inherited chronic diseases, such as diabetes, which occur as a result of more than one genetic mutation combined with environmental factors and as such are called **multifactorial diseases**. The natural or baseline risk of manifesting any heritable disease, including these chronic diseases, is high at 738,000 per million live births. The increased incidence per million children per gray of radiation to their parents for any heritable disease is approximately 4000 cases or 0.5% of the baseline rate [7].

Carcinogenic effects

The incidence of certain cancers—such as leukemia, head, neck, pharyngeal, thyroid, breast, and lung—historically has been shown to be increased following radiation exposure. Cancer induction following radiation disasters such as the bombing of Hiroshima, nuclear accidents and some medical procedures have been studied in an attempt to model and quantify risk. Because the data are fairly limited and the natural rate of cancer is so high (approximately 42% lifetime risk of developing cancer) it has been very difficult to precisely determine that risk and over the years, this has led to a great deal of disagreement and controversy.

In their most recent report the BEIR VII committee of the National Academy of Sciences examined all the available data and considered all leading hypotheses and models and concluded that the risk of developing cancer following exposure to low levels of radiation (<100 mSv) is linear with dose and that there is no threshold effect. This is referred as the **linear no-threshold** (LNT) **hypothesis**—no

threshold because the risk is assumed to be extrapolated down to the most minute dose and the risk, although proportionately minute (and virtually impossible to measure given the high background rate of cancer), is never zero. That is, radiation causes cancer and there is no "safe level" of radiation—every incidence of exposure carries a certain risk of producing cancer that is proportionate to the dose.

Calculating the risk of cancer induction given the radiation dose is not exactly straight-forward. For a given dose, the risk of cancer induction is higher in children for example than in adults. The risk of cancer induction in the elderly is lower due to the relatively long lag time to the onset of disease. And for reasons that are not entirely explained by increased expected lifespan, the risk of radiation induced cancer induction for women is higher than that for men. Overall the BEIR VII study estimates the average risk of developing cancer for the US population to be approximately 1% per 100 mSv [8].

To put this into context, suppose that a person representative of the average member of the US population agrees to undergo a CT examination of the pelvis as part of a research study. If the examination involves a dose of 10 mSv then the risk of that study causing cancer is 0.1% (1% × 10 mSv/100 mSv) or, to frame that in the context of overall risk of developing cancer, that person's lifetime risk of developing cancer was increased from 45% to 45.1% as a consequence of taking part in the study.

For patients, concern over the increased risk of cancer from diagnostic radiology and nuclear medicine tests must be weighed against the risk of delaying or "under" diagnosing disease. Judicious use of testing is always advisable; in addition, more attention is being given to balancing image resolution with radiation burden.

References

1. Hall EJ and Giaccia AJ. *Radiobiology for the Radiologist*, 8th edn. Philadelphia: Wolters Kluwer, 2019, p. 82.
2. Hall EJ and Giaccia AJ. *Radiobiology for the Radiologist*, 8th edn. Philadelphia: Wolters Kluwer, 2019, pp. 363, 367.
3. ICRP, 2007. The 2007 Recommendations of the International Commission on Radiological Protection. ICRP Publication 103. Ann. ICRP 37(2–4), p. 165.

4. ICRP, 2012. ICRP Statement on Tissue Reactions/Early and Late Effects of Radiation in Normal Tissues and Organs—Threshold Doses for Tissue Reactions in a Radiation Protection Context. ICRP Publication 118. Ann. ICRP 41(1–2), p. 6.

5. Hall, EJ and Giaccia, AJ. *Radiobiology for the Radiologist*, 8th edn. Philadelphia: Wolters Kluwer, 2019, p. 192.

6. ICRP, 2007. The 2007 Recommendations of the International Commission on Radiological Protection.

ICRP Publication 103. Ann. ICRP 37 (2–4), pp. 222–3.

7. ICRP, 2007. The 2007 Recommendations of the International Commission on Radiological Protection. ICRP Publication 103. Ann. ICRP 37 (2–4), p. 231.

8. National Research Council. *Health Risks from Exposure to Low Levels of Ionizing Radiation: BIER VII, Phase 2*. Washington DC: National Academies Press, 2006, p. 8.

Questions

1. Which of the following statements are correct for radionuclides used in nuclear medicine imaging:
   (a) The dose equivalent is ten times the absorbed dose.
   (b) The dose equivalent is equal to the absorbed dose for beta and gamma emitters.
   (c) The radiation weighting factor, or relative tissue damage per administered Gy of radiation, is larger for high-LET radiation than low-LET radiation.
   (d) All of the above.

2. True or false: Single strand DNA breaks which are caused by low-dose low-LET radiation are less likely to be repaired than double or multiple strand breaks which are caused by high-dose low-LET radiation or high-LET radiation.

3. Rank the following phases of the cell cycle from the most radiosensitive to the least radiosensitive:
   (a) Mitosis.
   (b) Interphase G_1.
   (c) Synthetic phase, S.
   (d) Interphase G_2 (latter part).

4. Which of the following are true?
   (a) Oxygen enhances DNA damage from high-LET radiation more than it enhances DNA damage from low-LET radiation.
   (b) The oxygen enhancement ratio for low-LET radiation is 1.
   (c) The oxygen enhancement ratio for high-LET radiation is 2.5 to 3.5.
   (d) All of the above.
   (e) None of the above.

5. Connect the following doses or risk factors with their estimated values:
   (a) Threshold dose in Gy below which radiation induced cataracts are unlikely.
   (b) Doubling dose (DD) that will increase the genetic mutation rate to twice the baseline rate.
   (c) Excess relative risk for cancer induction per sievert of low dose radiation exposure.

   Dose or risk factor value:
   (1) 0.5 Gy (50 rad).
   (2) 0.1%.
   (3) 1 Gy (100 rad).

6. Rank the following tissues in order from most radiosensitive to most radioresistant:
   (a) Lymphocytes.
   (b) Neural cells.
   (c) Spermatocytes.
   (d) Erythrocytes.
   (e) Intestinal crypt cells.

7. The highest risk for radiation induced severe mental retardation occurs during which stage of embryonic and fetal development?
   (a) Pre-implantation (weeks 0–2).
   (b) Embryogenesis (Organogenesis) (weeks 3–8).
   (c) Early fetal development (weeks 8–15).

8. True or false: In general, radiation exposure of the pre-implantation embryo will result in either survival without malformation or death.

Answers

1. (b) and (c). (a) is not true because the dose equivalent equals the absorbed dose times the weighting factor which is different for different types of emissions.

2. False. Double or multiple strand breaks are more difficult to repair.

3. (a), (d), (b), (c).

4. (e). (a) is incorrect since oxygen only enhances DNA damage from indirect action which is primarily caused by low-LET radiation; high-LET radiation causes damage primarily through direct action. (b) is incorrect, the OER for low-LET radiation is 2.5 to 3.5 and (c) is incorrect because the OER for high-LET radiation is 1.

5. (a) 1. (b) 3. (c) 2. For choice (3) please note that 1% per 100 mSv = 0.1% per sievert.

6. (a), (e), (c), (d), (b).

7. (c).

8. True.

CHAPTER 16

Radiation Dosimetry

Dosimetry is the calculation of the total absorbed radiation dose to individual organs or the whole body from internal and external radiation exposure. Absorbed doses for diagnostic procedures are relatively small and dosimetry is approximated using phantoms or standardized computer models of the human body and, in the case of nuclear medicine studies, radiopharmaceutical distribution studies. Therapeutic procedures involve much greater radiation doses and individual specific information, such as biodistribution of tracer doses and measuring organ mass based on imaging procedures, are frequently employed to more accurately estimate individual dosimetry.

This chapter will discuss some of the methods and terms used to represent dosimetry for diagnostic nuclear medicine procedures, which is largely the result of internal exposure, and computed tomography procedures, which involve external radiation exposure.

Nuclear medicine dosimetry

Internal dosimetry information is supplied with all radiopharmaceuticals, as shown for 18F-flourodeoxyglucose in Table 16.1. The table contains individual organ doses and the effective dose; in the following text we will briefly explore the derivation of these values.

Physical, biologic, and effective half-lives

The calculation of internal dosimetry relies on an understanding of the different types of half-lives used to describe radiopharmaceuticals. The **physical half-life** (T_p or $T_{1/2}$) is the time it takes for half of the nuclide atoms to become stable (see Chapter 1).

The **biologic half-life** (T_b) has nothing to do with radioactivity, but rather reflects the half-time for excretion of the material from the organ or whole body. For instance, the biologic half-life of ^{99m}Tc-MDP is the time it takes for one half of this radiopharmaceutical to be filtered and excreted by the kidneys and bladder. The **effective half-life** (T_e) is a measurement that combines the above two values; it is the time required for one half of the initial radioactivity to disappear from an organ or the body both by excretion and physical decay. The effective half-life is always shorter than either the physical or biologic half-life and is calculated using the formulas

$$\frac{1}{T_e} = \frac{1}{T_b} + \frac{1}{T_p}$$

Or

$$T_e = \frac{T_b \times T_p}{T_b + T_p}$$

Table 16.2 lists hypothetical values to demonstrate the relationship between the three types of half-lives. Table 16.3 lists actual values for selected radiopharmaceuticals, note that for many radiopharmaceuticals the biokinetics are relatively complex with more than one biological half-time for each organ.

Calculation of organ doses

Several systems are available for internal dosimetry calculations. Three of the more commonly used systems are the ICRP (International Committee for Radiation Protection), RADAR (Radiologic Dose Assessment Resource), and MIRD (Medical Internal

Essentials of Nuclear Medicine Physics, Instrumentation, and Radiation Biology, Fourth Edition.
Rachel A. Powsner, Matthew R. Palmer, and Edward R. Powsner.
© 2022 John Wiley & Sons Ltd. Published 2022 by John Wiley & Sons Ltd.

Table 16.1 Part of the estimated dosimetry for ^{18}F-FDG

Tissue	Absorbed dose (mGy/MBq)	Absorbed dose (rad/mCi)
Bladder wall	0.16	0.59
Heart	0.062	0.23
Kidneys	0.021	0.078
Red marrow	0.011	0.041
Effective dose (E)	0.019 mSv/MBq	

Adapted from ICRP Publication 80, 1998. Radiation Dose to Patients from Radiopharmaceuticals, Addendum to ICRP 53, 28(3), p. 49.

Table 16.2 Hypothetical physical, biologic, and effective half-lives

Tp (hours)	Tb (hours)	Te (hours)
1000	1	0.999
10	10	5
10	20	6.7
1	1000	0.999

Radiation Dose). Although the equations they employ for dosimetry calculations appear, at first glance, to be quite different, the underlying principles and components used in the calculations have much in common. The following is a discussion of one such approach, the MIRD (Medical Internal Radiation Dose) system, which, although one of the older models, is useful for demonstration purposes.

Using the MIRD system the dose delivered to an organ, $\bar{D}$, can be represented as product of the total (cumulated) activity within the organ, $\tilde{A}$, and S, a correction factor based on physiologic characteristics of the administered radionuclide and the organ of interest.

$$\bar{D} = \tilde{A} \times S$$

Description of terms

A_0, the **initial activity**, is the amount of injected activity that is in the organ immediately after injection. $A(t)$ is the activity within the organ as a function of time. The **cumulated activity**, $\tilde{A}$, is the summed total activity within the organ over the entire time the radioactivity remains within the organ. The uppermost plot in Figure 16.1 is a time activity curve; the activity at time 0 is A_0. The area under the curve, $\tilde{A}$, can be approximated with sequential thin rectangles (second uppermost panel). The cumulated activity can be calculated from the initial activity and the effective half-life, T_e, of the radiopharmaceutical as follows.

The **residence time**, τ, is the time over which the organ would receive the same total dose as if the amount of initial activity (A_0) were to remain constant, and then fall instantly to zero. If one were to rearrange the thin rectangles in the second panel of Figure 16.1 into a large rectangle which is equal to the area under the curve with height A_0, the width of this rectangle would be τ (lower panels).

Table 16.3 Sample physical, biologic, and effective half-lives

Radiopharmaceutical	T_p	T_b	T_e
^{99m}Tc-sulfur colloid (SC)[a]	6 hours	Infinite (not excreted)	6 hours
^{18}F-flourodeoxyglucose (FDG)[b]	1.83 hours	Infinite for 70% of the dose	1.83 hours for 70% of dose
		0.2 hours for 7.5% of dose	0.18 hours for 7.5% of dose
		1.5 hours for 22.5% of dose	0.82 hours for 22.5% of the dose
^{131}I-sodium iodide[c]	8 days	80 days for dose taken up by thyroid	7.3 days for the thyroid dose
		8 hours for remainder of dose	7.68 hours for the remainder of the dose

Sources:
[a] Annals of the ICRP. ICRP Publication 53, Radiation Dose to Patients from Radiopharmaceuticals, Pergamon, 1987, p. 179.
[b] Valentin J. Annals of the ICRP. ICRP Publication 106, Addendum 3 to ICRP Publication 53, Radiation Dose to Patients from Radiopharmaceuticals, Elsevier, October, 2007, p. 85.
[c] Annals of the ICRP. ICRP Publication 53, Radiation Dose to Patients from Radiopharmaceuticals, Pergamon, 1987, p. 259.

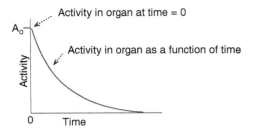

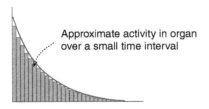

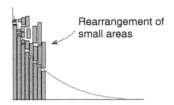

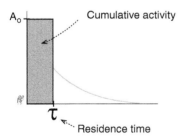

Figure 16.1 Time–activity curve, cumulative activity, and residence time.

$$\tilde{A} = \tau \times A_0$$

The residence time is related to the effective half-life (discussed above) by the equation

$$\tau = 1.44 \times T_e$$

It follows then that

$$\tilde{A} = 1.44 \times T_e \times A_0$$

S value: The radiation dose, $\bar{D}$, to any organ depends on the activity accumulated in that organ ($\tilde{A}$), on the size, shape, and density of the organ, and on the energy and type of radiation it contains and, for penetrating radiation, the energy and type of radiation emitted by accumulated activity in

---

Sample calculation of $\bar{D}$

A sample calculation of an absorbed dose may elucidate the above concepts. We will use a hypothetical case of ^{131}I sodium iodide ingestion with the lung as the target organ and the thyroid as the source organ. To simplify the calculation, we will assume that the thyroidal uptake of ^{131}I sodium iodide is instantaneous and that the 24-hour radioiodine uptake is 30%. The ingested dose is 37 MBq (1 mCi).

The initial activity in the thyroid is

$$A_0 = 7\,\text{MBq} \times 30\%\text{uptake}$$
$$= 11.1\,\text{MBq}\,(0.3\,\text{mCi})$$

The effective half-life for ^{131}I in the thyroid (see Table 16.2) is

$$T_e = 7.3\,\text{days}$$

The residence time is

$$\tau = 1.44 \times T_e$$
$$= 10.5\,\text{days}$$

The cumulated activity is

$$\tilde{A} = \tau \times A_0$$
$$= 10\,\text{days}\ 11.1\,\text{MBq} = 117\,\text{MBq days}$$
$$= 2800\,\text{MBq h}\,(75.6\,\text{mCi h})$$

The S value [1] for source thyroid and target lung is calculated as 2.9 × 10⁻⁶ rad/μCi/h. The absorbed dose to the lungs from the thyroid is

$$\bar{D} = \tilde{A} \times S = 75{,}600\,\mu Ci\,\text{h} \times 2.9 \times 10^{-6}\,\text{rad}/\mu Ci\,\text{h}$$
$$= 0.22\,\text{rad}\,(0.0022\,\text{Gy})$$

[1] Snyder, WS, Ford MR, Warner GG, Watson SB. MIRD pamphlet no. 11, Oak Ridge National Laboratory, Oak Ridge, Tennessee, p. 185.

other organs in the body (this will be covered in the next section). We have already discussed how cumulated activity can be calculated, but the calculation for the remaining factors is too complicated to pursue here. Fortunately, these calculations have been performed for most of the organs of the body and for the range of photon and particle energies emitted by the medically important radionuclides. These combined factors are referred to as the **S value**, which is available in standard tables.

Self-dose, target, and source organs: The term **self-dose** is used to describe the radiation dose to an organ from the radionuclide within it, for example, the dose to the liver from the accumulation of ^{99m}Tc–sulfur colloid within the liver. Moreover, the same approach can be applied for calculating the dose to any other organ of the body, the **target**, from the radioactivity of any other organ, called the **source** (for example, the dose to the thyroid from ^{99m}Tc sulfur colloid in the liver). The left side of Figure 16.2 depicts the liver as the source organ and all organs, including the liver, as target organs. In the figure on the right, the lung is the source organ following injection of ^{99m}Tc-MAA. The total dose to any organ as target is the sum of doses from all sources within the body. There are S values for each combination of source and target organs.

Effective dose

A value called **total body dose**, sometimes published in dosimetry tables for radiopharmaceuticals, is calculated as a ratio of the total energy deposited in the

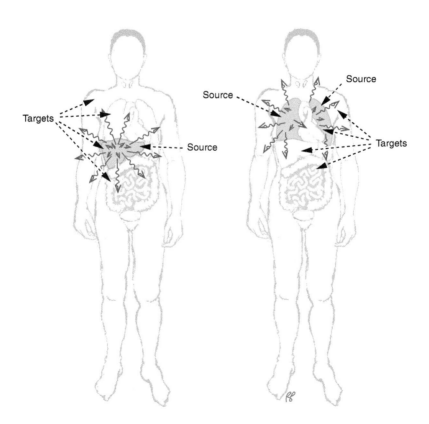

Figure 16.2 Source and target organs.

body divided by an average body mass. This calculation, however, does not factor in the relative radiosensitivity of organs in terms of relative risk of developing fatal cancers or heritable mutations following radiation exposure. As discussed in the preceding chapter, for a given absorbed dose, some organ systems such as the bone marrow are more likely to develop fatal cancers than other tissues such as cortical bone and brain. Similarly, radiation of gonadal organs increases the risk of transmitting a heritable mutation.

The parameter **effective dose** (*E* or *ED*) was developed to estimate these relative risks. Although originally applied to occupational dosimetry, effective dose is increasingly used to compare doses between different imaging modalities such as CT and nuclear medicine studies.

In order to calculate the effective dose for nuclear medicine procedures the **mean equivalent dose** (H_T) for tissue or organ T must be mentioned. H_T is the sum of the absorbed doses for each type of radiation multiplied by its radiation weighting factor (W_R) (see Chapter 15, Table 15.1):

$$H_T = \sum_R W_R \times D_{T,R}$$

Since the majority of radiopharmaceuticals in nuclear medicine are gamma, x-ray, or beta particles emitters their radiation weighting factor is 1 and therefore:

$$H_T = D_T$$

One can think of the effective dose as a sum of all of the "tissue-weighted" organ doses for the body.

$$E = \sum_T W_T \times H_T \text{ or}$$

$$E = \sum_T W_T \times D_T$$

where T is a specific type of tissue, such as liver or red marrow, D_T is the absorbed dose in the tissue, W_T is the tissue weighting factor.

Table 16.4 contains standard W_T values; higher values are applied to more radiosensitive organs or tissues.

CT dosimetry

CT patient dose is largely dependent upon the number and energies of the X-rays produced by the X-ray tube. The greater the number of X-rays (a function of the tube current measured in mAs) and the greater the maximum energy of the electrons (determined by the maximum voltage applied across the tube, measured in kVp) the greater the patient dose. As discussed in Chapter 9 the radiation dose to the patient is somewhat reduced by filtering out the lower energy X-rays in the spectrum. Many other scanner based factors contribute to patient dose and include beam collimation, detector efficiency, pitch, etc.

Absorbed dose in CT

CTDI
Absorbed doses from CT imaging are approximated by scanning phantoms containing dosimeters. The average absorbed dose at any point within a scanned slice of a standardized phantom (16 cm diameter for head estimates and 32 cm diameter for body estimates) is approximated by the **CTDIvol** (computed tomography dose index volume) which is frequently abbreviated as CTDI without a suffix. The CTDI is expressed in mGy.

DLP
CTDI values estimate the dose at point within a single slice of the phantom, but do not take into account the actual length of the CT scan. It would

Table 16.4 Tissue weighting factors (W_T)

Tissue (T)	Number of tissues	W_T	Total contribution
Lung, stomach, colon, bone marrow, breast, remainder	6	0.12	0.72
Gonads	1	0.08	0.08
Thyroid, esophagus, bladder, liver	4	0.04	0.16
Bone surface, skin, brain, salivary glands	4	0.01	0.04
			1

From: ICRP Publication 103, ICRP Annals of the ICRP, 37(2–4), 2007, p. 261.

make sense that the patient dose from a CT scan encompassing the chest, abdomen, and pelvis would be greater than the dose from a chest CT alone or from a scan of a single slice (assuming all scans were acquired with the same technique; kVp, mAs, etc.). To take into account the total length of the scan (L) another parameter, **DLP (dose length product)** is frequently reported and is calculated as

$$DLP\,(mGy-cm) = L\,(cm) \times CTDI_{vol}\,(mGy)$$

Estimation of relative risk: effective dose
Mathematical simulations of CT scans using computerized models of a body combined with scanner specific dose measurements are used to estimate organ doses. Then, in a similar fashion to the

calculation of effective dose described in the preceding section on nuclear medicine dosimetry, these organ doses are multiplied by organ specific weighting factors (W_T) and the results are summed to get the effective dose.

One simplification for estimation of effective dose, E, is achieved by multiplying the DLP for each region of the body: head, chest, abdomen, and pelvis by region specific conversion factors, also called **k factors** or **k conversion coefficients**. Sample k factors are 0.0021 mSv/mGy-cm for the head, 0.014 mSv/mGy-cm for the chest, and 0.015 mSv/mGy-cm for the abdomen and for the pelvis [1].

$$E\,(mSv) = DLP\,(mGy-cm) \times k\;(mSv/mGy-cm)$$

Derivation of CTDI$_{vol}$

Calculation of the CTDI$_{vol}$ begins with measurement of dose to standard CT phantoms containing thin dosimeters. Two standard phantoms are used to measure absorbed dose; one is larger in diameter to simulate the human torso and a smaller phantom approximates the dimensions of the human head.

A commonly used dosimeter is 100 mm long and the total dose measurement along the length of the dosimeter from scanning a single central slice is termed **CTDI100**. This dose comes from the X-rays that contribute to forming an image of the slice as well as the scatter radiation that is created within the rest of the phantom (Figure 16.3).

It was found that CTDI$_{100}$ measurements in the center of the scanned slice of the larger torso phantom were significantly less than the peripheral readings largely due to attenuation of

X-rays as they traverse the acrylic medium. Therefore, a modification, called the **CTDIw**, was devised which is a weighted average of peripheral and central dosimetry readings.

$$CTDI_W \times (2/3) \times CTDI_{100}\;at\;periphery + (1/3) \times CTDI_{100}\;at\;center$$

CTDI$_{vol}$ represents a further refinement of CTDI dosimetry calculations for helical acquisitions and is obtained when the CTDI$_W$ is divided by the pitch of the CT scan. This is because scans with greater pitch irradiate less of the body as there are "gaps" between each rotation (see Figure 9.11 in Chapter 9).

$$CTDI_{vol} \times CTDI_W / pitch$$

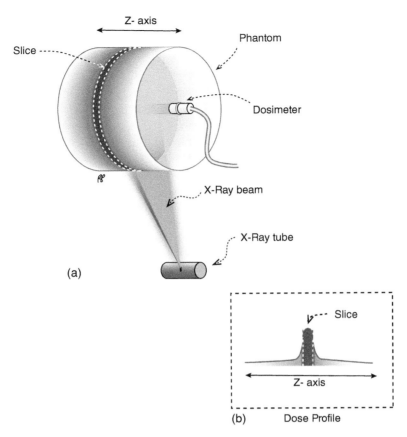

Figure 16.3 Measurement of CTDI. (a) A dosimeter placed in the center of the phantom measures the total dose over the length of the dosimeter from X-ray exposure to a single central slice. (b) Although the central slice receives the greatest dose, the remainder of the phantom receives significant dose from scatter of the X-rays within the phantom. The portion of the phantom immediately adjacent to the central slice receives an additional dose from the edges of the imperfectly collimated X-ray beam.

Reference

1. Christner, JA, Kofler, JM, McCollough, CH. Estimating effective dose for CT using dose-length product compared with using organ doses: consequences of adopting International Commission on Radiological Protection Publication 103 or dual-energy scanning. *Am J Roentgenol.* 2010; 194(4):881–9.

Questions

1. True or false: The effective half-life is always longer than either the physical or biological half-life.

2. What is the effective half-life of rubidium-86 which has a biological half-life of 45 days and a physical half-life of 18.8 days?

3. True or false: The biological half-life of a radiopharmaceutical labeled with ^{99m}Tc will be shorter than the same compound labeled with ^{111}In.

4. True or false: When calculating the total dose to a target organ the target organ should be included as one of the radiation sources.

5. Which measurement of dosimetry can be used to compare the relative risk for fatal cancer or heritable mutations as a result of radiation exposure from different types of diagnostic studies?
   (a) Dose equivalent (H_T).
   (b) Effective dose (E or ED).
   (c) Total absorbed dose.

6. True or false: In general absorbed dose values for diagnostic radiologic procedures are only estimates based on computer models and phantoms.

7. Which estimate of absorbed dose for CT procedures takes into account the length of the CT scan?
   (a) CTDI.
   (b) DLP.

Answers

1. False: The effective half-life is equal to, or shorter than either the physical or biological half-lives.
2. 13 days. $T_{eff} = (45 \times 18.8)/(45 + 18.8)$ days.
3. False, the biological half-life of a radiopharmaceutical is not affected by the physical half-life of the nuclide.
4. True.
5. (b). (a) and (c) do not take into account tissue radiosensitivity weighting factors.
6. True.
7. (b) DLP or dose length product.

CHAPTER 17

Radiation Safety

Rationale

The purpose of a radiation protection program is to monitor individuals' contact with radiation and to limit their exposure to as low a level as possible. Federal regulations are issued by the Nuclear Regulatory Commission (NRC) that outline acceptable levels of exposure. In addition, the government has set forth a general policy principle referred to as **ALARA**. To quote from Federal Register, Volume 56, No. 98:

> ALARA (acronym for "as low as reasonably achievable") means making every reasonable effort to maintain exposures to radiation as far below the dose limits . . . as is practical consistent with the purpose for which the licensed activity is undertaken.

Dose limits

Radiation dose may come from radiation sources outside the body (for example, an X-ray machine or radioactive material external to the body) or from radioactive material that has been taken into the body. These two modes of exposure to radiation are called **external exposure** and **internal exposure**, respectively. Table 17.1 lists the terms commonly used to describe radiation exposure.

Dose limits are separately prescribed for occupational workers (including the fetus of a pregnant worker) and the general public.

Occupational exposure

The prescribed limits for occupational exposure for radiation workers are listed in Table 17.2. Exposure limits to the embryo or fetus of a radiation worker can only be applied to workers who have voluntarily declared their pregnancy in written form.

Hospital workers

The maximal permissible exposure to hospital workers who are not classified as radiation workers is the same as the general public: 1 mSv/year (0.1 rem/year). If an individual is likely to receive over 10% of any of the occupational limits, they are classified as radiation workers and must be monitored (for example, by using a pen dosimeter or wearing a film and/or ring badge). For those individuals receiving less than this amount, their exposure is estimated. The limit refers only to cumulative exposure from the workplace and does not include contributing dose from background radiation, from any personal medical radiation exposure, etc.

Exposure to the general public

The estimated annual total effective dose equivalent (TEDE) for a member of the public should be less than 1 mSv (0.1 rem). The estimated exposure in an unrestricted area (such as the waiting room) must be less than 0.02 mSv/h (2 mrem/h). Exception to these limits is allowed under certain conditions for household contacts of patients receiving radioactive materials for treatment (see "Limiting Exposure to Family Members and the Public").

Background whole body radiation, at sea level, is approximately 3.6 mSv/year (360 mrem/year), including 2.0 mSv/year (200 mrem/year) from radon.

Essentials of Nuclear Medicine Physics, Instrumentation, and Radiation Biology, Fourth Edition.
Rachel A. Powsner, Matthew R. Palmer, and Edward R. Powsner.
© 2022 John Wiley & Sons Ltd. Published 2022 by John Wiley & Sons Ltd.

Table 17.1 Terms used to describe radiation exposure[a]

Term	Abbreviations	Units	Description
Absorbed dose	D	Gy (rad)	Energy deposited in a unit mass of irradiated material (such as tissue) following exposure to ionizing radiation
Weighting factor, radiation (quality factor)	W_R (Q)		Weighting factor which is multiplied by the absorbed dose to account for differences in biologic damage from different types of ionizing radiation. $W_R = 1$ for gamma, X-ray, beta radiation, $W_R = 20$ for alpha particles (see Chapter 15)
Dose equivalent	H_T (H)	Sv (rem)	Absorbed dose times radiation weighting factor: $H_T = D \times W_R$; for most nuclear medicine exposures $H_T = D$
Weighting factor, tissue	W_T		The weighting factor for organ T is the ratio of the risk of death from stochastic effects (cancer) from irradiation of organ T to the risk of stochastic effects if the same dose was distributed uniformly over the entire body; this value reflects both the relative radiosensitivity of the organ and the risk of fatality from irradiation; for example, the W_T for the thyroid is 0.04 (since thyroid cancer is generally treatable); in contrast, the W_T for bone marrow is 0.12 (due to its high radiosensitivity and the risk of leukemia) See Table 16.4 for a list of tissue weighting factors
Effective dose equivalent	H_E	Sv (rem)	$H_T \times W_T$ (calculated for all exposed organs and then summed)
Committed dose equivalent	$H_{T.50}$	Sv (rem)	Dose equivalent to organ T over the 50 years following intake of units of a quantity of radioactivity
Committed effective dose equivalent	$H_{E.50}$	Sv (rem)	$H_{T.50} \times W_T$ (calculated for all exposed organs and then summed)
Total organ dose equivalent	TODE	Sv (rem)	The total dose to an individual organ from both internal and external exposure $= H_{T.50} + H_d$
Total effective dose equivalent	TEDE	Sv (rem)	Sum of effective dose equivalent (external exposures) and the committed effective dose equivalent (internal exposures) TEDE $= H_E + H_{E.50}$ summed for all organs (except for the lens of the eye)
Measured			
Deep dose equivalent	H_d	Sv (rem)	External exposure to the whole body as measured by a whole body radiation monitoring badge at a tissue equivalent depth of 1 cm[a]
Shallow dose equivalent	SDE	Sv (rem)	External exposure to the skin measured by a whole body radiation monitoring badge at a tissue equivalent depth of 0.007 cm[a] or extremity measured by a ring badge
Lens dose equivalent	LDE	Sv (rem)	External exposure to the lens of the eye measured by a whole body radiation monitoring badge at a tissue equivalent depth of 0.3 cm[a]

Source: 10CFR Part 20, Standards for Protection Against Radiation, 20.1003, Definitions.
[a] Tissue depths are simulated by use of filters placed within the cases of the whole body radiation monitoring film or luminescent radiation badges; see Chapter 4 for a description of monitoring badges.

Methods for limiting exposure

Limiting occupational exposure

Limiting external exposure
The three methods of reducing external exposure relate to time, distance, and shielding.

Time: Minimize the time spent in the vicinity of a source of radiation. Work efficiently, but do not rush.

Distance: Maintain as large a distance from the source as practical. The radiation intensity from a source (patient or dose) diminishes rapidly as the distance from the source is increased. In Figure 17.1,

Table 17.2 NRC radiation dose equivalent limits for occupational exposure (abridged)

Organ/system	Limit in mSv/ year	Limit in rem/ year
Total effective dose equivalent (TEDE)[a]	50	5
Sum of DDE and $H_{T,50}$[a] (except for lens of eye)	500	50
Lens dose equivalent (LDE)[a]	150*	15*
Shallow dose equivalent to skin or extremity (SDE)[a]	500	50
Dose equivalent to embryo/fetus[b]	5 (0.5/ month)	0.5 (0.05/ month)
Dose equivalent to minors (<18 years)[c]	10% of adult limits	10% of adult limits

[a] 10CFR Part 20, Standards for Protection Against Radiation, 20.1201, Occupational dose limits for adults.
[b] 10CFR Part 20, Standards for Protection Against Radiation, 20.1208, Dose equivalent to an embryo/fetus (For workers who have declared their pregnancy).
[c] 10CFR Part 20, Standards for Protection Against Radiation, 20.1207, Occupational dose limits for minors.
*Recommended occupational limits from ICRP 118: 20 mSv/year (2 rem/year) averaged over 5 years with no year exceeding 50 mSv (5 rem) Ann. ICRP 41(1/2), p. 11.

the bird in the middle is closest to the source of the radiation (the bird on the left) and receives more radiation than the more distant bird on the right. The radiation dose decreases as the inverse square of the distance (r) from the source ($1/r^2$). Figure 17.2 illustrates areas of equal exposure at distances of (r) and ($2r$) from a source. At a distance r, the entire dose is spread over a sphere with a surface area of $4\pi r^2$. At twice this distance ($2r$), the dose is spread over a sphere with four times the area ($16\pi r^2$); the radiation dose at twice the distance ($2r$) is equal to one fourth of the dose at a distance (r).

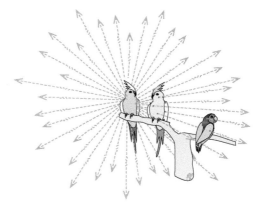

Figure 17.1 Exposure decreases as a function of distance from the source.

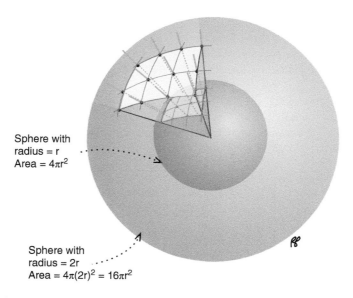

Sphere with
radius = r
Area = $4\pi r^2$

Sphere with
radius = 2r
Area = $4\pi(2r)^2 = 16\pi r^2$

Figure 17.2 Exposure decreases as the square of the distance from the source.

When handling radioactive doses, tools such as tongs can effectively reduce exposure to hands and forearms.

Shielding: When time and distance alone are not sufficient, shielding is usually used. Shields take many forms: syringe shields, vial shields, countertop shields (often with leaded glass), fixed and portable (on casters) lead barriers, as well as thinner shields of plastic that may be used for beta-emitting and very low-energy gamma-emitting sources. The use of lead or other dense materials as shielding for beta particles is discouraged because the dose will be increased owing to the bremsstrahlung effect (see Chapter 2).

Limiting internal exposure

Protection techniques are oriented mainly toward preventing the radioactive material from entering the body. Entrance is most commonly by inhalation, but ingestion, absorption through intact skin, and intake through skin puncture are also possible.

Limiting inhalation is accomplished by good laboratory design, including attention to adequate air replacement and good airflow patterns, use of fume hoods, and by other laboratory practices developed with the consideration of minimizing inhalation. For example, when working with a volatile radioactive source, the worker should be "up wind" of the source, that is to say, the source should be between the worker and an exhaust such as a hood. Although obvious, this practice is often not followed. The use of respirators to limit inhalation of airborne radioactive material is almost never required in a medical institution and should be considered only as a last resort.

Limiting ingestion is accomplished by good laboratory hygiene, such as wearing protective gloves and hospital coats when preparing doses or handling body fluids from a radioactive patient. It is strongly recommended that hands be washed after the removal of gloves as contamination can enter through unseen small holes in the gloves. To reduce the risk of inadvertent ingestion of radioactivity, eating, drinking, smoking, and applying makeup in radiation areas is strictly prohibited. Most compounds are not absorbed through intact skin. Because of their chemical composition, however, beta emitters such as ^{32}P and ^{131}I are absorbed readily through the skin. When dealing with these materials extra care should be taken to properly cover the hands, forearms, and other parts that could become contaminated.

Reducing the risk of contamination following a radiation spill

Careful handling of radioactive materials can reduce the risk of a spill. In the event of a spill it is important to reduce the spread of contamination. Any further spillage should be prevented (i.e. a leaking syringe should be re-capped) and the extent of the spill identified by surveying. All individuals in the vicinity should be notified that a spill has occurred. Individuals not in the room at the time of the spill should be kept out (except for a limited number of staff needed to help with the clean-up). Individuals in the room at the time of the spill should be kept away from the spill until they are surveyed for contamination and those that are contaminated should be decontaminated. The spill should then be carefully cleaned off the floor and equipment surfaces. The nuclear regulatory commission (NRC) classifies **major** versus **minor spills** based solely on the type of radionuclide and the estimated activity of the spill (see examples in Table 17.3) [1]. However, in practice, circumstances such as the presence of contaminated individuals and/or large numbers of involved individuals should be considered a more serious incident and response should be escalated to that of a major spill

Table 17.3 General guidance for differentiating minor versus major spills[a]

Radionuclide	Estimated activity (MBq)	Esitmated activity (mCi)
Flourine-18	3700	100
Gallium-67	370	10
Rubidium-82	370	10
Yttrium-90	37	1
Tc-99m	3700	100
Iodine-123	370	10
Iodine-131	37	1
Thallium-201	3700	100
Alpha emitters (Radium-223)	Any quantity	

[a] NUREG-1556, Vol. 9, Revision 3, Appendix N, Table N.1. Relative Hazards of Common Radionuclides in "Consolidated Guidance about Materials Licenses: Program-Specific Guidance about Medical Use Licenses", Sept, 2019, U.S. Nuclear Regulatory Commission.

even if the dose is below the limits in Table 17.3. In addition, a facility can identify a lower threshold of activity for designating a spill as major. Minor spills are controlled by practices described in the beginning of this section. Major spills require more aggressive additional measures, including covering, but not cleaning up the spill, marking the boundaries of the spill, and locking the room. In both cases the RSO must be notified of the event; in the event of a major spill the RSO must be notified immediately [1]. A report to the NRC may be required in the event of a major spill as defined in Table 17.3.

Employer and employee responsibilities in controlling risk

If an employee is likely to receive more than 10% of any annual limit, the employer is required to perform monitoring. In the case of external exposure, this is usually done with a personal dosimeter such as a film badge or other type of monitor. If the exposure is likely to be internal, for example, from vapors of liquid ^{131}I, monitoring thyroidal uptake is recommended to assess contamination. If the exposure is from ^{32}P, the radiation officer must assess the body burden by measurement of urine counts. A total dose should be estimated based on the effective half-life of the radioactivity.

At least annually, employers are required to notify each monitored employee of the employee's dose. Employers also are required to notify an employee in the event that any limit has been exceeded.

If an employee decides that the risks associated with occupational radiation exposure are too high, the employee may request a reassignment by the employer; however, the employer is not required to provide such a reassignment.

Employees should immediately notify their supervisor if they suspect that a work condition is unsafe or an NRC or state regulation or provision of the license has been violated. The NRC requires licensees to post Form NRC-3, which summarizes employee rights and responsibilities [2].

Limiting exposure to patients

Patient doses are calculated with the intention of reducing the exposure to as low a value as possible while performing a clinically useful diagnostic test or treatment. Special consideration must be given to the **pregnant patient**. The benefit of the test for the mother should be weighed against potential risk to the fetus. In general, limited diagnostic testing is possible. The administered dose should be reduced to the lowest feasible value. **Breast-feeding** should be discontinued until the maximum dose to the newborn infant is less than 1 mSv (0.1 rem) which is purposefully well below the allowed maximum of 5 mSv (0.5 rem) dose to a newborn infant or to a fetus. Guidelines been devised for breast-feeding mothers [3]. Examples are given in Table 17.4.

Limiting exposure to family members and the public

Education of patients and their family members is important particularly following the administration of beta emitters such as ^{131}I and ^{89}Sr. ^{131}I and ^{89}Sr are excreted through bodily fluids, predominantly via urine. To limit exposure to family members and members of the general public, patients must be carefully instructed on how to reduce contamination. Hygienic precautions, such as flushing the toilet twice after use, hand washing, and separate laundering of clothes and linen are necessary to prevent contact with radioactive urine, sweat, and saliva. In addition, following administration of ^{131}I which emits high energy gammas, patients and family must be educated on the rules of time and distance, as outlined above. Patients and family members should be given written guidelines on the preceding precautions for reference after treatment. Further discussion of radiation safety for radiopharmaceutical therapy can be found in Chapter 18.

Household contacts of patients receiving radioactive material should not receive more than 5 mSv (500 mrem) total effective dose equivalent from exposure to the patient. For children or pregnant women this limit is 1 mSv (100 mrem) [4]. Previously, to ensure exposures did not exceed these values, hospital admission was required for doses of sodium iodide ^{131}I that equaled or exceeded 1110 MBq (30 mCi). Patients can now receive higher activities as outpatients if, using dose calculations, it can be shown that the total effective dose equivalent to household contacts will not exceed 5 mSv (1 mSv for children and pregnant women). The procedure for the dose calculations is outlined in NUREG-1556 [5].

In general, though, hospitalization is still recommended for incontinent patients, or patients who cannot care for themselves. The hospital rooms used for admission must be designated for radiation

Table 17.4 Sample recommended times to discontinue breast-feeding following administration of common radionuclides to the mother[a]

Radiopharmaceutical	Administered Activity Above which Patient Instructions for Cessation are required in MBq (mCi)	Recommended Time to Discontinue Breast Feeding
I-131 NaI	0.01 (0.0004)	Do not resume breast feeding
I-123 NaI	20 (0.5)	3 days
I-123 MIBG	70 (2)	24 hours for 370 MBq (10 mCi)
Tc-99m DTPA	1000 (30)	24 hours
Tc-99m DISIDA	1000 (30)	24 hours
Tc-99m MIBI	1000 (30)	24 hours
Tc-99m MDP	1000 (30)	24 hours
Tc-99m MAG3	1000 (30)	24 hours
Tc-99m MAA	50 (1.3)	24 hours
Tc-99m Pertechnetate	100 (3)	24 hours
Tc-99m Sulphur Colloid	300 (7)	24 hours
Tc-99m PYP	900 (25)	24 hours
Tc-99m WBC	100 (3)	24 hours
Tc-99m RBC	400 (10)	24 hours
In-111 WBC	10 (0.2)	6 days
Tl-201 Chloride	40 (1)	4 days
F-18 FDG	Activity can be calculated using dose conversion factors[b]	4 hours
Ga-68 Octreotate	Activity can be calculated using dose conversion factors[b]	4 hours
Lu-177 Octreotate	Activity can be calculated using dose conversion factors[b]	Do not resume breast feeding
Ra-223 and all other alpha emitters	Activity can be calculated using dose conversion factors[b]	Do not resume breast feeding

Activities are rounded to 1 or 2 significant digits.
[a] NUREG 8.39, Revision 1, April 2020, USNRC, pp. 11–12.
[b] Reference given in NUREG 8.39, p. 22: Stabin M, "Internal Dosimetry in Pediatric Nuclear Medicine" *Pediatric Nuclear Medicine*, S. Treves (Ed.), Springer Verlag, New York, NY, pp. 556–81, 1995.

therapy and be monitored by the radiation safety staff to reduce staff, visitor, and other patient exposure.

Regulations

The Nuclear Regulatory Commission (NRC) regulations pertaining to the above text and other standard procedures performed in the routine practice of nuclear medicine are summarized in Appendix C.

References

1. NUREG-1556, Vol. 9, Revision 3, Appendix N, Table N.1, Relative Hazards of Common Radionuclides in "Consolidated Guidance about Materials Licenses: Program-Specific Guidance about Medical Use Licenses", Sept, 2019, U.S. Nuclear Regulatory Commission.
2. NRC Regulations Title 10, Code of Federal Regulations, 19.11 Posting of notices to workers, U.S. Nuclear Regulatory Commission, Aug 24, 2018.
3. US NRC Regulatory Guide 8.39 Revision 1, Release of Patients Administered Radioactive Materials, April, 2020, Table 3, p. 11.
4. NRC Regulation 10, part 35.75 Release of individuals containing unsealed byproduct material or implants containing byproduct material. Aug, 2017.
5. NUREG-1556, Vol. 9, Revision 2, Appendix U, "Consolidated Guidance about Materials Licenses: Program-Specific Guidance about Medical Use Licenses", Jan, 2008, U.S. Nuclear Regulatory Commission, p. U-2.

Questions

1. Associate the following annual exposures with the permissible maximum doses:
   (a) TEDE, total effective dose equivalent, for a member of the public.
   (b) Maximum permissible exposure to a hospital worker who is not a radiation worker.
   (c) Background whole body radiation at sea level.
   (d) Maximum permissible TEDE for a radiation worker.
      (1) 50 mSv (5.0 rem).
      (2) 3.6 mSv (0.36 rem).
      (3) 1.0 mSv (0.1 rem).

2. Select the three most effective ways to reduce exposure when working with radioactivity.
   (a) Reduce the time spent in the vicinity of a radioactive source.
   (b) Maintain the maximum possible distance from the source.
   (c) Shield the radioactive source.
   (d) All of the above.

3. A nursing mother should be instructed to permanently discontinue breast-feeding under which of the following circumstances?
   (a) After receiving any radiopharmaceutical.
   (b) After receiving an injection of 37 MBq of ^{99m}Tc MAA.
   (c) After ingesting 370 MBq of ^{131}I.

4. True or false: The maximum allowable exposure to the household contacts of a patient receiving radioactivity, including children and pregnant women, is 5 mSv.

5. True or false: Radionuclide spills are classified by the NRC as either major or minor spills based on the volume of fluid involved.

6. The embryo/fetus dose equivalent limits for radiation workers can be applied under which conditions?
   (a) For a radiation worker who is obviously pregnant but who has not declared her pregnancy in written form.
   (b) For a radiation worker who has declared her pregnancy in written form.
   (c) Both (a) and (b).

7. Bob is standing 2 meters away from a radioactive source; Phyllis is standing 4 meters away from the same source. Neither is shielded. Which of the following is true about Phyllis's exposure compared to Bob's exposure?
   (a) Phyllis's radiation exposure is equal to Bob's.
   (b) Phyllis's radiation exposure is half of Bob's.
   (c) Phyllis's radiation exposure is one-quarter of Bob's.

8. If the exposure rate for a point source is 1 R/h at 1 meter, what is the exposure rate at 3 meters?
   (a) 3 R/h.
   (b) 0.33 R/h.
   (c) 0.25 R/h.
   (d) 0.11 R/h.

Answers

1. (a) (iii). (b) (iii). (c) (ii). (d) (i).
2. (d).
3. (c).
4. False. It is 5 mSv for everyone except for children and pregnant women for whom the limit is 1 mSv.
5. False. The activity and type of radionuclide determines whether a spill is major or minor.
6. (b). The radiation worker must declare her pregnancy in written form before the limits on embryo/fetal dose can be applied.

7. (c). The dose from a source decreases by the inverse square of the distance from the source. So an additional 2 meters results in a decrease of $1/(2)^2 = ¼$. So, Phyllis's dose is ¼ that of Bob's.
8. (d). Exposure decreases by the inverse square of the distance from the source, so $1/(3)^2 = 1/9 = 0.11$ R/h.

CHAPTER 18

Radiopharmaceutical Therapy

This chapter is divided into two parts. The first part is a review of several common therapeutic radiopharmaceuticals and their biological mechanism of uptake.

The second part reviews radiation protection practices for handling and administering these radiopharmaceuticals.

Introduction

Radiopharmaceuticals are compounds composed of biologically active radioisotopes bound to another ion, or radioisotopes bound by a linker molecule to a carrier molecule that has high affinity for a special target or function in an organ or tissue (Figure 18.1).

If the radioisotope emits gamma rays, X-rays, or positrons it is diagnostic; if it emits alpha or beta particles it is therapeutic. Some radiopharmaceuticals can be both diagnostic and therapeutic.

Paired diagnostic and therapeutic radiopharmaceuticals

Most therapeutic radiopharmaceuticals are "paired" with a diagnostic radiopharmaceutical. This diagnostic agent is used to characterize the target tissue or organ, predict the uptake and estimate the dosimetry of its therapeutic counterpart prior to treatment.

Several therapeutic and diagnostic radiopharmaceuticals pairs are not structurally identical, but have similar or identical biologic uptake in an organ. Examples are ^{223}Ra-dichloride (therapeutic) and ^{99m}Tc-phosphonate compounds (diagnostic). Another example is ^{90}Y-microspheres (therapeutic) and ^{99m}Tc-macroaggregated albumin (^{99m}Tc-MAA—diagnostic).

When a **thera**peutic radiopharmaceutical and a diag**nostic** radiopharmaceutical are identical except for their radioisotopes, they are called **theranostic**. Examples are ^{123}I sodium iodide (diagnostic) paired with ^{131}I sodium iodide (predominantly therapeutic) and ^{68}Ga-dotatate (diagnostic) paired with ^{177}Lu-dotatate (predominantly therapeutic). In addition to beta particle emissions, both ^{131}I and ^{177}Lu also emit gamma photons that, while not ideal for imaging, permit assessment of their biodistribution following treatment.

Tissue-specific radiopharmaceutical treatments

The thyroid gland and radioiodine

The thyroid gland

The thyroid gland actively takes up iodide and sodium via the **sodium iodide symporter** cell membrane glycoprotein. Once inside the thyroid cells, the iodide atom combines with a portion of the protein **thyroglobulin** to make tyrosine derivatives (**mono**iodotyrosine (**MIT**) and **di**iodotyrosine (**DIT**) which are then combined to form the thyroid hormones, **T3** (**triiodothyronine**) and **T4** (**thyroxine**) (Figure 18.2). Thyroid hormones are crucial as they control the speed of metabolism of organs throughout the body.

Thyroid diseases treated with radioiodine:

Sodium iodide ^{131}I is one of the oldest therapeutic radiopharmaceuticals and was first used in the 1940s. It is used to treat overactive thyroid glands (hyperthyroidism), to eradicate residual thyroid tissue

Essentials of Nuclear Medicine Physics, Instrumentation, and Radiation Biology, Fourth Edition.
Rachel A. Powsner, Matthew R. Palmer, and Edward R. Powsner.
© 2022 John Wiley & Sons Ltd. Published 2022 by John Wiley & Sons Ltd.

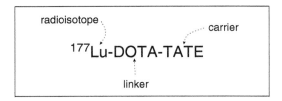

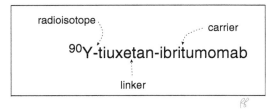

Figure 18.1 Radiopharmaceutical structure. Top: ^{131}I is part of an ionic compound "sharing" an outer shell electron with a Na atom. Middle and bottom: Radioisotopes are bound via a "linker" molecule to a carrier that interacts with cell receptors.

following thyroidectomy, and to treat recurrent or metastatic thyroid cancer.

Hyperthyroidism: Hyperthyroidism refers to an overactive thyroid gland which makes too much thyroid hormone. Overproduction of thyroid hormone can cause a myriad of unpleasant symptoms including difficulties with sleep, irritability, an overactive colon, weight loss, loss of bone mass, and arrhythmias. The two main causes of hyperthyroidism are an autoimmune disease called **Graves'** thyroiditis (in which the gland is diffusely overactive) and genetic mutations within the gland which cause hyperfunctioning nodules (a single overactive nodule is usually called a **toxic adenoma**, a gland with multiple hyperfunctioning nodules is called a **toxic multinodular goiter**).

Treatment of hyperthyroidism includes daily medication to suppress hormone production, ^{131}I sodium iodide administration, and/or surgery. Doses for treatment of hyperthyroidism range from approximately 5 mCi to 30 mCi (185 MBq to 1.1 GBq), with higher doses for specific situations such as a very large gland.

Thyroid cancer: There are many types of thyroid cancer. In differentiated thyroid cancers (papillary and follicular) the cells retain some of the function of normal cells and can usually take up

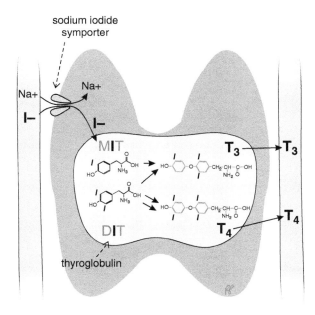

Figure 18.2 The thyroid incorporates iodide into thyroid hormones which are released into the blood stream.

131I sodium iodide (but to a lesser extent than normal thyroid tissue). Thyroid cancer restricted to the thyroid gland and nearby lymph nodes is removed surgically. Depending on the size and characteristics of the tumor 131I sodium iodide is used to eradicate the post-surgical remnants of the thyroid gland and any remaining tumor cells within this tissue. Once normal thyroid tissue is removed, serum blood tests, in particular thyroglobulin (Tgb), and total body 131I sodium iodide scans can be performed to assess for recurrent disease. Recurrent disease can be treated with surgery or 131I sodium iodide. Administered activity of 131I sodium iodide ranges from 2–5 mCi (7.4–18.5 MBq) for total body scans, up to 200 mCi (7.4 GBq) or more for metastatic disease treatment.

Radioiodine (131I and 123I sodium iodide)

131I and 123I sodium iodide are taken into the thyroid gland and processed just like stable sodium iodide (Figure 18.3).

131I: 131I is created in a nuclear reactor via fission of 235U or neutron irradiation of a tellurium target (Appendix A). 131I decays to 133Xe (Figure 1.22) by beta (electron) emission (606 keV and 192 keV are the maximum and mean energies of the most abundant beta emissions), and by gamma (364 keV) emission. The beta particles travel a mean distance of 0.4 mm in tissue [1].

123I: 123I is created in a cyclotron by proton bombardment of 124Xe. 123I decays to 123Te by electron capture causing emission of a characteristic 28 keV X-ray as an outer shell electron drops into

the new vacancy in the inner shell. The 123Te nucleus releases a 159 keV gamma photon as it drops to a more stable energy state with a half-life of nearly 10^17 years [2].

Uses of 123I and 131I in diagnostic imaging and therapy

Both isotopes can be used for imaging the gland and measuring the avidity of the gland for iodide (a gland that takes up more iodide is more metabolically active). The 159 keV photons emitted by 123I result in much better image quality than those derived from the 364 keV photons emanating from 131I. The latter high energy photons result in poorer image quality due to septal and crystal penetration. 123I results in a much lower radiation dose than 131I (7 mGy versus 777 mGy) to the thyroid for an administered dose of 3.7 MBq in a gland with 15% radioactive iodine uptake [3]. For this reason, it is exclusively used for standard diagnostic thyroid scans. For total body imaging to detect metastatic thyroid cancer, however, 131I is more commonly used.

223Ra-dichloride and treatment of bone metastatic disease

Bone physiology

Bone serves as a structural support for the body and a repository for minerals, particularly calcium. Bone marrow, found in cavities within bone, contains the progenitors of blood cells.

Bone is constantly remodeling in response to gravity and to muscle tension, but it also remodels at sites of fracture and around tumors within the bone. Bone remodeling is complex but can be simplified as the action of two types of bone cells: the

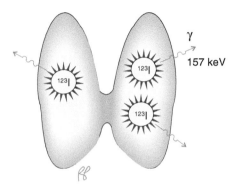
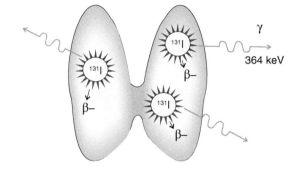

Figure 18.3 Left: The gamma emissions of 123I are used to create images of the thyroid gland. Right: The beta particles emitted by 131I destroy nearby thyroid tissue and the high energy gamma rays can be used for imaging as well.

osteoclasts, which break down bone tissue, and the **osteoblasts** which help create new bone by excreting a protein called **collagen**. The newly laid bone hardens as a molecule called **hydroxyapatite** adheres to the collagen. Hydroxyapatite contains, among other atoms, an abundance of calcium and phosphorus (Figure 18.4). Bone marrow is particularly radiosensitive given rapid cell formation during the production of blood cells.

^{223}Ra: ^{223}Ra is eluted from an ^{227}actinium/^{223}radium generator. ^{223}Ra has an 18.7 day half-life and during decay to stable ^{207}Pb emits primarily alpha particles (composed of two neutrons and two protons) which have a kinetic energy range of 5.8–7.53 MeV (Figure 18.5) [4].

^{223}Ra dichloride treatment
^{223}Ra dichloride is currently the most commonly used agent for the treatment of prostate cancer metastatic lesions within bone. The mechanism of incorporation into bone is the same as calcium. The alpha particles travel fewer than 100 microns in tissue due to their high LET (linear energy transfer—see Chapter 2) and cause more double-strand DNA breaks than beta particles (see Figure 15.3). The alpha particles destroy nearby bone surface cells such as osteoblasts, as well as tumor cells in close proximity to newly formed bone tissue (Figure 18.6 upper image). The short distance traveled by alpha particles in bone marrow dose is less than that the beta emissions from other bone directed therapeutic radiopharmaceuticals, ^{153}Sm EDTMP and ^{89}Sr chloride, which can travel 3 mm and 8 mm in soft tissue, respectively [5], [6].

Bone marrow suppression can, however, occur with ^{223}Ra dichloride. Prior to any treatment, blood cell counts must be monitored since decreasing counts reflect reduced bone marrow reserve. If counts are below the acceptable threshold, the

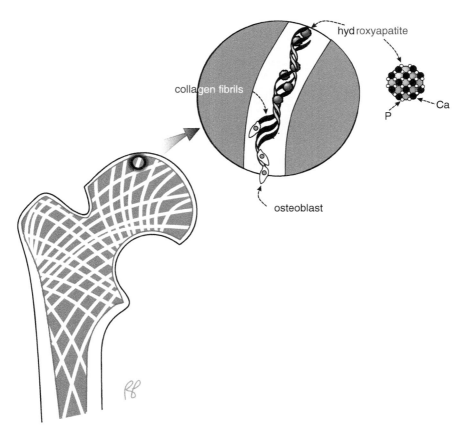

Figure 18.4 Collagen is secreted by osteoblastic cells. Hydroxyapatite is incorporated in the collagen matrix to create the hard structure of bone tissue.

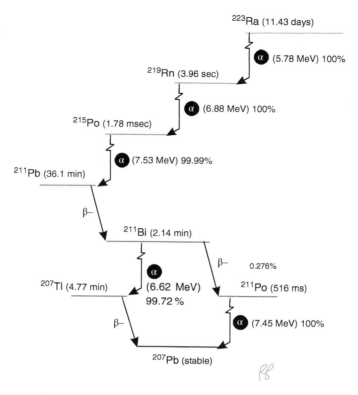

^{223}Ra (11.43 days)

α (5.78 MeV) 100%

^{219}Rn (3.96 sec)

α (6.88 MeV) 100%

^{215}Po (1.78 msec)

α (7.53 MeV) 99.99%

^{211}Pb (36.1 min)

β–

^{211}Bi (2.14 min)

β–   0.276%

α
(6.62 MeV)
99.72 %

^{207}Tl (4.77 min) ^{211}Po (516 ms)

β–   α (7.45 MeV) 100%

^{207}Pb (stable)

Figure 18.5 Decay scheme of ^{223}Ra.

subsequent dose should be delayed until there is adequate improvement.

^{223}Ra is a less than ideal imaging agent as decay produces few gamma emission (1.1% of total decay emissions with the most abundant emissions of energies ranging from 71–427 keV). Instead, ^{99m}Tc-diphosphonates, which are also incorporated into hydroxyapatite, are used to localize remodeling at sites of tumor metastases prior to treatment with ^{223}Ra dichloride (Figure 18.6b).

Radioactive ^{90}Y-microsphere treatment of liver tumors

Liver physiology
The liver performs many functions within the body including, but not limited to, metabolism of carbohydrates, fats, and proteins, synthesis of proteins such as albumin and clotting factors, and synthesis and excretion of bile. The **portal vein**, which supplies 80% of the blood and 50% of the oxygen to the liver, carries the breakdown products of food (the proteins, carbohydrates, and fats) and toxins from

the intestinal tract. The other 20% of blood supply (and 50% of the oxygen) comes from the common **hepatic artery** which splits into two major branches: the right hepatic artery, which supplies the right lobe of the liver; and the left hepatic artery, which supplies the left lobe of the liver (Figure 18.7).

Unlike normal liver tissue, some liver tumors are predominantly, or solely, supplied with blood from the hepatic artery and not the portal vein, allowing them to be treated by locally injecting radioactive materials through the branches of the hepatic artery.

^{90}Y: There are two means of production of ^{90}Y: elution from a ^{90}Sr/^{90}Y generator and neutron bombardment of stable ^{89}Y within a reactor.

Almost all of ^{90}Y decays (half-life of 64.1 hours) to ^{90}Zr by emission of beta particles with an average energy of 0.94 MeV and a maximum energy of 2.28 MeV that travel an average of 2.5 mm (maximum of 11 mm) in soft tissues. A very small amount of ^{90}Y decays to a higher energy "excited" state of ^{90}Zr which then decays to stable ^{90}Zr by pair

(a) ^{223}Ra

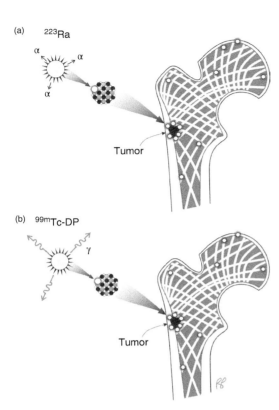

(b) ^{99m}Tc-DP

Figure 18.6 ^{223}Ra and ^{99m}Tc-DP compounds are incorporated into hydroxyapatite as calcium analogs. The alpha emissions of ^{223}Ra (a) destroy nearby tissue; the gamma emissions of ^{99m}Tc (b) are used to image newly formed bone.

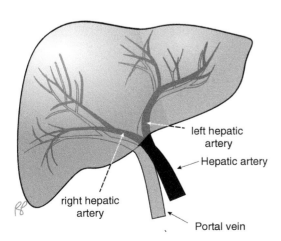

Figure 18.7 Hepatic artery and portal vein blood supply to the liver.

production (emission of an electron and positron, Figure 18.8). The pair production pathway occurs very rarely, yielding approximately one pair per 3.2×10^5 decays [7].

^{90}Y-microspheres

There are two forms of commercially available **^{90}Y-microspheres**. The first is made by incorporating ^{90}Y into a resin which is formed into microspheres ranging in diameter from 20–60 microns [8]. The second product is made by incorporating stable ^{89}Y into glass microspheres (20–30 microns in diameter) [9] which are then bombarded by neutrons converting the ^{89}Y into ^{90}Y. Small amounts of long-lived contaminants, such as ^{154}Europium (half-life of 8 years) are also created within the glass beads.

^{90}Y-microsphere treatment

Treatment is directed at either the right or left lobes of the liver, or at a portion (segment) of one of these lobes.

^{90}Y-microsphere therapy involves two steps: an imaging **mapping** procedure followed by a therapeutic procedure. In both cases particles are delivered through a long catheter which is inserted into the femoral artery and then advanced through the vessels until its tip is in position within the branch of the hepatic artery that supplies blood to the part of the liver containing the tumor (Figure 18.9).

The mapping procedure uses ^{99m}Tc-MAA (macroaggregated albumin) particles (Figure 18.10a) and imaging following injection is performed to verify that the particles are in the correct location in the liver and are not delivered to other organs, particularly the lung and gastrointestinal tract. The maximum dose to the lung for each treatment must be under 30 Gy, and the cumulative lung dose for more than one treatment must not exceed 50 Gy [9].

If the results of the ^{99m}Tc-MAA imaging are favorable, the patient proceeds to the therapeutic procedure with injection of the ^{90}Y-microspheres into the identical location in the hepatic artery (Figure 18.10b).

Distribution of the ^{99m}Tc-MAA and the ^{90}Y-microspheres within the liver is not identical, in large part because the MAA particles range in size from 10–150 microns (micrometers) with 90% of the particles in a MAA sample being 10–90 microns in size compared to 20–60 microns for the microspheres.

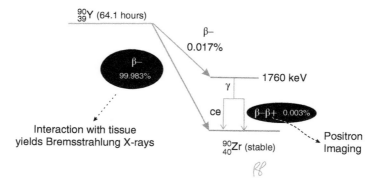

Figure 18.8 Decay scheme of ^{90}Y.

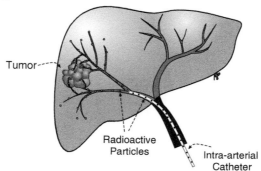

Figure 18.9 Introduction of radiolabeled microspheres through an intra-arterial catheter.

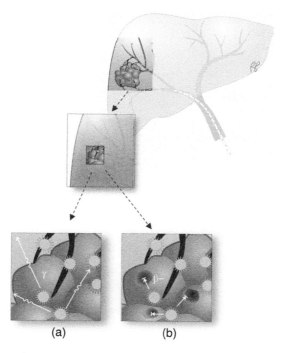

Figure 18.10 (a) ^{99m}Tc-MAA is used to simulate or "map" the future distribution of microspheres to ensure safety and effectiveness; (b) The beta particle emission from the ^{90}Y-microspheres destroy nearby tissues.

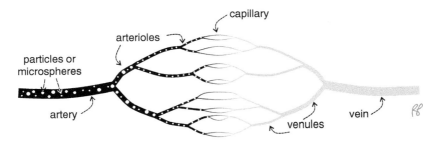

Figure 18.11 MAA particles and microspheres lodge in arterioles.

Both MAA particles and microspheres become lodged in the very small branches of the arteries, called **arterioles**, which have a diameter of approximately 10–100 microns (Figure 18.11).

Prescribed activity for ⁹⁰Y treatment

Although there are several methods for calculating the activity to be administered for resin ⁹⁰Y-microspheres, a common calculation is based on the patient's body surface area and the tumor, lobar, and whole liver volumes [8].

For ⁹⁰Y-glass microspheres the recommended dose range is 80–150 Gy³ to the treated lobe of the liver [9]. The treatment activity is based on the desired dose from this range and the mass of the lobe to be treated.

⁹⁰Y imaging

Bremsstrahlung: Even though ⁹⁰Y decay yields no significant gamma emissions, post-treatment images of the distribution can be obtained with gamma and PET cameras by utilizing two different decay products. The first is gamma camera imaging of the bremsstrahlung ("braking radiation") X-rays (Chapter 2) created through interaction of the beta particles with the nuclei of the atoms in tissues. A wide energy window must be used to capture the range of emitted X-ray energies yielding images with poor resolution.

Positron: Images with much better resolution are obtained when a PET-CT camera is used to image the 511 keV photons emitted during the annihilation of positrons ($\beta+$) from ⁹⁰Y decay. Due to the very low yield of positrons, these images take longer to acquire than standard ¹⁸F-FDG images.

Imaging and therapy targeting cancer cell membranes

Cancer cell targeting

Cancer cells can be targeted by radiolabeled molecules which attach to proteins on their cell membranes. Two of the common types of targeting are discussed below.

Monoclonal antibody targeting: **Radiolabeled monoclonal antibodies** bind to cell surface proteins (**antigens**) and this **antigen-antibody complex** remains on the surface of the cell. An example is ⁹⁰Y-ibritumomab tiuxetan [10] which attaches to an antigen called CD-20 expressed on the surface of normal B cells (a type of white blood cell), and to a greater extent on the surface of B-cell lymphomas (Figure 18.12). Therapy with radiolabeled monoclonal antibodies is called **radioimmunotherapy**.

Peptide receptor targeting: A second method of targeting is to radiolabel a small protein called a **peptide**, which attaches to a **receptor protein** on the cell surface (the peptide in this role is called a ligand) and this **ligand-receptor complex** is then taken inside the cell (Figure 18.13). This type of radionuclide therapy is labeled **PRRT**, an initialism of either **p**eptide **r**eceptor **r**adionuclide **t**herapy or **p**eptide **r**eceptor **r**adioligand **t**herapy.

¹⁷⁷Lutetium-dotatate and ⁶⁸gallium-dotatate for neuroendocrine tumors

Neuroendocrine cells: Neuroendocrine cells are stimulated by neurons (nervous system cells) to release hormones into the blood stream. Examples of neuroendocrine cells include medullary cells in the adrenal gland which release adrenalin, C-cells

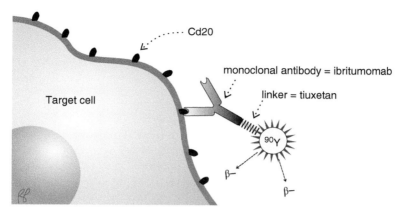

Figure 18.12 Therapeutic radiolabeled monoclonal antibody.

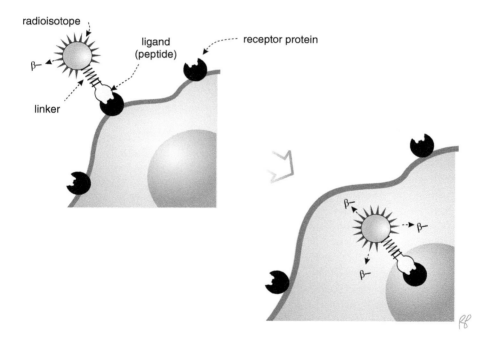

Figure 18.13 Therapeutic radiolabeled ligand.

in the thyroid which release calcitonin, and islet cells in the pancreas which release, among other hormones, insulin.

Tumors arising from neuroendocrine cells (**neuroendocrine tumors or NETs**), can retain the ability to secrete hormones causing debilitating symptoms. Examples include **carcinoid** tumors which produce excess serotonin causing flushing, rapid heart rate, and diarrhea, and **insulinoma** which secretes excess insulin causing hypoglycemia.

Somatostatin is a hormone that suppresses secretion of other hormones. Its man-made analog, octreotide, is used to treat the symptoms of neuroendocrine tumors. Somatostatin and octreotide bind to **somatostatin receptors** on the surface of neuroendocrine cells causing the cell to reduce hormone secretion. There are five different types of somatostatin receptors (SSTR1, SSTR2, SSTR3, SSTR4, and SSTR5). SSTR2 is the most common receptor.

Radiolabeled analogs of somatostatin are used for imaging and therapy of neuroendocrine tumors.

Examples of imaging agents are ^{68}Ga-dotatate (attaches to SSTR 2), and ^{68}Ga-dotatoc (attaches to SSTR 5). Theranostic therapeutic agents for these compounds are ^{177}Lu-dotatate and ^{90}Y-dotatoc. As ^{177}Lu is both a beta and gamma emitter, post-therapy gamma camera images can be obtained to assess distribution.

[177]*Lu dotatate administration:* [177]Lu has a physical half-life of 6.73 days and emits beta particles with maximum energy of 0.498 MeV, and a maximum soft-tissue penetration depth of 1.7 mm. In addition to the beta particles, ^{177}Lu has two gamma emissions at 113 keV and 208 keV with low relative abundance (6.2% and 10.4% respectively) [11].

[177]Lu-dotatate is administered every 8 weeks for a total of 4 doses, each measuring 7.4 GBq (200 mCi) [12].

Renal toxicity from this agent is a dose-limiting factor as 2–3% of the dose excreted by the kidneys is reabsorbed and retained in the **proximal tubule cells** by attaching to somatostatin and other cell receptors.

The kidney helps maintain overall fluid balance, regulates the quantity of many small particles (such as amino acids), and removes toxins from the blood stream. These actions are the result of filtration of blood products at the interface of the blood-containing **glomerulus** within the first part of the nephron, the **Bowman's capsule**. The fluids and small particles (filtrate) flow through the nephron into the ureter and eventually into the bladder (see Figure 18.14). Along the extent of the nephron, there are several sites of re-absorption and excretion of portions of the filtrate. To reduce the renal radiation dose, **amino acids** (in particular L-lysine and L-arginine) are infused before, during, and after the ^{177}Lu treatment. These amino acids are also ligands that compete with the ^{177}Lu-dotatate uptake by the receptors in the proximal renal tubule cells resulting in up to 50% [11] reduction in renal radiation dose (Figure 18.15).

Prior to each ^{177}Lu-dotatate administration, octreotide, the somatostatin analog discussed above is held for 24 hours for the short-acting form, and 4 weeks for the long-acting form of the drug. Blood cell counts and renal function must be measured prior to each treatment, and the administered ^{177}Lu-dotatate activity may need to be reduced or withheld if there is a severe reduction in these values.

Prostate-specific membrane antigen (PMSA) agents for prostate cancer

As several of these agents are still under development, or being tested in prospective clinical trials prior to final FDA approval, only a brief introduction follows:

Prostate-specific membrane antigen (PMSA): **Prostate-specific membrane antigen (PMSA)** is a **glycoprotein** (a molecule containing both amino acids and sugars) that is found on the surface of prostate cells, and cells of some other organs in the body such as the small intestine, kidneys, and salivary glands. Prostate cancer cells express up to 1000 times more of these glycoproteins than normal prostate cells.

Radiolabeled PMSA: -Although there are many different radiolabeled peptide ligands that target PMSA, the general convention is to include PMSA in their naming, for example: ^{68}Ga-PMSA-11 and ^{18}F-PMSA-1007 as imaging agents, and ^{177}Lu-PMSA-617 for therapy. The physical characteristics of the radionuclides ^{68}Ga and ^{177}Lu have been discussed earlier. [18]F is used widely in PET imaging, most notably as ^{18}F-FDG (fluorodeoxyglucose). [18]F is produced in a cyclotron by high energy proton bombardment of [18]O. [18]F has a half-life of 110 minutes and decays primarily (97%) by positron emission to stable [18]O.

Radiation protection

Special precautions must be taken when prescribing, handling, and administering radiopharmaceutical medications to patients in order to protect patients, their families, and staff from unnecessary radiation exposure.

Written directives

Written directives are required by the nuclear regulatory commission (10 CFR 35.4; see listing of regulations in Appendix D) for all ^{131}I sodium iodide doses greater than 1.1 MBq (30 microcuries) and all other therapeutic radiopharmaceuticals of any quantity. There are two parts of a written directive: the prescription which is completed prior to drug administration, and the documentation of administered activity which is completed immediately following treatment. The prescription must be signed by an authorized user and must contain the

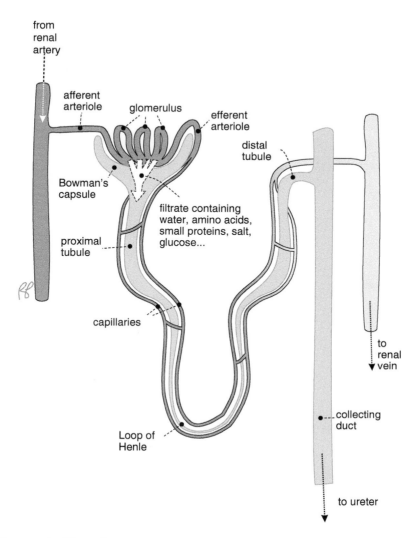

Figure 18.14 Components of the nephron.

patient's name, the complete name of the radiopharmaceutical (I-¹³¹I sodium iodide, for example), the prescribed activity, and the planned route of administration (intravenous, intra-arterial, intraperitoneal, or oral).

The documentation of the treatment must be signed by two qualified individuals. Both individuals must witness the dose calibrator reading, verify that the dose is being given in accordance with the prescription, and verify the patient's identification using two identifiers such as name and birthdate.

The administered dose must be within 20% of the prescribed dose. If the dose differs by more than 20% and the patient receives an absolute difference of more than 0.05 Sv (5 rem) effective dose equivalent or 0.5 Sv (50 rem) to an organ or tissue or skin than the prescribed dose, the incident must be reported as a medical event to the Nuclear Regulatory Commission (NRC). Licensees are also required by the NRC to establish a Quality Management Program (QMP) that includes regular chart review by a qualified person.

Dose preparation

Basic precautions for handling therapeutic radiopharmaceuticals are the same as those used for handling diagnostic radioisotopes and radiopharmaceuticals as described in Chapter 17,

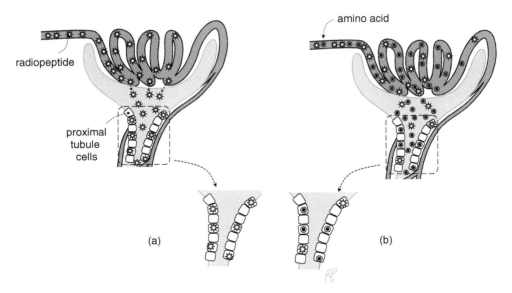

Figure 18.15 "Cold" amino acids competitively block the re-absorption of the ^{177}Lu-dotatate in the proximal tubule cells of the nephron.

Methods for limiting exposure. In addition, tongs are recommended for handling dose vials to reduce personnel exposure.

As with diagnostic radiopharmaceuticals, therapeutic doses should be manipulated behind lead bricks and leaded glass shields if there are significant gamma emissions (such as with ^{131}I). Plastic shields are recommended for beta or alpha emitters with little or no gamma emissions (such as ^{223}Ra or ^{90}Y).

Dose calibrator measurement of beta and alpha emitters

Dose calibrators are less than ideal for measuring alpha and beta emissions as these particles are easily blocked (see Chapter 4) by the surrounding liquid in which they are suspended, the glass containment vial, and the lining of the dose calibrator well. Most therapeutic agents, however, either emit small amounts of gamma radiation (such as ^{223}Ra) which can be measured by the dose calibrator, or in the case of "pure" beta emitters such as ^{90}Y, the beta particles interact with the surrounding materials to produce Bremsstrahlung X-rays (see Chapter 2) which can also be detected by the dose calibrator (Figure 18.16).

Prior to the first use of any therapeutic radiopharmaceutical, a **NIST** (National Institutes of Standards and Technology) standard of the agent is measured in the dose calibrator. The dial settings are adjusted until the measured activity matches the expected activity and then the settings are recorded and used to measure subsequent doses.

Dose administration

There are basic common radiation protection practices for therapeutic radiopharmaceutical administrations as well as additional recommended practices for specific agents. While administering a dose the precautions outlined above for dose preparation should be practiced. Rooms must also be prepared to minimize contamination. Additional recommendations for specific radiopharmaceuticals follow.

^{177}Lu-dotatate

Eye protection and shoe coverings are recommended for personnel caring for patients during ^{177}Lu-dotatate therapy which has a splash risk from contaminated vomitus. In addition, room preparation to reduce contamination requires posting the room as a radiation area, covering all or part of the floor and lower walls with disposable absorptive or waterproof materials. Door handles, sink handles, toilet seats, phones, and TV remote controls are covered with removable plastic. In room hospital scrubs and laundry and trash receptacles are placed for use by the patient. The patient should have a dedicated bathroom.

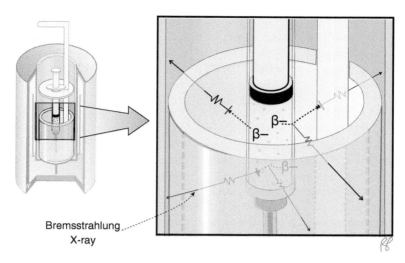

Figure 18.16 Bremsstrahlung X-rays resulting from the interaction of beta particles with the nuclei in surrounding materials are detected by the dose calibrator.

⁹⁰Y-microspheres

Careful handling of the catheter used to instill ^{90}Y-microspheres is required to ensure that there is no leakage of the microspheres into the room. Leakage of microspheres can cause easily spread contamination because of their shape and the effects of static electricity.

¹³¹I sodium iodide

Since ^{131}I emits a high energy gamma photon, increased distance and shielding and decreased time spent near the patient are particularly important. In addition, avoiding contamination is important as ^{131}I is readily absorbed through the skin.

Post-therapy radiation precautions

Following dose administration there are two sources of radiation exposure for individuals in contact with the patient: gamma and X-ray emissions from the patient and contamination with patient excretions containing radionuclides.

Gamma emissions

For the previously discussed therapeutic radiopharmaceuticals only ^{177}Lu-dotatate and ^{131}I sodium iodide have significant gamma emissions. Most patients can be discharged home immediately following treatment as long as the patient and family can follow instructions that reduce exposure such that the total effective dose equivalent to household contacts will not exceed 5 mSv (500 mrem) to adult family members and a maximum of 1 mSv (100 mrem) to children, pregnant women, and members of the general public. The procedure for calculating the maximum allowable activity for discharge is outlined in NUREG—1556, Vol. 9 Rev 2 (Appendix U) [13].

Pure beta emitters such as ^{90}Y, and alpha emitters such as ^{223}Ra rarely cause significant radiation exposure to other individuals as the majority of the energy of the beta and alpha emissions are absorbed by the patient's body.

Patients receiving ^{177}Lu-dotatate are instructed to sleep alone and remain at least 1 meter from adults for 7 days, this limit is increased to 15 days for children and pregnant women.

Patients receiving ^{131}I sodium iodide must physically distance from others for 1–7 days; the higher the dose, the longer the period of time. They can remain 1 meter from others for up to 1 hour per day and 2 meters from others for the remainder of the day, and they should sleep alone. For higher doses they must self-isolate for 1–2 days immediately after treatment.

If a patient receiving ^{131}I sodium iodide therapy cannot follow safety instructions, they should be admitted until they retain less than 30 mCi of ^{131}I or until the exposure at 1 meter from the patient is less than 7 mrem/h. Hospital stays are generally a minimum of 2–3 days to provide adequate time for excretion of ^{131}I in their urine (see below regarding contamination).

For inpatients, ^{131}I treatment precautions are designed to limit radiation exposure to staff, patients, and visitors as well as reduce the risk of contamination with ^{131}I from the patient's urine, sweat, and saliva. The inpatient rooms are prepared in a similar manner to the rooms used for administering ^{177}Lu-dotatate (see above). Hospital staff must don shoe covers, gowns, and gloves prior to entering the room and remove them immediately upon exiting the room. Medical staff are encouraged to limit the time spent in the patient's room, but there should be no hesitation to perform necessary medical procedures, particularly cardiac and pulmonary resuscitation, out of fear of radiation exposure. If care is taken to rotate staff performing CPR and unnecessary individuals are excluded from the room the staff exposure remains minimal.

Contamination

All radiopharmaceuticals (except for ^{90}Y glass microspheres) have some degree of excretion through urine and/or feces and care must be taken to ensure that other individuals are not contaminated. If possible, for [131]iodine therapy, patients should have a dedicated bathroom for use for 2–3 days immediately following treatment. Both ^{131}I and ^{177}Lu dotatate patients should increase fluid intake, sit on the toilet when urinating, flush the toilet twice, and wash their hands after use [14]. Following ^{131}I therapy clothes and linens used during the first 2–3 days should be washed separately. [131]Iodine is also found in saliva and sweat and because of this, sharing of dishware is discouraged and patients are encouraged to wear gloves while handling shared items such as phones.

[223]Ra is primarily excreted in the feces with minimal excretion in urine.

Written hygiene instructions

For all radiopharmaceutical administrations, the patient and family members must be educated on the rules of time and distance in order to reduce their exposure. Patients and family members should be given written specific guidelines on how to minimize exposure and contamination as a reference after treatment, and a copy of these instructions signed by the patient should be retained for their hospital records. It is also recommended that the patient carry a card or sheet of paper stating they have received a medical radionuclide on a specified date which also includes contact information for the treating clinician in case the patient triggers radiation alarms in public spaces.

References

1. Lin Y. Internal radiation therapy: a neglected aspect of nuclear medicine in the molecular era. *J Biomed Res.* 2015 Sep; 29(5): 345–55.
2. Laboratoire National Henri Becquerel website: www.lnhb.fr/nuclear-data/nuclear-data-table/
3. ICRP Publication 53. Radiation dose to patients from radiopharmaceuticals. *Annals of the ICRP.* 1987; (18):1–4, pp. 264 and 276.
4. Abou D, Ulmert D, Doucet M, et al. Whole-body and microenvironmental localization of radium-223 in naïve and mouse models of prostate cancer metastasis. *J Natl Cancer Inst.* (online) 2015 Dec 18;108(5):djv380. Print: *J Natl Cancer Inst.* 2016;108(5).
5. Quadramet Prescribing Information, Lantheus Medical Imaging, Inc., N. Billerica, Massachusetts, September 2017.
6. National Center for Biotechnology Information (2021). PubChem Compound Summary for CID 5388879, Strontium chloride SR-89. https://pubchem.ncbi.nlm.nih.gov/compound/Strontium-chloride-SR-89.
7. Pavel Dryák, Jaroslav Šolc. Measurement of the branching ratio related to the internal pair production of Y-90, applied radiation and isotopes (156), February 2020, https://doi.org/10.1016/j.apradiso.2019.108942.
8. Sirtex. SIR-SpheresY-90 resin microspheres (yttrium-90 microspheres). Package insert, Feb 2017, Sirtex Medical Limited, Australia, www.sirtex.com.
9. Therasphere yttrium-90 glass microspheres. Package Insert, Biocompatibles UK Ltd., Surrey, UK, BTG International Ltd., Rev. 14.

10. ZEVALIN (ibritumomab tiuxetan) 2009 Spectrum Pharmaceuticals, Inc. Irvine, CA. www.accessdata. fda.gov/drugsatfda_docs/label/2009/125019s0156. pdf

11. Zakun J, Bodei L, Mueller-Brand J, et al. The joint IAEA, EANM, and SNMMI practical guidance on peptide receptor radionuclide therapy (PRRNT) in neuroendocrine tumours. *Eur J Nucl Med Molec Imag.* 2013;40:800–816.

12. LUTATHERA® (lutetium Lu 177 dotatate) injection, for intravenous use. Highlights of Prescribing Information, Advanced Accelerator Applications USA, Inc. 2019.

13. NUREG-1556, Vol. 9, Revision 2, Appendix U, "Consolidated Guidance about Materials Licenses: Program-Specific Guidance about Medical Use Licenses", Jan, 2008, U.S. Nuclear Regulatory Commission.

14. LUTATHERA® (lutetium Lu 177 dotatate) Annex 1, Summary of Product Characteristics. Advanced Accelerator Applications. www.ema.europa.eu/en/ documents/product-information/lutathera-epar-product-information_en.pdf.

Questions

1. Match each of the following radiopharmaceuticals with their utility:
   (a) ^{131}I sodium iodide.
   (b) ^{123}I sodium iodide.
   (c) ^{177}Lu-dotatate.
   (d) ^{68}Ga-PMSA-11.
   (e) ^{90}Y-microspheres.
      (i) Sole use as a diagnostic agent.
      (ii) Sole use as a therapeutic agent.
      (iii) Can be used as a diagnostic and therapeutic agent.

2. True or false: Osteoclastic cells function to create new bone tissue by excreting a protein called hydroxyapatite.

3. True or false: The portal vein supplies more blood to normal liver tissue than the hepatic artery.

4. Why do ^{90}Y glass microspheres contain contaminants and ^{90}Y resin microspheres do not?

5. True or false: The amino acids L-lysine and L-arginine are infused along with ^{177}Lu-dotatate to reduce renal toxicity caused by ^{177}Lu-dotatate.

6. Which of the following items must be included in the written directive for a therapeutic radiopharmaceutical?
   (a) Signature of an authorized user.
   (b) The planned route of administration of the radiopharmaceutical.
   (c) The complete name of the radiopharmaceutical.
   (d) Patient identification using at least two means of identification by two different witnesses prior to administration of the dose.
   (e) Dose measurement verification by two different witnesses.
   (f) Signatures of the witnesses.
   (g) All of the above.

Answers

1. (a) (iii). (b) (i). (c) (iii). (d) (i). (e) (ii) or (iii) (like ^{177}Lu-dotatate post-therapy imaging is possible).
2. False. Osteoclasts break down bone tissue. Osteoblasts help create new bone tissue by laying down collagen. Hydroxyapatite binds to collagen.
3. True. The portal vein carries products from the intestinal tract to the liver and supplies 80% of the blood to the liver. The hepatic artery supplies 20% of the blood to the liver.
4. Because ^{90}Y is created by neutron bombardment of ^{89}Y atoms encased within glass microspheres; small amounts of contaminants produced by this process are trapped within the glass. ^{90}Y resin microspheres are created by incorporating pre-made ^{90}Y into the resin microspheres.
5. True. They directly compete with and block some of the uptake of ^{177}Lu-dotatate by the proximal renal tubule cells.
6. (g) All of the above.

CHAPTER 19

Management of Nuclear Event Casualties

Kevin Donohoe[1], Rachel A. Powsner, and *Edward R. Powsner*

[1] Beth Israel Deaconess Medical Center and Harvard Medical School, Boston, USA

Exposure to ionizing radiation may be accompanied by a range of physical manifestations, from no symptoms in the event of low-dose exposure, to rapid onset of nausea, vomiting and vascular collapse in the event of high-dose exposure. When exposures are sufficient to cause physical effects, the symptoms are not specific to radiation exposure, and therefore the cause of the symptoms may be difficult to diagnose if radiation exposure is not suspected. Unless the possibility of radiation exposure is considered, the diagnosis will be delayed, if made at all. In the case of a publicized exposure event it is likely that the number of people seeking assistance will be much greater than the number actually exposed. Because the number of people that were not exposed can easily overwhelm any health care system designed to treat acutely ill patients, it is important to plan not only for treatment of the injured, but also for triage of the "worried well".

This chapter begins with a brief discussion of the interaction of radiation with tissue. This is followed by a section on facility preparation for decontamination and treatment of victims of a radiation accident. A discussion of techniques for early dose assessment for appropriate triage is followed by a review of the acute radiation syndromes. The chapter concludes with an introduction to the treatment of internal contamination.

Interaction of radiation with tissue

Alpha particles

Alpha particles have a charge of +2 and a weight of 4 atomic mass units (amu). Because they are relatively heavy and have a +2 charge alpha particles

don't travel very far in tissue, depositing all their energy over a short distance (high LET; see Chapter 3). Alpha radiation travels only a few centimeters in air and only about 50 micrometers in tissue. A few layers of dead skin readily block alpha particles and they therefore cannot damage the viable dermal tissue beneath the dead layer of skin (Figure 19.1). On the other hand, the linings of the gastrointestinal and pulmonary system are susceptible to damage from ingested or inhaled alpha emitting atoms (Figure 19.2). The high LET of alpha particles means that all of their energy is deposited within these unprotected mucosal cells. Further, rapid cell turnover in tissues such as bronchial or gastrointestinal epithelium, means a greater proportion of cells are in the M or G_2 phases of mitosis which makes them relatively more vulnerable to radiation injury (see Chapter 15).

Beta particles

Beta particles have a charge of negative one and a mass of 0.00055 amu. They have a lower LET than alpha particles and therefore penetrate tissues further; they can travel as far as a few meters in air and a few millimeters in tissue. Unlike alpha particles, they can penetrate the dead cornified epithelium of the skin, and therefore may damage the living dermal cells beneath, causing signs of skin burn such as redness and blistering. Beta emitters, like all radiation, can also cause injury if ingested or inhaled in sufficient amounts.

Gamma rays and X-rays

Photons have no charge and no mass and therefore have relatively few interactions with air or tissue compared to particulate radiation. They can

---

Essentials of Nuclear Medicine Physics, Instrumentation, and Radiation Biology, Fourth Edition.
Rachel A. Powsner, Matthew R. Palmer, and Edward R. Powsner.
© 2022 John Wiley & Sons Ltd. Published 2022 by John Wiley & Sons Ltd.

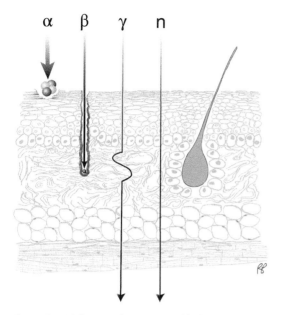

Figure 19.1 Alpha particles are stopped by layers of dead epidermis; high energy beta particles can penetrate short distances into skin; gamma photons and neutrons can penetrate into deep tissue.

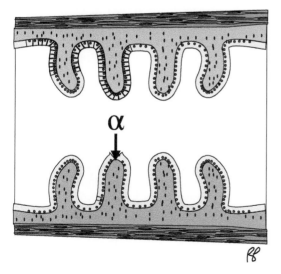

Figure 19.2 Alpha particles can damage the lining epithelium of the gastrointestinal tract or pulmonary system.

travel several kilometers in air and penetrate deeply into or through tissues. If photons interact with tissues they may cause both superficial and deep tissue injury.

Neutrons

Although exposure to neutrons is less commonly encountered in the practice of clinical medicine, it must be considered a possibility during unintentional radiation exposure. With this in mind, the discussion of the interaction of radiation with tissue has been expanded to include neutron radiation.

Neutrons are different from the preceding types of radiation in a number of ways. They have a finite existence with a half-life of 12 minutes in air, following which they decay into a proton, electron, and neutrino. They have a mass of 1 amu and have no charge. Since they have no positive or negative charge they lack the great attractive or repellant forces in their interactions with atoms that we have seen with charged particles (alphas and betas). For this reason, as well as for differences in mass, the interactions of neutrons are limited to interaction with atomic nuclei.

Also, like photons, neutrons can penetrate and pass through tissue; they differ from photons in that they have mass and as a result can interact directly with the hydrogen nuclei in tissue through a process called **elastic scattering** (Figure 19.3).

In this process some of the kinetic energy of the neutron is transferred to the proton and the proton is separated from its atom. The proton thus becomes a moving charged particle which can damage surrounding tissue. Exposure to neutrons can result in both superficial and deep tissue injury.

While the different radiations described above have different LETs and may interact with the atoms in tissue in different ways, the resulting tissue damage is similar, resulting from ionization and creation of free radicals in tissue (see Chapter 15).

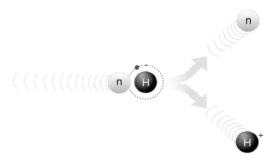

Figure 19.3 Elastic scattering of proton following neutron interaction with a hydrogen atom nucleus.

Table 19.1 Selected radionuclides used for occupational applications and/or identified in fallout from the Chernobyl power plant accident

Nuclide	Physical half-life	Emissions
^{3}Hydrogen (tritium)	12 years	β^{-}
^{14}Carbon	5.7×10^{3} years	β^{-}
^{32}Phosphorus	14.3 days	β^{-}
^{60}Cobalt	5.27 years	β^{-}, γ
^{90}Strontium	28 years	β^{-}
^{125}Iodine	60.1 days	γ
^{131}Iodine	8 days	β^{-}, γ
^{137}Cesium	30 years	β^{-}, γ
^{192}Iridium	74 days	β^{-}
^{235}Uranium	7×10^{8} years	α, γ
^{238}Uranium	4.5×10^{9} years	α, γ
^{238}Plutonium	88 years	α, γ
^{239}Plutonium	2.4×10^{4} years	α, γ
^{241}Americium	458 years	α

Derived in part from Soloviev V, et al. [1], IAEA, Safety Report Series, No. 2, p. 5 [2], and REAC/TS [3].

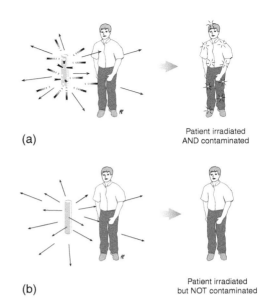

(a) Patient irradiated AND contaminated

(b) Patient irradiated but NOT contaminated

Figure 19.4 Exposure and contamination.

Radionuclides

Table 19.1 lists radionuclides that are more commonly used for research, military, or industrial applications as well as some of the nuclides that were identified in radioactive fallout from the Chernobyl nuclear power plant accident.

Hospital response to a radiation accident

In the event of a radiation accident there may be large numbers of people presenting to the hospitals for evaluation. It is likely that the majority of these individuals will not require acute medical care. Triage of a large number of individuals for contamination and possible radiation exposure can overwhelm limited hospital resources which are better suited to provide acute medical care. Establishing a **screening and decontamination facility** at an off-site location and re-directing people without acute injury to that location may help to provide victims with the most appropriate care. Alternatively, an on-site decontamination facility separate from the hospital, such as a large tent or peripheral building may suffice. A prepared hospital emergency department can then be reserved for medical treatment and decontamination of the injured and critically exposed.

Exposure and contamination

Radiation accidents can result in partial or whole body irradiation. If aerosolized radionuclides are released during the accident an individual's skin, respiratory tract, and/or clothing can become **contaminated** (Figure 19.4a). A contaminated individual is a potential source of radiation exposure not only to themselves, but also for other patients and hospital personnel. Exposure of those in the vicinity of the contaminated individual is rarely hazardous; however, the goal is always to minimize or eliminate unnecessary exposure and contamination. Even small amounts of contamination of a health care facility may result in loss of use of the contaminated areas and the need for costly decontamination procedures. In contrast, an irradiated, noncontaminated person is NOT a source of radiation exposure for others (Figure 19.4b).

Hospital facilities

Decontamination facility

In preparation for a large number of contaminated, but well individuals, some hospitals have designated an area such as a tent or peripheral hospital building with easily controlled access, clothing collection hampers, multiple showers with large waste-water collection tanks, replacement clothing, and survey meters. When needed, these facilities should be staffed by properly clothed (see below) personnel with knowledge of the use of survey meters. In most cases, removal of clothing will eliminate 95% of external contamination. Decontamination of other areas of the body, such as hands and face, can often be done with a damp cloth. While flushing contaminated areas with water may also remove contamination, the contaminated water will then become a waste hazard that is more difficult to control than a contaminated towel or washcloth.

Treatment/decontamination room for seriously wounded individuals

The treatment of life-threatening wounds or medical conditions takes priority over decontamination. Patients with these conditions may be cared for in a previously designated combination treatment/decontamination room in the emergency department. Ideally this room should have immediate access to the outside so that transportation of a contaminated individual into the room does not risk contamination of the rest of the emergency department. A **buffer zone** should be established for decontamination and monitoring of personnel and patients leaving the treatment room prior to entering uncontaminated areas of the hospital. If there is adequate notification prior to patient arrival, the treatment room may be prepared with a secure floor covering with a nonskid surface to aid in room decontamination. Several large plastic-lined waste containers should be present, and any equipment present in the room which is not needed should be removed prior to arrival of the victim or covered to help prevent contamination. A shielded area or a location away from the treatment area should be identified for containment of solid radioactive debris such as shrapnel from a wound. A pair of long-handled tongs for handling metal fragments should be available.

After the patient is medically stabilized decontamination can proceed.

External decontamination

Although the standard practice of having emergency room or ambulance personnel remove and isolate a victim's clothing in plastic bags will often accomplish the majority of the surface decontamination, further decontamination may be required.

Prior to decontamination swab samples of contaminated areas should be obtained and placed in carefully labeled plastic specimen tubes for later analysis. Swabbing of orifices, such as the nose and mouth, will help for later determination of the amount of material inhaled or ingested.

Decontamination should proceed in the following order: wounds, orifices, and intact skin. Contaminated wounds can be flushed with water; however, using a damp washcloth or even the application of minimal water will help to avoid spreading contamination and producing large volumes of contaminated fluids. Draping the area around the wound will prevent contamination of surrounding skin. Abrasion of skin or wounds during decontamination damages the skin and may cause systemic absorption of superficial contamination. Therefore, gentle wiping with a soapy or damp cloth, followed by a survey for residual radioactivity is recommended.

If contaminated, the eyes and ears can be gently flushed with water or saline. Oral cavity contamination can be reduced by repeated rinsing and by brushing teeth. The nasal cavity can usually be cleared by simply having the patient blow his/her nose.

If the hair is contaminated, shampooing with gentle shampoos without conditioners prior to skin-washing is recommended. Conditioners are discouraged as they may bind particulates to hair.

Use of soft cloths and lukewarm water and soap is recommended for skin cleansing; alternatively diaper wipes or the equivalent can be used. Cleansing of the skin should be gentle to avoid abrasion.

Patient radiation survey

An accurate survey of patients and an accurate determination of the radiation dose received is critical for subsequent health care. While the goal is always to minimize radiation exposure as much as possible, the health effects of low-dose exposure are debatable, and rarely require acute intervention, while high-dose exposures are more consequential and may require more acute attention to decontamination and more acute health care. Therefore, an accurate survey of the patient for residual contamination and a history of exposure at the accident site are critical.

Following removal of clothing and prior to decontamination the patient should be **surveyed** for baseline measurement of contamination. When performing surveys, it is important to move the probe slowly and to keep a fixed distance from the body. If possible careful records of distribution of contamination and readings at sites of contamination should be recorded. A cartoon diagram of a patient is often adequate for mapping areas and amounts of contamination.

Following washing, the survey should be repeated using the same technique used for the initial survey. Decontamination should proceed until no more contamination can be removed and should be stopped if the skin becomes irritated. Skin that remains contaminated can be swathed in plastic to encourage sweating to remove additional local contamination. The plastic should be removed periodically and the area redressed as needed.

Survey meter

A standard **Geiger–Müller survey meter** (see Chapter 4) with a **frisking or pancake probe** (Figure 19.5) is adequate for monitoring decontamination progress. The very thin mica window behind the protective wire mesh will allow detection of gamma photons, alpha, and some beta particles.

This method of surveying is limited by the inability of **low-energy betas** (with energies lower than 60 keV) such as those from tritium to penetrate the

mica [4]. Although most commonly encountered alpha particles are of high enough kinetic energy to penetrate the mica window (>3 MeV), **alpha particles** have a short range in air and can only be detected with the probe placed very close to the area to be surveyed (Figure 19.6). However, one must not actually touch the surface to avoid contamination of the probe itself.

Covering the probe with a glove to prevent its contamination may also block alpha particles and prevent their detection. Probes are available that are more efficient for the detection of alpha particles and low energy beta particles, but most hospitals do not have these specialized detectors available.

A rough **discrimination of alpha, beta, and gamma emissions** can be determined by comparing the reading directly from the source with that obtained with an intervening piece of paper to block alpha particles and then with an intervening piece of aluminum or plastic to block both alpha and beta particles (Figure 19.7).

Personnel

Personal protection

Wearing protective coverings will greatly reduce the risk of contamination of hospital staff involved in patient care. Caps or hoods (particularly for individuals with long hair), eye protection, masks, gowns, double gloves (with the inner glove taped to the gown sleeve), and plastic shoe covers are recommended for personnel directly involved with decontamination. Plastic is preferable to paper for shoe covers for durability and resistance to liquids. Gowning and gloving with materials that are readily available in the surgical suite is often perfectly acceptable. Using standard surgical clothing also

> ### Survey meter quality control
>
> Prior to use a battery check and source check should be performed on the survey meter. The inspection sticker on the side of the meter should be checked to verify that the yearly calibration is up-to-date. For more detailed information on the calibration of survey meters see Chapter 14.

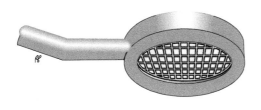
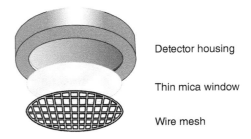

Detector housing

Thin mica window

Wire mesh

Figure 19.5 Frisking (pancake) probe for attachment to survey meter.

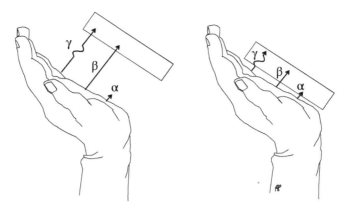

Figure 19.6 Detector proximity is necessary for alpha detection.

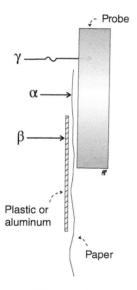

Figure 19.7 Paper and plastic or aluminum can be placed between the radioactive source and the detector to aid in differentiating alpha, beta, and gamma emissions.

insures that the clothing needed is always available and in adequate supply.

If there is a credible risk of contamination from radioactive iodine (^{131}I), medical personnel should be treated with oral potassium iodide as soon as possible prior to exposure to radioiodine.

Reducing exposure

The standard practices for minimizing total exposure are reducing the **time** of exposure, increasing the **distance** from the source of the radiation, and when feasible, placing **shielding** between the radiation source and personnel. These fundamentals remain applicable when treating radiation accident victims. When treating heavily contaminated patients, rotate staff to reduce the time any one individual spends with the patient, if possible. Nuclear medicine technologists or radiation safety personnel trained to use survey meters can be invaluable for helping to contain contamination and to monitor exposures to those treating the victim. In most cases, exposures to health care personnel will be minor, yet low exposures cannot be assumed. Active monitoring of exposures will go far towards maintaining safety and reassuring healthcare personnel. When not directly caring for a contaminated patient, staff should try to remain a reasonable distance away from the patient. Historically, hospital-based medical personnel treating radiation accident victims, including those who treated victims from the Chernobyl accident, received only minimal radiation exposures.

Dosimeters

Personnel should be supplied with direct reading dosimeters, such as pocket dosimeters, so that immediate readings are available at the time of exposure. Depending on the device used, these devices may not provide a means of permanent record keeping and may not discriminate between types or energies of radiation. All personnel should, therefore, wear film badges, thermoluminescent dosimeters (TLDs), or optically stimulated luminescent detectors (OSLs) in addition to direct reading dosimeters. For a more detailed description of these devices please refer to Chapter 4.

Evaluation of the radiation accident victim

An initial history of the event obtained from the victim or credible witness is essential for understanding the radiation exposure and extent of medical trauma. Distance from the radiation source at the time of exposure, evidence of trauma and type and time of onset of symptoms are examples of information that are helpful during initial triage of patients. If radiation exposure is suspected, a complete blood count with differential, blood for **HLA typing**, urinalysis, skin, oral, nasal, and wound swabs as well as urine and fecal samples should be obtained as soon as possible. The **initial lymphocyte counts** can be used with subsequent counts, obtained every 6 hours, to estimated absorbed dose.

HLA (human leukocyte antigen) typing can be used for future transfusions and stem cell or bone marrow transplants, if needed. The swabs and blood, urine and fecal samples can be used to estimate quantity and type of internal contamination. A 24-hour post-exposure blood sample should be sent for analysis of **lymphocyte chromosomal abnormalities** for more accurate dosimetry.

The symptoms and medical course of an accident victim are determined by the type of radiation, the absorbed radiation dose, the distribution of the absorbed dose (whole body versus localized) and the route of exposure (external, internal). For example, exposure of intact skin, which is protected by several layers of dead skin cells, to a nonabsorbable alpha emitter causes relatively little injury whereas ingestion of the same quantity of material can be fatal. Similarly, a single exposure of 10 Gy of gamma radiation to the hand will result in severe local burns and tissue damage but survival is likely; a whole body dose of 10 grays from a gamma emitter will be lethal.

Early estimation of whole-body radiation exposure

It is important to identify those patients requiring hospital admission, monitoring, and treatment following radiation exposure. Radiation survey measurements from the site of the radiation accident, patient symptoms and time of onset, and blood lymphocyte counts can be used to estimate absorbed doses.

Symptoms and time of onset following exposure

An absorbed whole-body dose greater than approximately 1 Gy may cause **radiation sickness** characterized by specific signs and symptoms. The severity of the signs and symptoms and the rapidity of their onset increase with increasing absorbed dose. The most commonly sought data for early estimation of absorbed dose is the time of onset of **nausea and vomiting** following the radiation accident. Unfortunately, nausea and vomiting are also commonly seen in people involved in a sudden traumatic event that are not exposed to radiation. These symptoms may be caused by abdominal or head trauma or merely by anxiety surrounding the event. It is important that the treating physician be made aware that exposure to radiation occurred so that they can consider the importance of the symptoms.

Table 19.2 summarizes the signs and symptoms of radiation sickness and recommended patient disposition at increasing estimated whole body doses.

Blood count estimates of exposure

Neutrophil, platelet, and lymphocyte counts decrease following radiation exposure. Lymphocytes are relatively more radiosensitive and their counts drop more rapidly following exposure. There are several techniques for estimating dose from lymphocyte counts obtained in the early hours or days following exposure. Dose can be estimated from the minimal lymphocyte count within the first 48 hours following exposure [6], from a plot of the lymphocyte counts from frequent sampling during the first 12 hours post exposure [7], or by the percent drop in the lymphocyte counts in the first 24 hours [5].

It should be noted, for all dose estimates based on white blood cell counts and particularly those based on a single measurement, that lymphocyte and neutrophil counts can be adversely affected by many factors including stress and underlying illness.

Chromosomal aberrations

Quantitation of chromosomal aberrations in lymphocytes is considered to be the most reliable biological marker for dosimetry measurements. These tests, although highly accurate for estimating exposures,

Table 19.2 Signs, symptoms, and recommended disposition of exposed patients

Estimated whole body dose (Gy)	Onset of vomiting	Percent of cases	Diarrhea severity and onset	Percent of cases
<1	None	–	None	–
1-2	>2 h	10–50%	None	–
2-4	1–2 h	70–90%	None	–
4-6	<1 h	100%	Mild 3–8 h	<10%
6-8	<30 min	100%	Heavy 1–3 h	>10%
>8	<10 min	100%	Heavy <1 h	100%

Estimated whole body dose (Gy)	Headache severity and time of onset	Percent of cases	Fever (hours)	Percent of cases	Level of consciousness
<1	None	–	None	–	Normal
1–2	Slight	–	None	–	Normal
2–4	Mild	–	Mild 1–3 h	10–80%	Normal
4–6	Moderate 4–24 h	50%	Moderate to high 1–2 h	80–100%	Normal
6–8	Severe 3–4 h	80%	High <1 h	100%	May be reduced
>8	Severe 1–2 h	80-90%	High <1 h	100%	Unconscious—may be for only seconds or minutes (greater than 50 Gy incidence is 100%)

Estimated whole body dose (Gy)	Recommended disposition
<1	Outpatient with 5-week follow-up of blood labs, skin examinations
1–2	Outpatient with antiemetic therapy, and frequent laboratory and physical exam follow-up or general admission for symptomatic treatment and observation
2–4	Admission with supportive care and hematology consult[a]
4–6	Admission to tertiary care facility with intensive supportive care including fluid management, hematology care, infectious disease consults
6–8	Admission to tertiary care facility with intensive supportive care including fluid management, hematology care, infectious disease consults
>8	Likely lethal, although with intense medical support may survive up to 12 Gy exposure

Adapted with permission from the International Atomic Energy Agency Safety Report Series, No. 2, Diagnosis and Treatment of Radiation Injuries, Table VIII, p. 16 [2], with additional information from Cosset JM, Girinsky T, Helfre S, Gourmelon P. Medical Management During the Prodromal and Latent Periods [5].

[a] For estimated whole body doses ≥ 2 Gy early treatment with colony-stimulating factors is recommended. The Medical Aspects of Radiation Incidents, p. 14 [3].

are not widely available and can take several days to complete. However, techniques for more rapid assessment of chromosomal aberrations with adequate dose estimate accuracy have been developed [3].

Early estimation of local radiation exposure

The early biologic consequences of radiation exposure to a portion of the body or the whole body can be helpful in determining the radiation dose. The time of onset of **initial erythema** of the skin (so-called to distinguish it from the later episodes of more intense reddening of the skin) can be used to estimate absorbed local dose and guide subsequent

patient management. Table 19.3 summarizes these findings as they pertain to localized body exposure.

Acute radiation sickness

Acute radiation sickness following whole body exposure is often divided into four stages. The **prodromal stage** (or syndrome) includes symptoms of anorexia, nausea, vomiting, and easy fatiguability. The greater the dose the shorter the duration of the prodromal stage before advancing to the next stage, but the more severe the symptoms. Immediate diarrhea, fever, headache, and hypertension are

Table 19.3 Estimated local radiation dose and recommended patient management based on time of onset of early erythema

Estimated skin dose (Gy)	Time of onset of initial erythema and/or abnormal skin sensation	Recommended patient management
<6	None	Outpatient with 5-week follow-up of blood labs and examinations
6–8	1–2 days[a]	
8–15	12–24 hours	Admission to general ward for observation
15–30	8–15 hours	Admission to surgical burn ward with hematology consult
>30	3–6 hours Edema of mucosa can also be seen	Admission to tertiary care facility with intensive surgical (burn) and hematology support

Adapted in part with permission from the International Atomic Energy Agency Safety Report Series, No. 2, Diagnosis and Treatment of Radiation Injuries, Table III, p. 7 [2].
[a] Cosset JM, IAEA, p. 14 [5].

seen only in doses above the lethal threshold. During the **latent period** the patient may have few or no symptoms in the presence of ongoing organ damage. **Manifest illness** is marked by symptoms related to the involved organ (see syndromes listed below). The **recovery phase** may extend from weeks to years if the radiation dose is not acutely lethal. The overall duration of these stages is dependent on the dose the patient received and the specific tissue that has been injured.

Acute radiation syndromes

The course of illness following exposure to a single whole-body dose of greater than 2 Gy is directly related to the absorbed dose. The acute radiation syndromes may be divided into three categories:

1. Hematopoesis: doses greater than 1–2 Gy.
2. Gastrointestinal: doses greater than 6–8 Gy.
3. Central nervous system (CNS)/cardiovascular: doses greater than 20–30 Gy [8].

Hematopoetic syndrome

The prodrome consists of nausea, vomiting, diarrhea, headache, fever, and possible decreased level of consciousness presenting within 6 hours of exposure and lasting for days. During the latent period of 2–3 weeks, the patient will feel relatively well, but the number of circulating red blood cells, white blood cells, and platelets will be steadily decreasing. Following the latent phase, the manifest illness is characterized by infection and hemorrhage.

Gastrointestinal syndrome

The prodrome consists of the same symptoms of acute radiation sickness seen in the hematopoetic syndrome with nearly universal decrease in level of consciousness beginning within minutes of exposure and lasting days. Latency is approximately one week, during which time the patient feels relatively well. However, during the latency period the intestinal tract lining is sloughing which leads to the manifest gastrointestinal illness stage when the patient is likely to expire from fluid loss, electrolyte imbalance, and sepsis.

Central nervous system (CNS) and cardiovascular syndrome

The patient will suffer nearly immediate nausea, vomiting, hypotension, ataxia, convulsions, and loss of consciousness. There is no latency period and death is likely within days.

Treatment of acute radiation sickness

Approximately 50% of those patients exposed to an acute whole-body dose of 3.5 Gy will succumb within 2 months without medical treatment ($LD_{50/60}$); with intensive medical treatment 50% survival may be achieved after exposure to as much as 8 Gy (REAC/TS, p. 17) [3]. For doses above 2 Gy, hospitalization with isolation and close observation is recommended. The medical management of acute radiation sickness requires a multidisciplinary approach. Specialists in burn care, intensive care, infectious disease, hematology, and radiation safety often need to be closely involved in patient care.

Treatment of internal contamination

Patients can become contaminated internally with radiation by ingestion, inhalation, or absorption of specific nuclides through intact skin or open wounds.

Internal contamination with radiation is treated by blocking gastrointestinal absorption, blocking organ specific uptake of the radionuclide, and/or promoting excretion of the contaminants. The treatment is directed at the element and is independent of the specific isotope of that element. For example, the treatment of ingestion of all isotopes of strontium is the same. The process of reducing the amount of internal contamination is sometimes referred to as **decorporation**.

Examples of decorporation include the use of chelating agents such as CaDTPA for binding plutonium (the chelated compound is more readily excreted in urine), increasing oral intake of water to dilute and increase urinary excretion of tritium, and the ingestion of potassium iodide soon after exposure to radioactive iodine to block thyroid uptake of the radionuclide. A detailed table of treatment procedures for internal contamination can be found in an International Atomic Energy Agency publication: Generic procedures for medical response during a nuclear or radiological emergency [9].

Local radiation injury to the skin

The clinical signs of local radiation injury to the skin may be similar to those of thermal burns, but time of onset is dose dependent. With doses of 10–18 Gy there may be an initial phase of erythema occurring within 12–24 hours. Whether or not there is an episode of erythema within 12–24 hours there is a later phase erythema occurring at 12–20 days. This is compared to doses greater than 80 Gy for which the first signs of erythema occur at 1–2 hours post-exposure followed by a second episode of erythema within the first 4 days (Table VI, p.11, IAEA) [2].

Two characteristic skin findings following radiation exposure at higher doses are dry desquamation and wet desquamation. **Dry desquamation** is a reddened, dry, flaking, itchy skin due to partial damage of the basal layer. It occurs above a threshold of 8–12 Gy, typically 25–30 days following exposure. **Moist desquamation** is characterized by blistering, redness, pain, and a weeping discharge resulting from the complete damage of the basal layer of the skin. Moist desquamation begins on day 20–28 at a threshold of 15–20 Gy.

Further damage in the form of ulceration in the skin can occur at doses greater than 20 Gy, (beginning at 14–21 days post exposure), or, with deeper penetration, necrosis can be seen at doses greater than 25 Gy (beginning 21 days or longer following exposure) (Table V, p. 10, IAEA) [2].

Medical and industrial accidental overexposure

Much of this chapter is addressed toward accidental or unwanted exposures of large populations, such as with nuclear power plant accidents and terrorist-related exposures (e.g., a "dirty bomb"). While these sources of exposure are attention-getting and of public concern, by far the largest source of accidental overexposures currently are seen in industry and in medical procedures involving radiation. Overexposures in these settings are frequently defined as unintended (1) whole body exposure of 1 Gy or more; (2) local skin exposure of 3 Gy or more; (3) individual organ exposure of 5 Gy or more; or (4) presenting clinical symptoms suspicious for unintended radiation exposure [10]. It should also be noted that these higher dose exposures in medicine are almost exclusively seen in patients already scheduled for radiation exposure. Overexposures more typically occur in therapeutic procedures such as radiation therapy or radiopharmaceutical therapy, and in complex vascular fluoroscopy procedures such as coronary angiograms, but can occur in other diagnostic procedures such as CT imaging [11]. Care for individual patients with over-exposure will typically be similar to that described above.

It should be noted that medical and industrial overexposures more typically affect individuals or small groups, rather than large populations.

As with any accidental overexposures, unless there are overt physical manifestations, a medical overexposure may never be detected, so the true number of overexposures is not known. Fortunately, diligent quality control and reporting of medical overexposures has resulted in a decline in the incidence of these events [12].

References

1. Soloviev V, Ilyin L, Baranov, et al. Chapter 9. Radiation accidents in the former U.S.S.R. In: Gusev IA, Guskova AK, Mettler FA (eds). *Medical Management of Radiation Accidents*, 2nd edn. Boca Raton, FL: CRC Press, 2001, pp. 157–65.
2. International Atomic Energy Agency. *Diagnosis and Treatment of Radiation Injuries.* Jointly sponsored by the International Atomic Energy Agency and The World

Health Organization. Safety Report Series, No. 2, Vienna, 1998. www.pub.iaea.org/MTCD/publications/PDF/P040_scr.pdf.

3. Oak Ridge Institute for Science and Education. *The Medical Aspects of Radiation Incidents.* Radiation Emergency Assistance Center/Training Site (REAC/TS), Oak Ridge, TN. www.orise.orau.gov/reacts, revised July, 2017.

4. Steinmeyer G-M. Pancake detectors: everything you've wanted to know (but were afraid to ask). *RSO Mag.* 2005; 10(5):10.

5. Cosset JM, Girinsky T, Helfre S, Gourmelon P. Medical management during the prodromal and latent periods. In: Ricks RC, Berger ME, O'Hara FM (eds). *The Medical Basis for Radiation-Accident Preparedness, The Clinical Care of Victims.* Proceedings of the Fourth International REAC/TS Conference on The Medical Basis for Radiation-Accident Preparedness, March 2001, New York: Parthenon, 2001, pp. 45–51.

6. Mettler FA, Voelz GL. Major radiation exposure—what to expect and how to respond. *New Engl J Med.* 2002; 346(20):1554–61.

7. Goans RE, Holloway EC, Berger ME, Ricks RC. Early dose assessment following severe radiation accidents. *Health Phys.* 1997; 72(4):513–518.

8. Waselenko JK, MacVittie TJ, Blakely WF, Pesik N, et al. Medical management of the acute radiation syndrome: Recommendations of the strategic national stockpile radiation working group. *Ann Intern Med.* 2004; 140(12):1037–51.

9. International Atomic Energy Agency. Generic procedures for medical response during a nuclear or radiological emergency. Vienna, Austria, April 2005, pp. 70–72.

10. Coeytaux K, Bey E, Christensen D, Glassman ES, Murdock B, Doucet C. Reported Radiation overexposure accidents worldwide, 1980–2013: A systematic review. *PLoS One.* 2015; 10(3). https://doi.org/10.1371/journal.pone.0118709.

11. Radiation Overdoses Despite F.D.A. Warnings – Graphic – NY Times.com https://archive.nytimes.com/www.nytimes.com/interactive/2011/03/05/health/radiation-overdoses-despite-FDA-warnings.html.

12. Emery RJ, Valizadeh F, Kennedy V, Shelton AJ. An analysis of variables influencing the number of radiation overexposure events in Texas from 1970 to 2000. *Health Phys* 2005; 89(1):46–52. https://doi.org/10.1097/00004032-200507000-00004.

Questions

1. True or false: Removing clothing and washing with soap and water generally removes the majority of external radioactive contamination.

2. Which of the following are true about the interaction of neutrons with matter?
   (a) They have a positive charge so they interact with outer shell electrons.
   (b) Like photons they can pass through matter without transferring energy.
   (c) The neutron can transfer some of its kinetic energy to a proton causing its ejection from the atom.

3. True or false: A patient who has been irradiated by photons, but not contaminated, is still a radiation risk for hospital staff.

4. When using a Geiger counter with a pancake probe as a survey meter for unknown contaminants which of the following practices are recommended?
   (a) A battery check should be performed prior to use.
   (b) Keep the probe at least one meter away from the patient or object being surveyed.
   (c) Ascertain that the meter calibration is up to date.
   (d) Place a glove over the pancake probe to prevent contamination of the probe.
   (e) (a) and (c).
   (f) (b) and (d).
   (g) All of the above.

5. Which of the following is true about the use of a Geiger survey meter fitted with a thin mica window?
   (a) It can be used to detect most commonly encountered alpha particles.
   (b) Only lower energy beta particles (less than 60 keV) can be detected.

6. What are effective ways to reduce your total exposure when working with a radioactive patient:
   (a) When not actually tending to the patient try to keep as close to the patient as possible.
   (b) When feasible keep radiation shielding between yourself and the patient.
   (c) Try to reduce the total amount of time you spend near the patient.
   (d) (a) and (b).
   (e) (b) and (c).
   (f) All of the above.

7. Which of the following clinical findings have been used for an initial radiation dose estimate for an accident victim?
   (a) The time of onset of nausea and vomiting.
   (b) Chest pain.
   (c) Lymphocyte counts within the first 48 hours.
   (d) Time of onset of initial skin erythema.
   (e) Palpitations.
   (f) Presence of fever.

8. Associate the following statements with the appropriate acute radiation syndrome:
   (a) Occurs at absorbed doses greater than 20 Gy.
   (b) A 2–3 week latency period during which the patient's blood counts are decreasing.
   (c) No discernible latency period and death usually occurs within days of exposure.
   (d) A one week latency followed by fluid loss, electrolyte imbalance, and sepsis.

   Syndrome:
   (1) Hematopoetic syndrome.
   (2) Gastrointestinal syndrome.
   (3) CNS and cardiovascular syndrome.
   (4) Pulmonary-hepatic syndrome.

Answers

1. True.
2. (b) and (c). (a) is incorrect—they have no charge.
3. False.
4. (e) is correct. The probe should be used close to, but not touching, the skin or object to allow detection of alpha and beta particles. A glove will block detection of alpha particles, so it should not be used to cover the probe.
5. (a) only. (b) is not correct as only beta particles with energies higher than 60 keV can be detected.
6. (e). (a) is incorrect; when not tending to the patient increase the distance between yourself and the patient.
7. (a), (c), (d), and (f).
8. (a) (3). (b) (1). (c) (3). (d) (2).

APPENDIX A

Common Nuclides

Nuclide	Production method	Half-life (s = secs m = mins h = hours d = days y = years)	Decay mode	βmax or α energies in keV[a]	γ energies in keV[a]	Decay product	Half-life of decay product
^{11}C	^{11}B(p,n)^{11}C	20 m	β^+	961	511[b]	^{11}B	Stable
^{13}N	^{16}O(p,α)^{13}N	10 m	β^+	1198	511[b]	^{13}C	Stable
^{15}O	^{14}N(d,n)^{15}O	124 s	β^+	1735	511[b]	^{15}N	Stable
^{18}F	^{18}O(p,n)^{18}F	109 m	β^+	634	511[b]	^{18}O	Stable
^{22}Na	^{19}F(α,n)^{22}Na	2.6 y	β^+, EC, γ	546	511[b] 1274	^{22}Ne	Stable
^{57}Co	^{60}Ni(p,α)^{57}Co	272 d	EC, γ		122	^{57}Fe	Stable
^{64}Cu	^{64}Ni (p,n) ^{64}Cu	12.7 h	β^-, EC, β^+	β^- 579 β^+ 653	511[b]	^{64}Zn ^{64}Ni	Stable Stable
^{67}Ga	^{66}Zn(d,n)^{67}Ga	78 h	EC, γ		93 185 300 393	^{67}Zn	Stable
^{68}Ga	^{67}Zn(p,γ)^{68}Ga ^{68}Ge$\rightarrow$^{68}Ga	68 m	β^+	1899	511[b]	^{68}Zn	Stable
^{81m}Kr[c]	^{81}Rb $\rightarrow$ ^{81m}Kr	13 s	IT		191	^{81}Kr	2.3×10^5 y
^{82}Rb	^{82}Sr $\rightarrow$ ^{82}Rb	1.3 m	β^+, EC	3381 2604	511[b]	^{82}Kr	Stable
^{89}Sr	^{88}Sr(n,γ)^{89}Sr	51 d	β^-	1495		^{89}Y	Stable
^{90}Y	^{90}Sr $\rightarrow$ ^{90}Y	64 h	β^-	2279		^{90}Zr	Stable
^{99}Mo	^{98}Mo(n,γ)^{99}Mo ^{235}U(n,f)^{99}Mo	66 h	β^-, γ	1215 437	140	^{99}Tc	2×10^5 y
^{99m}Tc	^{99}Mo $\rightarrow$ ^{99m}Tc	6 h	γ		140	^{99}Tc	2×10^5 y
^{111}In	^{112}Cd(p,2n)^{111}In	67 h	EC, γ		171 245	^{111}Cd	Stable

(Continued)

Essentials of Nuclear Medicine Physics, Instrumentation, and Radiation Biology, Fourth Edition.
Rachel A. Powsner, Matthew R. Palmer, and Edward R. Powsner.
© 2022 John Wiley & Sons Ltd. Published 2022 by John Wiley & Sons Ltd.

Nuclide	Production method	Half-life (s = secs m = mins h = hours d = days y = years)	Decay mode	βmax or α energies in keV[a]	γ energies in keV[a]	Decay product	Half-life of decay product
^{123}I	^{121}Sb$(\alpha,2n)^{123}$I	13 h	EC, γ		159	^{123}Te	10^{12} y
^{131}I	^{130}Te$(n,\gamma)^{131m}$Te ^{131m}Te$(\beta^-)^{131}$I ^{235}U$(n,f)^{131}$I	8 d	β⁻, γ	606	364	^{131}Xe	Stable
^{133}Xe	^{235}U$(n,f)^{133}$Xe	5.2 d	β⁻, γ	346	81	^{133}Cs	Stable
^{133}Ba	^{132}Ba$(n,\gamma)^{133}$Ba	10.5 y	EC, γ		356	^{133}Cs	Stable
^{137}Cs	^{235}U$(n,f)^{137}$Xe	30 y	β⁻, γ	514	662	^{137}Ba	Stable
^{153}Sm	^{152}Sm(n,γ) ^{153}Sm	46 h	β⁻, γ	635 705 808	70 103	^{153}Eu	Stable
^{177}Lu	^{176}Lu$(n,\gamma)^{177}$Lu	6.6 d	β⁻, γ		208	^{177}Hf	Stable
^{201}Tl	^{203}Tl$(p,3n)^{201}$Pb ^{201}Pb $(9.33h) \rightarrow {}^{201}$Tl	3 d	EC, X-ray		X-ray: 69–83	^{201}Hg	Stable
^{223}Ra	^{227}Ac $\rightarrow {}^{227}$Th $\rightarrow {}^{223}$Ra	11.4 d	α	5640 5710 5852		^{219}Rn	Stable

Primary source: Bé M, Chisté V, Dulieu C, et al. *Table of Radionuclides*. Bureau International Des Poids et Mesures, Pavillon de Breteuil, F-92310 SÈVRES, PARIS, 2004.

[a] The most abundant particulate or photon emissions are listed.

[b] Annihilation photons.

[c] Yano,Y, McRae, J, and Anger, H,Lung Function Studies Using Short-Lived 81mKr and the scintillation camera. J Nuc Med.1970; 11(11): 674–679.

APPENDIX B

Major Dosimetry for Common Pharmaceuticals

Radiopharmaceutical	Effective dose mSv/MBq (rem/mCi) adult	Principal target organ absorbed dose mGy/MBq (rads/mCi)
^{18}F-flourodeoxyglucose (FDG)	0.019 (0.07)	Urinary bladder wall 0.13 (0.48)
^{18}F-flouride	0.017 (0.063)	Urinary bladder wall 0.15 (0.56)
^{68}Ga-citrate	0.1 (0.37)	Bone surfaces 0.63 (2.3)
^{82}Rb-chloride	0.0011 (0.0041)	Kidneys 0.0093 (0.034)
^{99m}Tc DMSA (dimercaptosuccinic acid)	0.0088 (0.033)	Kidneys: 0.18 (0.67)
^{99m}Tc HMPAO (ceretec)	0.0093 (0.034)	Kidneys: 0.034 (0.35)
^{99m}Tc RBC	0.007 (0.026)	Heart wall: 0.023 (0.085)
^{99m}Tc MAG3 (mertiatide, mercaptoacetyl glycine)	Normal function: 0.007 (0.026) Reduced function: 0.0061 (0.023)	Urinary bladder wall: 0.11 (0.41) Urinary bladder wall: 0.083 (0.31)
^{99m}Tc non-absorbable (such as DTPA or SC) for oral gastric emptying	Liquid: 0.019 (0.07) Solids: 0.024 (0.089)	Upper large intestinal wall: 0.12 (0.44) Upper large intestinal wall: 0.12 (0.44)
^{99m}Tc pertechnetate	0.013 (0.048)	Upper large intestinal wall: 0.056 (0.21)
^{99m}Tc-DTPA (pentetate) intravenous	0.0049 (0.018)	Urinary bladder wall: 0.062 (0.23)
^{99m}Tc-IDAs (iminodiacetic acid gallbladder imaging agents such as DISIDA, PIPIDA, etc)	0.016 (0.059)	Gallbladder: 0.11 (0.41)
^{99m}Tc-MAA (macroaggregated albumin)	0.011 (0.041)	Lung: 0.066 (0.24)
^{99m}Tc-labeled phosphates and phosphonates (MDP and HDP)	0.0049 (0.018)	Urinary bladder wall 0.047 (0.17)
^{99m}Tc-Myoview (tetrofosmin)	Rest: 0.008 (0.03) Exercise: 0.0069 (0.026)	Gallbladder: rest: 0.036 (0.13) Gallbladder: exercise: 0.027 (0.1)
^{99m}Tc-labeled large colloids (such as sulfur colloid)	0.0091 (0.034)	Spleen: 0.074 (0.27)
^{99m}Tc-Sestamibi	Rest: 0.009 (0.033) Exercise: 0.0079 (0.029)	Gallbladder: 0.039 (0.14) Gallbladder: 0.033 (0.12)
^{99m}Tc-WBC (HMPAO)	0.011 (0.041)	Spleen: 0.15 (0.56)

(Continued)

Essentials of Nuclear Medicine Physics, Instrumentation, and Radiation Biology, Fourth Edition.
Rachel A. Powsner, Matthew R. Palmer, and Edward R. Powsner.
© 2022 John Wiley & Sons Ltd. Published 2022 by John Wiley & Sons Ltd.

Radiopharmaceutical	Effective dose mSv/MBq (rem/mCi) adult	Principal target organ absorbed dose mGy/MBq (rads/mCi)
[111]In Octreotide	0.054 (0.2)	Spleen: 0.57 (2.1)
^{111}In-WBC (Oxyquinoline)[2]	0.59 (2.2)	Spleen: 5.5 (20)
[111]InCl-DTPA (intrathecal)[2]	0.14 (0.52)	Spinal column: 0.95 (3.5)
[123]I MIBG (meta-iodobenzylguanidine)[2]	0.018 (0.067)	Liver: 0.071 (0.26)
[123]I Sodium iodide (oral intake)	Low thyroid uptake: 0.15 (0.056) Medium thyroid uptake: 0.22 (0.81) High thyroid uptake: 0.3 (1.1)	Thyroid: Low thyroid uptake: 2.5 (9.3) Medium thyroid uptake: 4 (15) High thyroid uptake: 5.6 (21)
[131]I NP-59 (6-B-iodomethyl-19-norcholesterol)[2]	1.5 (5.6)	Adrenals: 4 (15)
[131]I Sodium iodide (oral intake)	Thyroid: Low thyroid uptake: 14 (52) Medium thyroid uptake: 22 (81) High thyroid uptake: 29 (107)	Thyroid: Low thyroid uptake: 280 (1000) Medium thyroid uptake: 430 (1600) High thyroid uptake: 580 (2100)
[131]I Metaiodobenzylguanidine (MIBG)[2]	0.2 (0.74)	Liver 0.83 (3.1)
[133]Xe (xenon gas) rebreathing for 5 minutes	0.00073 (0.0027)	Lungs 0.0011 (0.0041)
[201]Tl (thallous chloride)	0.14 (0.52)	Kidneys: 0.48 (1.8)
[123]I ioflupane (DATscan) (with thyroid blocking)[1]	0.021 (0.078)	Large intestine: 0.04 (0.15)

[1] GE Healthcare prescribing information for DaTscan Ioflupane ^{123}I injection. General Electric Company, 2015.
[2] ICRP 53 1998.
All others are adapted from:
ICRP, 2015. *Radiation Dose to Patients from Radiopharmaceuticals: A Compendium of Current Information Related to Frequently Used Substances.* ICRP Publication 128. Ann. ICRP 44(2S). Sage Publications.

APPENDIX C

Guide to Nuclear Regulatory Commission (NRC) Publications

Title 10, "Energy", Code of Federal Regulations (10CFR) [1]

Title 10 of the Code of Federal Regulations contains the regulations governing the use of nuclear materials by all individuals and organizations with an NRC license. Three parts of this document are relevant to the practice of nuclear medicine: Part 19: Notices, Instructions, and Reports to Workers: Inspection and Investigations; Part 20: Standards for protection against radiation; and Part 35: Medical Use of Byproduct Material.

NUREG – 1556, Vol. 9, Revision 3, Consolidated Guidance About Materials Licenses [2]

This document is a detailed guide for filling out an NRC license application for the medical use of radionuclides. The appendices contain model procedures for several of the regulations outlined in 10CFR20 and 35.

Sections of these documents relating to routine practice are organized for reference in the following table:

Table D.1 Selected sections of 10CFR Parts 19, 20, 35, and NUREG-1556, Vol. 9

Topic	10CFR Part Section	NUREG-1556, Vol. 9, Revision 3 Model Procedures
Required postings: NRC Form 3 "Notice to Employees" and regulations in 10CFR parts 19 and 20	19.11	
Required instructions to workers concerning risks associated with exposure to radiation	19.12	
Requirement for reporting exposure data to individual workers	19.13	Appendix M covers occupational dose monitoring program Appendix Y covers reporting requirements
Definitions of terms for Part 20	20.1003	
Requirement for development of radiation protection program to comply with regulations and ALARA and to perform reviews of the program at least annually.	20.1101	Appendix L outlines medical license audit Appendix N includes model spill clean-up procedures and other emergency procedures Appendix T covers procedures for safe use of unsealed licensed material
Occupational dose limits for adults	20.1201	
Occupational dose limits for minors	20.1207	
Dose equivalent to embryo/fetus	20.1208	
Public dose limits	20.1301	

(Continued)

Essentials of Nuclear Medicine Physics, Instrumentation, and Radiation Biology, Fourth Edition.
Rachel A. Powsner, Matthew R. Palmer, and Edward R. Powsner.
© 2022 John Wiley & Sons Ltd. Published 2022 by John Wiley & Sons Ltd.

Table D.1 (*Continued*)

Topic	10CFR Part Section	NUREG-1556, Vol. 9, Revision 3 Model Procedures
Minimum exposure threshold for monitoring individual workers	20.1502	
Requirement for room ventilation or other controls to reduce inhalation of airborne radiation	20.1701 and 20.1702	
Security and surveillance of radioactive materials	20.1801 and 20.1802	
Requirements for posting radiation signs	20.1901, 20.1902	
Criteria for exemptions to labeling requirements	20.1905	
Requirements for receiving and opening packages	20.1906	Appendix O covers receiving Appendix P covers opening
Rules for waste disposal and records of waste disposal	20.2001 and 20.2108	Appendix W
Record keeping for individual monitoring results	20.2106	
Requirements for form and maintenance of record keeping	20.2110 and 35.5	
Quantities of licensed material requiring labeling	Part 20, Appendix C	
Provisions for protection of human research subjects	35.6	
Application for license, amendment, or renewal	35.12	
Written directives with procedures for administration	35.40 and 35.41	Appendix S includes procedures for developing, maintaining, and implementing written directives
Training requirements for radiation safety officers, medical physicists, authorized users, nuclear pharmacists.	35.50–35.59	
Use and calibration of the dose calibrator	35.60	Appendix G covers dose calibrator calibration
Calibration of survey instruments	35.61	Appendix K includes instrument specifications and calibration program
Methods for determination of dosages of unsealed byproduct material for medical use	35.63	
Requirements for possession of sealed sources	35.67	Appendix Q includes model procedures for leak testing
Labeling of vials and syringes	35.69	
End of day surveys	35.70	Appendix R
Criteria for release of individuals following radioactive doses	35.75	Appendix U includes additional sources of information
Use of unsealed radioactive materials for imaging studies for which no written directive is required	35.200	
Training requirements for imaging and localization studies	35.290	
Use of unsealed radioactive materials for which a written directive is required	35.300	
Training requirements for use of unsealed radioactive material for which a written directive is required	35.390–35.396	

Table D.1 (*Continued*)

Topic	*10CFR Part Section*	*NUREG-1556, Vol. 9, Revision 3 Model Procedures*
Records of written directives and procedures for administration	35.2040 and 35.2041	Appendix X covers record keeping requirements
Dose calibrator calibration records	35.2060	
Radiation survey instrument calibration records	35.2061	
Records for unsealed source patient doses	35.2063	
Records for leak test and inventory of sealed sources	35.2067	
End of day survey records	35.2070	
Records for release of individuals containing radioactive materials	35.2075	
Records of decay-in-storage	35.2092	
Report and notification of a medical event	35.3045	Appendix Y outlines reporting requirements
Report and notification of doses to embryo/fetus or nursing child	35.3047	
Report of leaking source	35.3067	

References

1. Title 10, Code of Federal Regulations (10CFR). Office of the Federal Register National Archives and Records Administration. Part 19: last reviewed August 24, 2018. Part 20: 20.1003-20.1301, last reviewed August 24, 2018. 20.1502-Appendices, last reviewed November 1, 2018. Part 35: 35.12, 35.59-35.200, 35.2040-35.2092, 35.3067, last reviewed August 29 2017. 35.40-35.57, 35.290-35.390, last reviewed January 16, 2019. 35.3045-35.3047, last reviewed August 17, 2020. Government Printing Office.

2. NUREG–1556, Vol. 9, Rev 3 Consolidated Guidance About Materials Licenses. Program-Specific Guidance About Medical Use Licenses. Final Report September 2019. Prepared by M. Burkhart, A. Cockerham, J. Cook, et al. Office of Nuclear Material Safety and Safeguards, U.S. Nuclear Regulatory Commission, Washington, D.C. 20555-0001.

APPENDIX D
Recommended Reading by Topic

Review of Basic Physics

Kuhn KF, Noschese F. *Basic Physics: A Self-Teaching Guide*, 3rd edn. Hoboken, NJ: Jossey-Bass, (Wiley), 2020.

Nuclear Medicine

Mettler FA, Guiberteau MJ. *Essentials of Nuclear Medicine and Molecular Imaging*, 7th edn. Philadelphia: Elsevier, 2019.

Basic Nuclear Medicine Physics and Instrumentation

Cherry SR, Sorenson JA, Phelps ME. *Physics of Nuclear Medicine*, 4th edn. Philadelphia: Elsevier Saunders, 2012.

PET Technology

Zhang J, Knopp MV (eds). *Advances in PET: The Latest in Instrumentation, Technology, and Clinical Practice.* Switzerland: Springer Nature, 2020.

CT Technology

Goldman LW. Principles of CT and CT technology. *J Nucl Med Technol.* 2007;35(3):115–28.

Goldman LW. Principles of CT: radiation dose and image quality. *J Nucl Med Technol.* 2007;35(4):226–8.

Goldman, LW. Principles of CT: multislice CT. *J Nucl Med Technol.* 2008;36(2):57–68.

MRI Technology

Levitt MH. *Spin Dynamics: Basics of Nuclear Magnetic Resonance*, 2nd edn. (Chapters 1 and 2). Oxford: Wiley, 2008.

Weishaupt D, Koechli VD, et al. *How Does MRI Work?: An Introduction to the Physics and Function of Magnetic Resonance Imaging*. New York: Springer, 2006.

DICOM and Information Technology

Pianykh OS. *Digital Imaging and Communications in Medicine (DICOM): A Practical Introduction and Survival Guide*, 2nd edn. New York: Springer, 2012.

NEMA Medical Imaging and Technology Alliance. Resource page: http://medical.nema.org/

Nuclear Medicine Quality Control

Zanzonico P. Routine quality control of clinical nuclear medicine instrumentation: a brief review. *J Nucl Med.* 2008;49:1114–31.

AAPM Report No. 126. *PET/CT Acceptance Testing and Quality Assurance*. The Report of AAPM Task Group 126, October 2019.

Radiobiology

Hall EJ, Giaccia AJ. *Radiobiology for the Radiologist*, 8th edn. Hoboken, NJ: Wolters Kluwer, 2019.

Radiation Dosimetry

Stabin MG. *The Practice of Internal Dosimetry in Nuclear Medicine* (Series in Medical Physics and Biomedical Engineering). CRC Press, Taylor and Francis Group, 2017.

RADAR—Radiation Dose Assessment Resource. www.doseinfo-radar.com/

NRC Regulations

NRC Regulations Title 10, Code of Federal Regulations: Parts 19 (August 2018), 20 (August and November, 2018), and 35 (January, 2019 and August, 2020). www.nrc.gov/reading-rm/doc-collections/cfr/

Essentials of Nuclear Medicine Physics, Instrumentation, and Radiation Biology, Fourth Edition.
Rachel A. Powsner, Matthew R. Palmer, and Edward R. Powsner.
© 2022 John Wiley & Sons Ltd. Published 2022 by John Wiley & Sons Ltd.

Consolidated Guidance About Materials Licenses. Program-Specific Guidance About Medical Use Licenses, Final Report (NUREG-1556, Vol 9, Rev 3), September 2019. www.nrc.gov/reading-rm/doc-collections/nuregs/staff/sr1556/v9/

Therapeutics in Nuclear Medicine

Sgouros G, Bodei L, McDevitt MR, Nedrow JR. Radiopharmaceutical therapy in cancer: clinical advances and challenges. *Nature Rev Drug Discov.* 2020;19:589–608. www.nature.com/articles/s41573-020-0073-9/

Radiation Accidents

Oak Ridge Institute for Science and Education. *The Medical Aspects of Radiation Incidents*, 4th edn. Oak Ridge, TN: Radiation Emergency Assistance Center/Training Site (REAC/TS), Revised 7/2017. https://orise.orau.gov/resources/reacts/documents/medical-aspects-of-radiation-incidents.pdf/

Index

Page locators in **bold** indicate tables. Page locators in *italics* indicate figures. This index uses letter-by-letter

Essentials of Nuclear Medicine Physics, Instrumentation, and Radiation Biology, Fourth Edition.
Rachel A. Powsner, Matthew R. Palmer, and Edward R. Powsner.
© 2022 John Wiley & Sons Ltd. Published 2022 by John Wiley & Sons Ltd.